T0296553

A HISTORY OF
EMBRYOLOGY

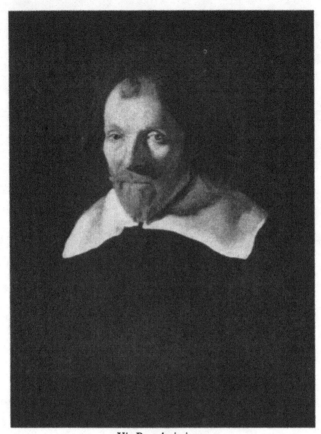

Vir Praeclarissimus
GULIELMUS HARVEY
Mysterii Generationis Indagator Diligens.

[*Frontispiece*

A HISTORY OF
EMBRYOLOGY

JOSEPH NEEDHAM, F.R.S.

*Fellow of Gonville & Caius College,
and Sir William Dunn Reader in Biochemistry
in the University of Cambridge*

SECOND EDITION
REVISED WITH THE ASSISTANCE OF

ARTHUR HUGHES, Ph.D

*Lecturer in Anatomy in the
University of Cambridge*

CAMBRIDGE
AT THE UNIVERSITY PRESS
1959

CAMBRIDGE
UNIVERSITY PRESS

University Printing House, Cambridge CB2 8BS, United Kingdom

Cambridge University Press is part of the University of Cambridge.

It furthers the University's mission by disseminating knowledge in the pursuit of
education, learning and research at the highest international levels of excellence.

www.cambridge.org
Information on this title: www.cambridge.org/9781107475540

© Cambridge University Press 1959

First edition 1934
Second edition 1959
First published 1959
First paperback edition 2014

A catalogue record for this publication is available from the British Library

ISBN 978-1-107-47554-0 Paperback

DII LABORIBUS OMNIA VENDUNT

*Nobilissimo juveni Medico Philippo
de Glarges, amicitiae ergo libenter
Gulielmus Harveus scripsit, Anglus,
Med. Reg. et Anat. Prof. Londin.
Mai 8, 1641*

From the commonplace book
of Philip de Glarges

Not to prayse or disprayse: all did well.

William Harvey's MS notes,
Canones Anatomiae Generalis, 6

CONTENTS

Chapter Three

EMBRYOLOGY IN THE SEVENTEENTH CENTURY

Chapter Four

EMBRYOLOGY IN THE EIGHTEENTH CENTURY

PLATES

NOTE

The use of the shortened and (&) indicates
collaboration between two or more authors

PRELIMINARY NOTE

THE contribution to the history of science contained in the following four chapters first appeared as the opening part of a treatise on Chemical Embryology, published in 1931. They were delivered in the form of lectures about the same time at the University of London under the title "Speculation, Observation and Experiment as illustrated by the History of Embryology." The munificence of that University assured their appearance in separate, and amplified, form.[1]

I suppose that the study of the history of science needs no apology. If at first sight the discussion of what was thought in the past rather than what is known now appears to be of merely antiquarian value, a deeper consideration will admit, with Louis Choulant, that the history of science is the guarantee of its freedom. The mistakes of our predecessors remind us that we may be mistaken; their wisdom prevents us from assuming that wisdom was born with us; and by studying the processes of their thought, we may hope to have a better understanding, and hence a better organisation, of our own. Theoretical errors, such as the final cause, preformationism or phlogiston; practical errors, such as the divorce between speculation and technique in the Hellenistic age, are always able to show us a more excellent way.

The present contribution does not claim, what probably no historical work can truly deserve, the ascription of a complete lack of bias in its presentation. Designed as it was to introduce a discussion of the border-line between embryology and biochemistry, it sought rather to lay bare the roots of chemical embryology in history, than to collect data indiscriminately on all the interesting aspects of the subject. Its title, "The Origins of Chemical Embryology," made no secret of this. And no obvious disadvantage attaches to such a plan, except the difficulty of deciding when to leave off. For although it is possible in reasonable space to try to do justice to all aspects of embryology before 1800, after that date the number of investigators and the variety of problems attacked becomes too great to handle conveniently on the same scale as before.[2]

[1] By embryology we mean in this book the embryology of animals exclusively. The history of the embryology of plants has been fully written only in Russian, by Baranov, but there is a shorter work by Souèges in French.
[2] Cf. the valuable work of Studnička; Florian; Dogelb; Oppenheimer; Fischer & Schopfer; and others.

Bifurcation begins; the spheres of morphology and physiology more obviously separate, and in the latter division chemical researches play an ever-increasing part. It is now hoped that a group of workers will soon be able to continue the story in a companion volume through the nineteenth century under a number of separate headings.

No exhaustive treatise on the history of embryology as yet exists.[1] The nearest approach to it is the very valuable memoir of B. Bloch with its epitome, but this only covers the era of the Renaissance with thoroughness. Hertwig's account, which he printed at the beginning of his great *Handbuch der Entwicklungslehre*, does not deal very fully with any aspect of the subject before 1800, nor do the much shorter ones of Henneguy and Minot. The latter paper is interesting in that it ends with an emphasis on the need for physico-chemical work in the future. The introduction to Keibel's book is much slighter, but contains some useful information. There are various monographs and papers on special points, such as Pouchet's rather untrustworthy treatment of the embryology of Aristotle, and Lones' discussion of it, which is worse. Camus' notes are still the best commentary on the *Historia Animalium*. Again, useful information on some cultural points is to be had from the treatise of Ploss & Bartels. The introductions to certain books also contain valuable information, and in this class comes Dareste's remarkable book on teratology. The bibliographies contained in von Haller's eighth volume and in the books of Schurig and Heffter are naturally of the greatest assistance. The valuable books of F. J. Cole and Thadeusz Bilikiewicz on seventeenth-century embryology appeared too late for use in the first preparation of this book, but have contributed to its revision.[2]

In 1939 there appeared a work, *The Rise of Embryology*, by the learned Californian anatomist A. W. Meyer, author of numerous periodical publications on our subject, some of which are referred to in the bibliography. His book stands to mine in much the same relation as the second volume of David Eugene Smith's notable *History of Mathematics* to the first; the one adopting a basically chronological treatment, the other a topical form in which separate subjects are chosen in succession for consideration. However, Meyer devotes the bulk of his work to

[1] Here we cannot attempt to provide a bibliography of the most important modern works dealing with the subject itself. Yet in case scientific men or historians of other fields might appreciate some helpful introduction to embryology, mention may be made of the popular books of Rostand, Waddington and Guttmacher. An engineer or an historian of astronomy might then proceed to the recent surveys of Waddington, Barth, or Willier *et al.*
[2] Certain minor works on the history of embryology have proved inaccessible— Beseke; Eccleshymer; H. Fasbender; Favaro; Ferckel; Gilis; Hopf; Ottow. Other articles deserving mention are those of Gerber; Keller; du Bois.

the eighteenth and nineteenth centuries, passing over the earlier periods in his first thirty pages. His treatment of the nineteenth century is interesting indeed, though nothing could supersede the remarkable work of E. S. Russell, *Form and Function*. Particular interest attaches to L. A. Blacher's monograph on *Embryology in Russia in the 18th and 19th Centuries* (1955), since so much of the classical work centring around 1800 was done or published in that country.

These observations made, the principal reviews of the subject are chiefly to be found in histories of science in general, such as Sarton's; histories of biological theory, such as Rádl's; histories of obstetrics, such as von Siebold's, Spencer's and E. Fasbender's; histories of gynaecology, such as McKay's; and histories of anatomy, such as Singer's and von Töply's. Histories of medicine as a whole are numerous and good: I have found those of Garrison and Neuburger-Pagel most useful. Those which deal with special periods are also of assistance, such as Schrutz and Browne on Arabian, I. Bloch on Byzantine, and Harnack on Patristic medicine. Histories of chemistry provide no help, for ancient chemistry was so oriented towards "practical" results, such as the *lapis philosophorum* and *elixir vitae*, that the egg was only considered as a raw material for various preparations. The investigation of its change of properties during the development of the embryo did not occur to the alchemists. Detailed studies of particular subjects, such as those contained in Singer's two excellent volumes, *The History and Method of Science*, may also be of some assistance. Again, there are books which give a wonderful orientation and an articulate survey of vast tracts: of these Clifford Allbutt's *Greek Medicine in Rome*, with its mass of references, is among the most valuable. And Miall's *Early Naturalists* must not be omitted, for, apart from the peculiar charm of style which marks it, it contains some singularly helpful bibliographical data.[1] But the study of the original sources, so far as that is possible, is a duty which cannot be avoided, and in what follows I have been careful to copy down no statement from a previous review when it was possible to read the actual words of the writer himself. This practice of going to the originals is made peculiarly necessary in a case such as the present one, when the history of a subject is regarded from a rather new angle.

The arrangement of my chapters I adopted in the first edition, and now preserve, only on the ground that it is suitable enough in the present state of historical knowledge. Little was then said about embryology in China because at that time I could find out little about it, but it will be thoroughly treated in the eighth volume of my work on the

---

[1] A fine beginning has been made on the bibliographies of seventeenth-century men of science by Keynes and Fulton.

history of science in general in that great culture, *Science and Civilisation in China*. Nor am I content with the short section on embryology in India, but here there are special difficulties owing to the absence of an established chronology for ancient and mediaeval Indian texts, and an adequate account of it must be left for others to give. No permanent framework for historical facts is proposed in what follows; I only attempt to bring them together, and to reveal some of the relationships between them. If the traditional pattern turns out to be badly distorted—and there are many signs that it may—the facts can be rearranged.

But in whatever way this may turn out to be desirable, one necessity must constantly be kept before the mind's eye, namely the knowledge of the relations between scientific thought and technical practice at any given period. For embryology this knowledge is difficult to acquire, since up to the time of the Renaissance obstetrics remained a part of primitive folk-medicine rather than of serious medical science. We see, however, in the publication of the Hellenistic gynaecological treatises in the sixteenth century (Bauhin, Spach; see p. 109) the satisfaction of a new demand, even though it took the typical Renaissance form of what might be called palaeolatry. It was part of that movement to rationalise obstetrics which included Harvey's *De Generatione* and Malpighi's *De Formatione Pulli* and culminated in the celebrated man-midwives of the eighteenth century.[1] Again, the relation of the early systematists—Belon, Rondelet, Aldrovandus, Ray—to the beginnings of mercantile expansion is fairly clear, for the mediaeval bestiary could not cope with the influx of new animals and plants from hitherto unknown regions, any one of which might prove to be an exploitable commodity.

The Hellenistic divorce between scientific thought and empirical technique is an important case in point. Greek life was divided strictly into θεωρία and πρᾶξις. The latter was not thought fitting for a man of good birth. "Antiquity," says Diels, "was entirely aristocratic in attitude. Even prominent artists, such as Pheidias, were classed as artisans, and were incapable of bursting through the barrier separating the workers and peasants from the upper class. A second cause of the slight technical progress in antiquity was its slave-holding system, which led to a lack of any impulse to develop the machine as a substitute for manual labour."[2] Xenophon in the *Oeconomicus* held the industries in poor repute.[3] "Men engaged in the mechanical arts," he says, "must ever be

[1] E.g. the Chamberlens, Palfyn (see Stein), Mauriceau, William Smellie, John Burton of York ("Dr Slop"), and Joseph Needham of Devizes; see the articles of Rosenthal and Mengert. The dissertation of Caspar Bose (1729) is a typical attack on the midwives of the time.
[2] See Ciccotti.　　　　　[3] IV, 3; VI, 13–16.

both bad friends and feeble defenders of their country." He troubled himself little with those skilful in carpentry, metallurgy, painting and sculpture, but was always anxious to meet a "gentleman" (καλός τε κἀγαθός). The results of this were inevitable. Classical surgery and obstetrics benefited practically nothing from the speculations of the biologists from Alcmaeon to Herophilus (see pp. 29 ff.). Surgeons and midwives remained members of the painter-cobbler-builder group, the group of base-born "mechanicks", entirely distinct from the astronomer-mathematician-metaphysician-biologist group, the group familiar with courts and tyrants.

Only the greatest broke away from this tradition: Aristotle, when he conversed with fishermen, Archimedes perhaps, when he constructed his mechanical devices. For the rest, it was too strong. Down to the end of the Roman period the artillery in use remained precisely what it had been six hundred years before, although the Empire was crumbling under barbarian pressure, and would have given anything, one would imagine, for an improved artillery capable of withstanding the Gothic armies. It is strange, as has been acutely said, that the Romans never invented anything so much in the Roman taste as a railway. So far as Hellenistic empirical industrial chemistry was concerned, the Democritean and Epicurean atoms might never have existed. And in medicine, the only effect of the brilliant Greek atomic speculations was to give rise to the Methodic school of Roman physicians, described by Allbutt, whose influence was never strong, and who contributed relatively little to the main stream of therapeutics originating with Hippocrates.

In sum, we must not dissociate scientific advances from the technical needs and processes of the time, and the economic structure in which all are embedded. We shall never understand the failure of Greek science if we consider it in abstraction from the environment which sterilised its speculation. The history of science is not a mere succession of inexplicable geniuses, direct Promethean ambassadors to man from heaven. Whether a given fact would have got itself discovered by some other person than the historical discoverer had he not lived, it is certainly profitless and probably meaningless to enquire. But scientific men do not live in a vacuum; on the contrary, the directions of their interest are ever conditioned by the structure of the world they live in. Further historical research will enable us to take into account the social and economic status of the investigator himself (cf. Chambers for the Hellenistic artist, and Yearsley for the sixteenth-century physician).

It would thus be of the greatest interest to know accurately the sources of the emoluments of embryologists at different times.[1] From Orn-

[1] On this, cf. Cumston and Dittrick.

stein's admirable book on the scientific societies of the Renaissance, the suspicion arises that their royal patronage was dictated not only by a purely disinterested passion for abstract truth, but by a desire to profit as much as possible by the new techniques which the decay of the anti-usury doctrines, the willingness of the rising mercantile class to make industrial "ventures," and the far-ranging thought of the scientific men were combining to produce. In England's Royal Society, indeed, the preoccupation of the early Fellows with the "improvement of trade and husbandry" is patent to anyone acquainted with its early history (cf. Thomas Sprat's account of it).[1] Thus Dr Jasper Needham, elected in 1663, read only one paper before the Society—not, as might have been expected from his profession, on the transfusion of blood or the anatomy of the brain; but on the value and use of "China Varnish". However, it is probable that for the most part the embryologists whose work we shall have to discuss were practising physicians, free or relatively free from the ancient tradition, and conscious that to understand the mystery of generation would be to advance the science and art of medicine.

In this connection it is of interest that the Church in the seventeenth and eighteenth centuries provided a certain source of demand for embryological research. Of this Swammerdam and Malebranche (see p. 169) provide interesting examples, and the conviction, then widely held, that research into the nature of generation would throw light on orthodox theological doctrines, such as that of original sin, led to an economic situation of value for biological development. Finally, it would be rash to minimise the factor of pure curiosity in seventeenth-century science. The recreational quality of Leeuwenhoek's investigations is, as Baas-Becking says, too obvious to be overlooked.[2]

The history of single forms of scientific knowledge is in a way happier because containing more of continuity than that of civilisation as a whole. The assiduity with which men of different periods in the rise and decline of a culture pursue the different forms of human experience may, as Spengler has shown, vary much, but those forms remain fundamentally the same, even if their manifestations are profoundly changed.

[1] And the very interesting letter of Robert Boyle to a friend, Marcombes, quoted by Fulton. "The other humane studies I apply myself to" (1646) "are natural philosophy, the mechanics, and husbandry, according to the principles of our new philosophical college, that values no knowledge, but as it hath a tendency to use. And therefore I shall make it one of my suits to you, that you would take the pains to enquire a little more thoroughly into the ways of husbandry etc. practised in your parts; and when you intend for *England*, to bring along with you what good receipts or choice books of any of these subjects you can procure; which will make you extremely welcome to our *invisible college*, which I had now designed to give you a description of." Fulton remarks that this statement of its aim was inadequate, but we may take leave to think it was not so inadequate as many would suppose.
[2] The full scope of Leeuwenhoek's discoveries is now appearing, thanks to the labours of van Rijnberk and his collaborators.

That science, at any rate, does maintain some sort of continuity whatever gaps there may be between the phases of its progress, is a belief agreeable with all the available facts, and one which no criticism will easily shake.

It only remains to record my indebtedness to those who have assisted me in the preparation of this work. Primarily I am grateful to Dr Charles Singer, who annotated my typescript with valuable comments and lent me many papers and pictures, and to Professor R. C. Punnett, who placed unreservedly at my disposal his knowledge of the history of generation and his library of old and rare biological books. To Dr Arthur Peck I am indebted for the correction of my Greek, and it was Professor A. B. Cook who introduced me to the embryology of the ancients. For guidance on Talmudic and Jewish matters I thank Dr Walter Pagel, the late Dr Louis Rapkine and Dr H. Loewe. Without the assiduous backing of Mr Powell, the Librarian of the Royal Society of Medicine, and his assistants, and of Mr H. Zeitlinger, I should have dealt much more inadequately than I have with papers and books which cannot be consulted in Cambridge. And in addition to those mentioned above, the following friends kindly read through and criticised the proofs: Professor Reuben Levy, the late Professor F. M. Cornford, the late Sir William Dampier, Mr Gregory Bateson, Professor Roy Pascal and the Rev. W. L. Elmslie.

To the Master of Gonville and Caius College I am indebted for permission to reproduce the portrait of William Harvey (attributed to Rembrandt) which hangs in our Senior Combination Room. Although the authenticity of this is not accepted by Keynes in his recent study of the portraits of Harvey, it has been in the possession of the College since 1798, when it came to us from the Earl of Leicester. After comparison with other portraits of Harvey, many feel unable to concur in its rejection.

J. N.

CHAPTER I

EMBRYOLOGY IN ANTIQUITY

1. Ideas of Primitive Peoples

SINCE biological science as a whole was little cultivated in ancient Egypt and the ancient civilisations of Babylonia, Assyria[1] and India, the study of embryology was equally little pursued. Doubtless the un-developed embryo, whether in egg or uterus, carried with it, for these persons of remote antiquity, some flavour of the obscene in the literal sense of the word. But embryology stands in a peculiar relation to the history of humanity, in that even at the most remote times children were being born, and, though the practitioners of ancient folk-medicine might confine their ideas for the most part to simple obstetrics,[2] they yet could hardly avoid some slight speculation on the growth and forma-tions of the embryo. Figure 1 illustrates this level of culture. It is a painted and carved door from a house in Dutch New Guinea, taken from de Clercq's book; the original was of yellowish brown wood. The male embryo is clearly shown, but the artist evidently had a hazy con-ception of the umbilical cord. The line passing from the uterus to the head may or may not be merely ornamental. The movement of the foetus *in utero* played and still plays a large part in the folklore of prim-itive peoples, as may be read in the exhaustive treatise of Ploss & Bartels. For information concerning god-embryos in primitive religion see Briffault.[3] The works of Hutton and of Ashley Montagu may be con-sulted for a mass of information regarding primitive philosophies of life and its development.

2. Egyptian Antiquity

Egyptian medicine did not venture on embryological speculation, or so it would seem from the writings which have come down to us—the Ebers medical papyrus does not once mention the embryo (Brugsch).[4] But there are points of interest as regards Egypt in this connection. One particular aspect of Egyptian thought is certainly of embryological

[1] See Zervos.   [2] See R. F. Spencer.   [3] Vol. 1, p. 96.
[4] A general account of ancient Egyptian gynaecology and obstetrics is given by Reinhard.

18

interest, namely the theory of the placenta, recently investigated by Murray.

In Frazer's *Folk-Lore in the Old Testament* there is a chapter entitled "The Bundle of Life" in which he discusses the idea of the external soul, and the various receptacles used to contain it. He draws attention to the compliment which Abigail paid to David at their first meeting: "And though man be risen up to pursue thee, and to seek thy soul, yet the soul of my lord shall be bound in the bundle of life with the Lord thy God; and the souls of thine enemies, them shall he sling out, as from the hollow of a sling." This implies, as he says, that the souls of living people could be tied up for safety in a bundle, and that on the contrary, when the souls were those of enemies, the bundle might be undone and the souls scattered to the winds.

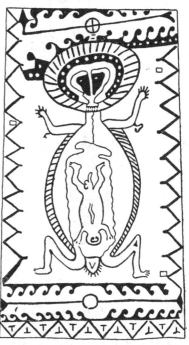

Fig. 1: *Painted and carved door from Dutch New Guinea (de Clercq).*

Murray explains that this was a distinctively Egyptian doctrine, since Syria was an Egyptian province and had been so for centuries. She discovered among the titles of the Egyptian royal officials the significant "Opener of the King's Placenta." Other evidence demonstrates that the fate of the placenta, at any rate in the dynastic families, was regarded as of great importance, since it was thought to be the especial seat of the external soul. Although the above-mentioned title (which had ten holders, all related to the royal house, in the fourth, fifth and sixth dynasties) ceased to exist towards the end of the Old Kingdom, a standard representing the royal placenta was carried before the Pharaoh down to the time of the Ptolemies. Murray conjectures that the term "Opener" originated from some actual or forgotten ritual king-murder, the bundle of life containing the placenta being ceremonially opened at the conclusion of the reign.

The standard (Murray & Seligman) is here illustrated (Fig. 2 A, B), as are also bundles of life (Fig. 2 C–F).

Reverence for the placenta and umbilical cord is also noted in various

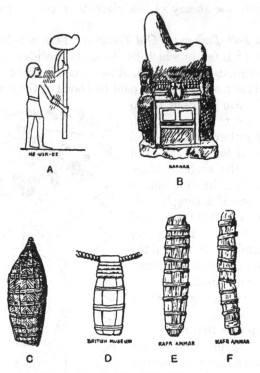

Fig. 2: The Bundle of Life (Murray).

African tribes (Roscoe). The whole subject is of interest as being a definite theory, even if pre-scientific, about the nature of an easily observed biological phenomenon, namely the placenta.[1]

Ancient Egypt supplies the starting-point for another and profounder train of thought which recurs constantly throughout the history of embryology, and to which I shall have to refer again more than once. This was concerned with the problem of deciding at what point the immortal constituent universally regarded as existing in living beings took up its residence in the embryo. Some fragments of ancient Indian philosophy assure us that the Vedic writers occupied themselves with

---

[1] To be compared with this preservation of the placenta is the care taken in the disposal of the umbilical cord by primitive peoples, including the early Greeks. Cook shows, with much detail (vol. 2, pp. 169 ff.), that the stone called "Omphalos," which was a cult-object at many temples, especially that of Delphi, though exoterically supposed to represent the navel of the earth (and in this way connected with a pillar supporting the heavens), was probably also intended to mark the burial-place of the umbilical cord of the priest-king, or perhaps of Zeus. Modern Greek folklore, too, includes special cares in the bestowal of the umbilical cord. "Omphalos" has been the subject of special monographs by Roscher.

this question, and according to Crawley the *Avesta* theorises upon it. But as early as 1400 B.C., i.e. during the eighteenth dynasty in Egypt, something was said regarding this, for we have extant at the present day a very beautiful hymn to the sun-god, Aton, written by no less a person than Akhnaton (Nefer-kheperu-Ra Ua-en-Ra, Amenhetep Neter heq Uast), generally known as Amenophis IV or the "heretic" king, who abandoned the traditional worship of the Theban god Amen-Ra and established an Aton-cult, as

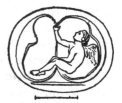

Fig. 3. Eros hatching from the cosmic egg. (A Hellenistic gem described by A. B. Cook, vol. 3, p. 1033.)

has been described by Baikie and others. One of his hymns, which bears considerable resemblance to the one hundred and fourth psalm, runs as follows (in Breasted's translation):

(The sun-god is addressed)

> Creator of the germ in woman,
> Maker of seed in man,
> Giving life to the son in the body of his mother,
> Soothing him that he may not weep,
> Nurse (even) in the womb.
> Giver of breath to animate every one that he maketh
> When he cometh forth from the womb on the day of his birth.
>
> Thou openest his mouth in speech,
> Thou suppliest his necessity.
>
> When the fledgeling in the egg chirps in the shell
> Thou givest him breath therein to preserve him alive.
> When thou hast brought him together
> To the point of bursting out of the egg,
> He cometh forth from the egg
> To chirp with all his might.
>
> He goeth about upon his two feet
> When he hath come forth therefrom.

Here no distinction is made between life and soul. At this early period there is no trace of the notions which appear later, such as the idea that embryos are not alive until the time of birth or hatching, or the idea that the soul is breathed into the embryo at some particular point in development. But in later times these considerations carried great weight, and with the rise of theology a definite stand had to be taken about them, for otherwise no ethical status could be assigned to abortion. Speculation on these matters has continued without cessation since the time of Akhnaton, reaching a climax perhaps in Christian times with Cangiamila's *Embryologia Sacra*, and living on embedded in Roman Catholic theology up to our own era.[1] In the last century the subject seems to have had a special fascination for Ernst Haeckel, who frequently mentioned it.[2] But the future holds no place for the discussion of such themes, and what has been called "theological embryology" is already dead, though we may perhaps descry its successor, psychological embryology, in such researches as those of Teuscher, Cesana, y Gonzalez, Swenson, Kuo Zing-Yang and Coghill.[3]

3. Artificial Incubation

The Egyptians were responsible for one of the greatest helps in systematic embryological study, namely the discovery of the artificial incubation of the eggs of birds.[4] The success of this process was to have so obvious an effect on embryology, and the abortive attempts to bring it to completion were so frequent in the West right up to the nineteenth century A.D.[5] that it is remarkable to find artificial incubation practised "probably," in Cadman's words, "as far back as the dawn of the Old Kingdom, about 3000 B.C." It is doubtful whether the very remote date could be supported by Egyptological evidence; for, according to Hall and Lowe, hens were not introduced into Egypt from Mesopotamia or India until the time of the eighteenth dynasty (*ca.* 1400 B.C.) when there was much intercourse with the East (cf. Queen Tiy and the Tel-el-Amarna correspondence): before then the Egyptians had only goose or duck eggs. Artificial incubation is certainly as old as Diodorus Siculus and Pliny, for both of them refer to the practice, the latter in connection with a curious piece of ancient sympathetic magic.

---

[1] See below, pp. 65–6, 75 and 204, also the interesting note of Vorwahl. Here might also be mentioned the probability that embryos (aborted or of other origin) were used in antiquity as substitutes for human sacrifice. The literature on this can be reached through the short discussion of Partington, p. 294, who mentions the habitual burial of foetuses under glass-furnaces in his history of chemical technology. More recently the subject has been thoroughly investigated by Eliade, pp. 75 ff.

[2] *Evolution of Man*, vol. 2, p. 355; *Riddle of the Universe*, ch. 8.

[3] The large mass of modern work on the psycho-neural development of the foetus has been brought together in admirable monographs by Carmichael; Detwiler, and Gesell & Amatruda. The great classic on physiological embryology is of course the book of W. Preyer in 1885, and it was this which stimulated the present writer to produce his *Chemical Embryology* forty-six years later.

[4] An excellent history of the technique in all cultures has recently been written by Landauer.

[5] Cf. pp. 202 ff.

Livia Augusta, the Empresse [says Pliny], wife sometime of Nero, when she was conceived by him and went with that child (who afterwards proved to be Tiberius Caesar) being very desirous (like a young fine lady as she was) to have a jolly boy, practised this girlish experiment to foreknow what she should have in the end; she tooke an egge, and ever carried it about her in her warme bosome; and if at any time she had occasion to lay it away, she would convey it closely out of her own warme lap into her nurses for feare it should chill. And verily this presage proved true, the egge became a cocke chicken, and she was delivered of a sonne. And hereof it may well be came the device of late, to lay egges in some warme place and to make a soft fire underneath of small straw or light chaffe to give a kinde of moderate heate; but evermore the egges must be turned with a mans or womans hand, both night and day, and so at the set time they looked for chickens and had them.[1]

Pliny also says:

Over and besides there be some egs that will come to be birds without sitting of the henne, even by the worke of Nature onely, as a man may see the experience in the dunghills of Egypt. There goeth a pretty jeast of a notable drunkard of Syracusa, whose manner was when hee went into the Taverne to drinke to lay certaine egges in the earth, and cover them with moulde, and he would not rise nor give over bibbing untill they were hatched. To conclude, a man or a woman may hatch egges with the very heate onely of their body.

This story occurs also in Aristotle.

The Emperor Hadrian—*curiositatum omnium explorator*, as Tertullian calls him—writing from Egypt in A.D. 130 to his brother-in-law, L. Julius Servianus, says, "I wish them no worse than that they should feed on their own chickens, and how foully they hatch them, I am ashamed to tell you."[2] In the *Description de l'Égypte*, written by the members of the scientific staff of Napoleon's Egyptian expedition, and published at Paris in 1809, Rozière & Rouyer wrote on the artificial incubation of the Egyptians.[3] They conjecture very probably that Hadrian was shocked owing to a misunderstanding shared by Aristotle, Pliny, de Pauw[4] and de Réaumur, namely that the *gelleh* or dung was used to heat the eggs by its fermentation, and not, as is and was actually the case, by being slowly burnt in the incubation ovens. Baÿ gave an account of the ovens in modern times, but the best one is that of Lane, written in 1836:

The Egyptians have long been famous for hatching fowls' eggs by artificial heat. This practice, though obscurely described by ancient authors, appears to

---

[1] Philemon Holland's translation.
[2] Gregorovius, p. 124.
[3] Vol. 1, p. 203.
[4] Vol. 1, p. 204.

have become common in ancient Egypt from an early time. In Upper Egypt there are over fifty establishments, and in Lower Egypt more than a hundred. The furnace is constructed of sundried bricks and consists of two parallel rows of small ovens and cells for fire divided by a narrow vaulted passage, each oven being about 9 or 10 feet long, 8 feet wide and 5 or 6 feet high, and having above it a vaulted fire-cell of the same size but rather less in height. The eggs are placed upon mats or straw, one tier above another usually to the number of three tiers and the burning fuel is placed upon the floors of the fire-cells above. The entrance of the furnace is well closed. Each furnace consists of from twelve to 24 ovens and receives about 150,000 eggs during the annual period of its continuing open, one quarter or one third of which generally fail. The peasants supply the eggs and the attendants examine them and afterwards generally give one chicken for every two eggs that they have received. The general heat maintained during the process is from 100 to 103° of Fahrenheit's thermometer. The manager, having been accustomed to the art from his youth, knows from long experience the exact temperature that is required for the success of the operation without having any instrument like our thermometer to guide him. The eggs hatch after exactly the same period as in the case of natural incubation. I have not found that the fowls produced in this manner are inferior in point of flavour or in other respects to those produced from the egg in the ordinary way.[1]

Plate IA (opposite), taken from Cadman, shows the interior of a modern peasant's incubator. There is reason to believe that its construction and operation vary very little, if at all, from that of the ovens used in dynastic Egypt.

When Baÿ visited the rustic incubators in 1912 he took with him a flask of lime water and a thermometer. The former showed a large precipitation of calcium carbonate and the latter stood at 40° C. He was led to speculate on the value of a high CO_2 tension in the atmosphere, and concluded that it must have a beneficial effect, since the loss in the traditional incubator was not more than 4 per cent., while that in the oil-heated agricultural incubators of his time was as much as 40 per cent. Cadman, writing in 1921, suggests that the well-known non-sitting instinct of Egyptian poultry is an effect of the ancient practice of artificial incubation. But enough has been said of the Egyptian *Ma'mal al-katakeet*, or chicken factories. In spite of the remarkable opportunity thus afforded for acquiring facts in experimental embryology, no use was apparently ever made of it, though there seems to be a certain amount of traditional information current among the peasant operators, as, for example, that the *rūḥ* or life enters into the egg at the eleventh day. It would be interesting to investigate this aspect of the subject further.

[1] *Manners and Customs*, p. 287.

24

PLATE I

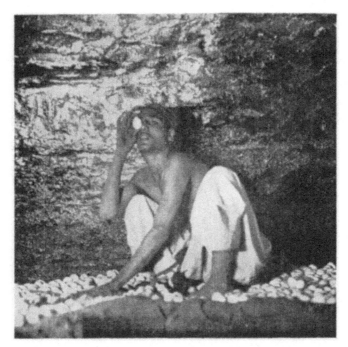

(A) Egyptian peasant incubator (from Cadman).

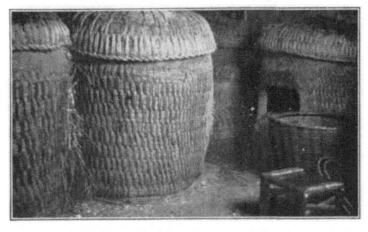

(B) Chinese peasant incubator (from King).

In China also it would appear that artificial incubation was successfully carried on in antiquity, if we may judge by the account given by
King.[1] Incubation in China is carried on in wicker baskets, heated with
charcoal pans (Plate IB, facing page 24). The attendants sleep in the
incubator itself, and use the same thermometer as the Egyptians,
namely their eyelids, to which they apply the blunt end of the egg.
The Egyptian success was known generally in the West in later times,
though it could not be imitated. "The Aegyptians," said Sir Thomas
Browne, "observed a better way to hatch their Eggs in Ovens, than the
Babylonians to roast them at the bottom of a sling, by swinging them
round about, till heat from motion had concocted them; for that con-
fuseth all parts without any such effect." Browne's slightly rueful tone
suggests that he tried it himself. It is interesting that this quaint experiment was the cause of a controversy between Sarsi, who asserted on the
authority of Suidas that it was possible, and Galileo, who thought the
idea ridiculous.[2] Modern work on the instability of albumen solutions,
such as that of Harris, lends some colour to the legend.[3]

4. Indian Antiquity

Ancient Indian embryology achieved a relatively high level. Structures such as the amniotic membrane are referred to in the *Bhagavad-
Gītā*.[4] The *Suśruta-saṃhita* says[5] that the embryo is formed of a mixture
of semen and blood,[6] both of which originate from chyle. In the third
month commences the differentiation into the various parts of the body,
legs, arms and head; in the fourth follows the distinct development of
the thorax, abdomen and heart; in the sixth are developed hair, nails,
bones, sinews and veins; and in the seventh month the embryo is furnished with any other things that may be necessary for it. In the eighth
there is a drawing of the vital force (*ojas*) to and from mother and
embryo, which explains why the foetus is not yet viable.[7] The hard parts
of the body are derived from the father, the soft from the mother.
Nourishment is carried on through vessels which lead chyle from mother
to foetus.[8]

The outstanding work on Indian embryology is now that of Dasgupta,
who in his chapter "Speculations in the medical schools" deals with the
Āyur veda, that great body of medical texts extending over more than

[1] *Farmers* . . . p. 157.
[2] *Frammenti e Lettere*, p. 66.
[3] See Needham (1931), p. 275.
[4] *Ca.* 2nd century B.C.
[5] The oldest parts of this *corpus* are now considered to date from the first two or
three centuries A.D.
[6] As we shall see, this is a very Greek idea.
[7] Perhaps this is comparable with the Hippocratic ἕλκειν.
[8] For further details, see Vullers and Esser.

twenty centuries in its composition. Both the *Atharva veda* and the *Āyur veda* deal with the curing of disease, but the former only by means of magic and incantations.

The factors going to the production of the foetus were (*a*) the father's semen, (*b*) the mother's blood (*śoṇita*), (*c*) the *ātman*, or subtle body, (*d*) the *manas* or mind, united to a particular embryo by reason of its *karma*. The subtle body consisted of fire, earth, air and water in the proper proportions. On these elements the Buddhist writers laid especial stress, adding to them two more, the principle of knowledge (*vijñāna-dhātu*) and the semen-blood substratum mentioned above, and thus obtaining the six constituents (*ṣaṇṇāṃ dhātūnāṃ samavāyāt*). Elsewhere the blood in question is specifically referred to as menstrual (*ārtava*), both by Suśruta and Caraka. This is of great interest in view of the Aristotelian doctrine described on pp. 42–3 of the present work, which it precisely resembles. The theory may, of course, have arisen quite independently in Greece and India, but it is perhaps more likely to have passed in one direction or the other, in which direction it is hard to say (cf. also the cheese analogy discussed on p. 50).

In this connection it is of interest that, according to Stopes,[1] the Hindu theologians considered it a crime for a girl to menstruate before going to her husband's house from her father's. Webb, in his *Pathologica Indica*, expressly states[2] that the regrettable institution of child marriage (cf. Rathbone) originated from the belief that the menstrual blood was the *materia prima* of the embryo and that to lose any before the first entry of sperm amounted to child murder. "If an unmarried girl has the menstrual secretion in her father's house, he incurs a guilt equal to the destruction of the foetus." Was it a mere chance that this interpretation of Aristotelian doctrine did not occur to the West? Other semi-superstitious beliefs about the catamenia certainly flourished there, as Crawfurd, Feis and others show.

Ḍalhaṇa, writing about A.D. 1100, says: in the first month the foetus has a jellylike form (*kalala*), in the second month, the material constituents of the body having undergone a chemical change (*abhiprapacyamāna*) due to the action of cold, heat and air (echo of Hippocrates?), the foetus becomes hard (*ghana*). Differentiation of limbs takes place in the third and fourth months, the appearance of consciousness and intelligence later. The controversies in the West about the priority of appearance of the limbs and organs (see pp. 28 ff.) have apparently their exact, and equally barren, counterpart in India. Thus the head appears first, according to Kumāraśiras and Śaunaka; the heart, according to Kṛtavīrya; the navel, according to Pārāśara; etc., etc.

---

[1] *Contraception*, p. 256.   [2] Pp. 259, 278.

The comparison of the formation of the embryo with the clotting of milk into cheese, first noted in Aristotle (see pp. 50, 84–5), occurs also in Indian embryology. The *Suśruta-saṃhita* says that as the semen and blood undergo chemical changes through heat, seven different layers of skin (*kalā*) are formed, like the creamy layers (*santānikā*) formed in milk. This concept occurs again in a Sūtra on embryology originally written in Sanskrit, translated into Chinese (first MS. A.D. 1104), and now into German by Hübotter. "Development, O Ananda," Buddha is made to say, "is comparable to a vessel of milk, like as this ferments and forms a kind of *kefir* or cheese." The rest of this text contains an account of the harmonious collaboration of many factors ("winds" with different names; a typically Buddhist characteristic) in the formation of the foetus.[1]

In which direction did all these theories travel along the Graeco-Indian line of communication?

5. Hellenic Antiquity; the Pre-Socratics[2]

Ancient Greek thought shows many evidences of appreciation of the mystery of embryonic growth, as for example in the Orphic cosmogonies, which had their origin about the seventh or eighth century B.C. In these religious and legendary descriptions of the world, which have been exhaustively discussed by A. B. Cook and F. Lukas, the cosmic egg plays a large part, and has been shown to occur also in the ancient cosmogonies of Egypt, India, Persia and Phoenicia (see Fig. 3, page 21). A familiar reference to this cosmic egg,[3] out of which all things were produced at the beginning of the world, is in Aristophanes' comedy *The Birds*, where the owl, as leader of the Chorus, says in the Parabasis (Sir John Sheppard's translation):

Chaos was first, and Night, and the darkness of Emptiness, gloom tartarean, vast;
Earth was not, nor Heaven, nor Air, but only the bosom of Darkness; and there with a stirring at last

---

[1] Hammett and I. Fischer have assembled some material dealing with ancient Indian ideas on heredity.

[2] In the ensuing sequence of sections, the material is treated, as throughout this book, chronologically. Balss (1936), however, gives a valuable summary of embryology from the pre-Socratics to Galen inclusive, arranged under subject-headings. So also does A. W. Meyer (1940).

[3] Perhaps another reference to the place of the egg in ancient cosmogony occurs in *The Arabian Nights*, where Aladdin's request for a roc's egg is treated as a blasphemy by the genie. In the visions of St Hildegard, too (see on, p. 84), the cosmic egg appears, according to Liebeschütz. And the tenacity of life of this notion may be gauged from the fact that C. Fourier at the end of the eighteenth century, and C. H. Rice (in *Psyche*, 1929!) entertained it. It also influenced early theories of mineral formation (Adams).

Of wings, though the wings were of darkness too, black Night was inspired
  a wind-egg[1] to lay,
And from that, with the turn of the seasons, there sprang to the light the
  Desired,
Love, and his wings were of gold, and his spirit as swift as the wind when it
  blows every way.
Love moved in the Emptiness vast, Love mingled with Chaos, in spite of
  the darkness of Night,
Engendering us, and he brought us at last to the light.

The pre-Socratic philosophers nearly all seem to have had opinions
upon embryological phenomena, many of which are worth referring to.[2]
These investigators of nature who lived in Greece from the eighth
century onwards are only known to us through the writings of others, or
in some cases in the form of fragments, for all their complete books have
perished. Diels' collection of the *Fragmente der Vorsokratiker* is the
most convenient source for what is left, but the assembling of their
opinions has not been left to modern times, for a collection of them
occurs in the writings of Plutarch of Chaeronea[3] (3rd century A.D.). It
is necessary to make use of some caution in describing their views, for
Aristotle, as an instance, frequently gives the most unfair versions of the
views of his predecessors. The account which follows is based upon
Plutarch, in Philemon Holland's translation,[4] and Diels. Empedocles of
Acragas, who lived about 444 B.C., believed that "the embryo derives
its composition out of vessels that are four in number, two veins and
two arteries, through which blood is brought to the embryo." He also
held that the sinews are formed from a mixture of equal parts of earth
and air, that the nails are water congealed, and that the bones are formed
from a mixture of equal parts of water and earth. Sweat and tears, on
the other hand, are made up of four parts of fire to one of water.
Empedocles also had opinions about the origin of monsters[5] and twins,

[1] Infertile eggs were commonly called "wind-eggs" in antiquity (see below, pp. 52
and 67). The notion of animals being impregnated by the wind has been investigated
by Zirkle.
[2] See the recent monograph by Lesky.
[3] It is now certain that this collection is not by Plutarch himself but by an earlier
compiler, Aetios (see Burnet). The embryological material is in Bk. v of *De Placitis*.
[4] In certain cases, Holland's translation (1603) has been modified so as to make it
agree with Diels' text. My thanks are due to Mr H. C. Baldry in connection with this.
[5] As this is the first mention made so far of monsters, I may take the opportunity of
remarking that apart from cursory references from time to time (see below, e.g. pp.
81, 88, 103, 112, 178, 194, 204, 210 and 218), the ramifications of the history of
teratology have not here been seriously pursued. The monographs of Ballantyne,
Dareste and C. J. S. Thompson contain much material on this subject. Ballantyne
points out that perhaps the oldest explanation of them was that the gods were playing,
as in the phrase attributed to Heraclitus, Ζεὺς παίζει, hence "lusus naturae," "Natur-
spiel," and our own "sport." He also considers the relation of ancient teratology to
augury, and figures an interesting Chaldean teratoscopic tablet. In later times the

and asserted that the influence of the maternal imagination upon the embryo was so great that its formation could be guided and interfered with.[1]

Empedocles [says Plutarch] saith that men begin to take forme after the thirtie-first day and are finished and knit in their parts within 50 daies wanting one. Asclepiades saith that the members of males because they are more hot are joynted and receive shape in the space of 26 daies, and many of them sooner, but are finished and complet in all limbes within 50 daies but females require two moneths ere they be fashioned, and fower before they come to their perfection, for that they want naturall heat. As for the parts of unreasonable creatures they come to their accomplishment sooner or later, according to the temperature of their elements. . . . Empedocles alloweth it to be a creature animall, howbeit that it hath no breath within the bellie, mary the first time that it hath respiration is at the birth, namely, when the superfluous humiditie which is in such unborne fruits is retired and gone, so that the aire from without entreth into the void vessels lying open.

Anaxagoras of Clazomenae (500–428 B.C.) may have said that the milk of mammals corresponded to the white of·the fowl's egg, but that observation is also attributed to Alcmaeon of Crotona. It is more certain that he spoke of a fire inside the embryo which set the parts in order as it developed, and that the head was the part to be formed first in development. This thesis was supported by Alcmaeon, and by Hippo of Samos, a Pythagorean, in the fifth century B.C., but Diogenes of Apollonia maintained about the same time that a mass of flesh was formed first, and afterwards the bones and nerves were differentiated. Plutarch remarks about this: "Alcmaeon affirmeth that the head is first made as

application of the Aristotelian system of causation to monsters gave occasion for much waste of human ingenuity, as in the treatises of Schott (1662) and Licetus (1616), where all four causes have to operate on three levels, divine, natural and diabolical. In 1578 Michel de Montaigne took a very modern view of terata, as described by Debrunner. An embryologist and an art historian in parabiosis, so to say, have written an interesting introduction to the subject (Hamburger & Born).

Schatz has gone about to prove, not unconvincingly, that much of mythology arose from the observation of developmental abnormalities. Thus a cyclops foetus may have suggested Polyphemus, a sympodial one Siren, and a diprosopous one Janus. The idea of Centaur may have originated from a hydrocephalic calf, and the Gorgon head from an acormic placental parasite. Occipital encephalocoele would have produced Atlas, foetal exomphalos Prometheus, and achondroplasia Egyptian Ptah. The likelihood of these surmises increases on careful consideration. Cf. *Science and Civilisation in China*, vol. 3, for parallel Asian data.

When visiting the famous Buddhist cave-temples at Tunhuang, Kansu, in China, in 1943 I observed several frescoes of guardian deities (*lokapāla*) with arms coming forth from their eyes, and bearing distal eyes on the palms of these supernumerary limbs (Plate II, facing page 30). It occurred to me to wonder whether some monk pacing the seashore had chanced upon a spontaneous example of heteromorphosis in a crustacean. These forms commonly regenerate an eye-stalk instead of an antenna, or an antenna instead of a limb.

[1] See below, p. 215.

being the seat of reason. Physicians will have the heart to be the first, wherein the veines and arteries are. Some thinke the great toe is framed first, others the navill."

The other contributions of Diogenes to this primitive embryology were the recognition of the placenta as an organ of foetal nutrition, and the view that the male embryo was formed in four months but the female not till five months had elapsed—a notion similar to that found in Asclepiades and Empedocles, as we have seen. He also associated heat with the generation of little animals out of slime, and compared this with the heat of the uterus. He considered that the embryo was not alive. "Diogenes saith that infants are bred within the matrice inanimate, howbeit in heat, whereupon it commeth that the inborn heat, so soon as ever the infant is turned out of the mother's wombe, draweth the cold into the lungs."[1] But the principal pre-Socratic embryologist was, as Zeller points out,[2] Alcmaeon of Crotona, who lived in the sixth century B.C., a disciple of Pythagoras, though apparently an independent one. He is said to have been the first man to make dissections. The fragments of Alcmaeon (not to be confused with Alcman, the Lacedaemonian poet) have been collected together by Wachtler; the most important are XVII and XIX. Athenaeus in the *Deipnosophists* says, in his usual chatty way, "Now with respect to eggs Anaxagoras in his book on natural philosophy says that what is called the milk of the bird is the white which is in the eggs." This may be a wrong ascription; it may refer to Alcmaeon, for Aristotle says in his book on the generation of animals,[3]

Nature not only places the material of the creature in the egg but also the nourishment sufficient for its growth, for since the mother-bird cannot protect the young within herself she produces the nourishment in the egg along with it. Whereas the nourishment which is called milk is produced for the young of vivipara in another part, in the breasts, Nature does this for birds in the egg. The opposite, however, is the case to what people think and what is asserted by Alcmaeon of Crotona. For it is not the white that is the milk, but the yolk, for it is this that is the nourishment of the chick, whereas they think it is the white because of the similarity of the colour.

Whether Aristotle was led to this conclusion because of his erroneous ideas about the part played in foetal nutrition by yolk and white respectively or whether he recognised a similarity between yolk and milk on account of their fatty nature, we cannot tell. In any case, his correction of Alcmaeon was in the right direction; and the comparison of the

[1] Another emendation of Holland has been necessary here for the reason given on p. 28.
[2] Vol. I, p. 522. [3] 752b 19.

PLATE II

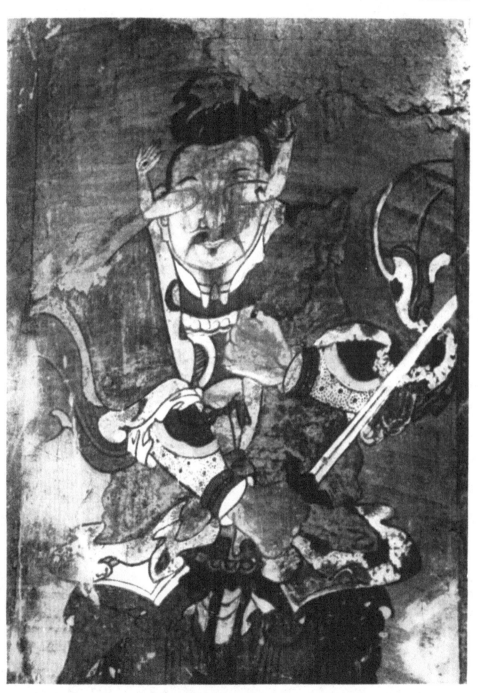

Heteromorphosis in a guardian deity (lokapāla) *depicted in a fresco on the wall of one of
the cave-temples at Ch'ien-Fo-Tung, Tunhuang, Kansu province, China.*
(Original photograph, 1943.)

amino-acid distribution in the two phosphoproteins, the casein of milk and the vitellin of yolk (Abderhalden & Hunter) shows their similarity.

Parmenides asserted a connection between male embryos and the right side of the body and between female embryos and the left side of the body—an idea which, considering its total lack of foundation, had a very long lease of life in the world of thought.[1] There was much controversy on the question of how foetal nutrition went on; the atomists, Democritus (born about 460 B.C.) and Epicurus (born about 342 B.C.), said that the embryo ate and drank *per os*. "Democritus and Epicurus hold," says Plutarch, "that this unperfect fruit of the womb receiveth nourishment at the mouth; and thereupon it cometh that so soon as ever it is borne it seeketh and nuzzeleth with the mouth for the brest head or nipple of the pappe: for that within the matrice there be certain teats; yea, and mouths too, whereby they may be nourished. But Alcmaeon affirmeth that the infant within the mother's wombe, feedeth by the whole body throughout for that it sucketh to it and draweth in maner of a spunge, of all the food, that which is good for nourishment." It would appear also that Democritus believed the external form of the embryo to be developed before the internal organs were formed.

6. Hippocratic Embryology and the Doctrine of the Two Seeds

But the foregoing fragments of speculation do not really amount to much. The first detailed and clear-cut body of embryological knowledge is associated with the name of Hippocrates, of whom nothing certain is known save that he was born probably in the forty-fifth Olympiad, about 460 B.C., that he lived on the island of Cos in the Aegean Sea, and that he acquired greater fame as a physician than any of his predecessors, if we may except the legendary names of Aesculapius, Machaon and Podalirios. It has not been believed for many centuries past that all the writings in the collection of Hippocratic books were actually set down by him, and much discussion has taken place about the authenticity of individual documents.

Most of the embryological information is contained in a section which in other respects (style, etc.) shows homogeneity. We are therefore rather interested in the unknown biological thinker who wrote the books in this class, for he could with considerable justice be referred to as the first embryologist. Littré discusses his identity, but there is no good evidence for any of the theories about it, though perhaps the most likely one is that he was Polybus, the son-in-law of Hippocrates. That the

---

[1] Thus it occurs as one of the few ideas contained in the *Callipaedia* of Claudius Quilletus, which ran through many editions in the eighteenth century.

writings on generation are only slightly later than the time of Hippocrates is more or less clear from the fact that Bacchius knew of them, and
actually mentions them.

For the most part the embryological knowledge of Hippocrates is
concerned with obstetrical and gynaecological problems.[1] Thus in the
Aphorisms, ἀφορισμοί, the books on epidemics, ἐπιδημίαι, the treatise
on the nature of women, περὶ γυναικείης φύσιος, the discussions of
premature birth, περὶ ἑπταμήνου, the books on the diseases of women,
περὶ γυναικείων, and the pamphlet on superfoetation, there are many
facts recorded about the embryo, but all with obstetrical reference.
There are some curious notions to be found there, such as the association
of right and left breasts with twin embryos and a prognostic dependent
on this.[2]

But the three books which are most important in the history of
embryology are the treatise on *Regimen*, περὶ διαίτης, the work on
generation, περὶ γονῆς, and the book about the nature of the infant,
περὶ φύσιος παιδίου. The two latter really form one continuous discussion, and it is not at all clear how they came to be split up into
separate books. In the *Regimen* the writer expounds his fundamental
physiological ideas, involving the two main constituents of all natural
bodies, fire and water. Each of these is made up of three primary
natures, only separable in thought and never found isolated, heat, dryness and moisture, and each of them has the power of attracting (ἕλκειν)
their like, an important feature of the system. Life consists in moisture
being dried up by fire and fire being wetted by moisture alternately;
τροφή, the nourishment (moisture) coming into the body, is consumed
by the fire so that fresh τροφή is in its turn required.

It is important to note that the Hippocratic school was far more akin
in its general attitude to living things to modern physiology[3] than the
Aristotelian and Galenic physiology. For no considerations of final
causes complicate the causal explanations of the Hippocratic school, and
the author of the περὶ διαίτης indeed devotes seven chapters to a detailed comparison of the processes of the body (*a*) with the processes of
the inorganic world both celestial and terrestrial, and (*b*) with the
processes used by men in the arts and crafts, such as iron-workers,
cobblers, carpenters and confectioners. These discussions present
strongly mechanistic features.

---

[1] The treatises *On Semen* and *On the Development of the Child* have recently been
translated by Ellinger.
[2] Special treatment of the opinions in the Hippocratic *corpus* on heredity will be
found in Johannsen and Hommel, and on scientific methodology in Senn.
[3] And to Democritean physiology. Wellmann has discussed the relation between the
pre-Socratic atomists and the Hippocratic *corpus*.

He then in Section 9 sets forth his theory of the formation of the embryo.

Whatever may be the sex which chance gives to the embryo, it is set in motion, being humid, by fire, and thus it extracts its nourishment from the food and breath introduced into the mother. First of all this attraction is the same throughout because the body is porous but by the motion and the fire it dries up and solidifies (ὑπὸ δὲ τῆς κινήσιος καὶ τοῦ πυρὸς ξηραίνεται καὶ στερεοῦται); as it solidifies, a dense outer crust is formed, and then the fire inside cannot any more draw in sufficient nourishment and does not expel the air because of the density of the surrounding surface. It therefore consumes the interior humidity. In this way parts naturally solid being up to a point hard and dry are not consumed to feed the fire but fortify and condense themselves the more the humidity disappears—these are called bones and nerves. The fire burns up the mixed humidity and forwards development towards the natural disposition of the body in this manner; through the solid and dry parts it cannot make permanent channels but it can do so through the soft wet parts, for these are all nourishment to it. There is also in these parts a certain dryness which the fire does not consume, and they become compacted one to another. Therefore the most interior fire, being closed round on all sides, becomes the most abundant and makes the most canals for itself (for that was the wettest part) and this is called the belly. Issuing out from thence, and finding no nourishment outside, it makes the air pipes and those for conducting and distributing food. As for the enclosed fire, it makes three circulations in the body and what were the most humid parts become the *venae cavae*. In the intermediate part the remainder of the water contracts and hardens forming the flesh.

In this account of the formation of the embryo, which seems at first sight a little fantastic, there are several interesting things to be remarked. Firstly, there is to be noted throughout it a remarkable attempt at causal explanations and not simply morphological description. The Hippocratic writer is out to explain the development of the embryo from the very beginning on machine-like principles, no doubt unduly simplified, but related directly to the observed properties of fire and water. In this way he is the spiritual ancestor of Gassendi and Descartes. The second point of interest is that he speaks of the embryo drying up during its development, a piece of observation which anyone could make by comparing a fourth-day chick with a fourteenth-day one, but which we express to-day in graphical form.[1] Thirdly, the ascription of the main driving force in development to fire has doubtless no direct relation to John Mayow's discovery,[2] two thousand years later, that

[1] The water-content of the chick embryo drops from 95 per cent. at the fifth day to 80 per cent. at hatching. See Fig. 4.
[2] 1672.

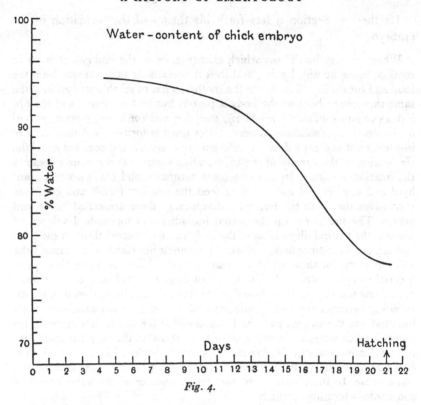

Fig. 4.

there is a similarity between a burning candle and a living mouse each in its bell-jar, and may mean as much or as little as Sir Thomas Browne's remark,[1] "Life is a pure flame, and we live by an invisible sun within us." Yet the essential chemical aspect of living matter is oxidation, and the development of the embryo no less than the life of the adult is subject to this rule, so that what may have been a mere guess on the part of the Hippocratic writer may also have been a flash of insight due to the simple observation which, after all, it was always possible to make, namely, that both fires and living things could be easily stifled.

Preformationism is perhaps foreshadowed in Section 26 of the same treatise.

Everything in the embryo is formed simultaneously. All the limbs separate themselves at the same time and so grow, none comes before or after other, but those which are naturally bigger appear before the smaller, without being formed earlier. Not all embryos form themselves in an equal time but some earlier and some later according to whether they meet with fire and

[1] 1645.

34

food, some have everything visible in 40 days, others in 2 months, 3, or 4. They also become visible at variable times and show themselves to the light having the blend (of fire and water) which they always will have.

The work on *Generation* is equally interesting. The earlier sections deal with the differences between the male and female seed, and the latter is identified with the vaginal secretion.[1] Purely embryological discussion begins at Section 14, where it is stated that the embryo is nourished by maternal blood, which flows to the foetus and there co-agulates, forming the embryonic flesh. The proof alleged for this is that during pregnancy the flow of menstrual blood ceases; therefore it must be used up on the way out.[2] In Section 15 the umbilical cord is recognised as the means by which foetal respiration is carried on. Section 17 contains a fine description of development with a very interesting analogy. "The flesh," it is said, "brought together by the breath (τὸ πνεῦμα) grows and divides itself into members, like going to like, dense to dense, flabby to flabby, humid to humid. The bones harden, coagulated by the heat." Then a demonstration experiment follows:

Attach a tube to an earthen vessel, introduce through it some earth, sand, and lead chips, then pour in some water and blow through the tube. First of all, everything will be mixed up, but after a certain time the lead will go to the lead, the sand to the sand, and the earth to the earth, and if the water be allowed to dry up and the vessel be broken, it will be seen that this is so. In the same way seed and flesh articulate themselves. I shall say no more on this point.

Here again was an attempt at causal explanation, rather than morphological description.

Section 22 contains a suggestive comparison between seeds of plants and embryos of animals, but the identification of stalk with umbilical cord leads to a certain confusion. Perhaps the most interesting passage of all is to be found in Section 29.

Now I shall speak [says the unknown Hippocratic embryologist] of the characters which I promised above to discuss and which show as clearly as human intelligence can to anyone who will examine these things that the seed is in a membrane, that the umbilicus occupies the middle of it, that it alternately draws the air through itself and then expels it, and that the members are attached to the umbilicus. In a word, all the constitution of the foetus as I

---

[1] This doctrine of the two seeds, reinforced by Epicurean support, competed for many centuries with the Aristotelian doctrine that only the male contributed seed while the female provided blood (cf. pp. 39-40, 43, below). In 1870 the great morphologist Wilhelm His saw the importance of this saecular controversy for the history of biology and sketched its development in an interesting paper, too little known.

[2] This was the essence of Aristotle's doctrine, see below, pp. 42 ff.

have described it to you, you will find from one end to the other if you will use the following proof. Take 20 eggs or more and give them to 2 or 3 hens to incubate, then each day from the second onwards till the time of hatching, take out an egg, break it, and examine it. You will find everything as I say in so far as a bird can resemble a man. He who has not made these observations before will be amazed to find an umbilicus in a bird's egg. But these things are so, and this is what I intended to say about them.

We see here as clearly as possible the beginnings of systematic embryological knowledge, and from this point onwards, through Aristotle, Leonardo, Harvey and von Baer, to the current number of the *Archiv f. Entwicklungsmechanik*, the line runs as straight as Watling Street.

In Section 30 there is an important passage in which the author discusses the phenomena of birth.

I say that it is the lack of food which leads to birth, unless any violence has been done; the proof of which is this—the bird is formed thus from the yolk of the egg, the egg gets hot under the sitting hen and that which is inside is put into movement. Heated, that which is inside begins to have breath and draws by counter-attraction another cold breath coming from the outside air and traversing the egg, for the egg is soft enough to allow a sufficient quantity of respiration to penetrate to the contents. The bird grows inside the egg and articulates itself exactly like the child as I have previously described. It comes from the yolk but it has its food from and its growth in, the white. To convince oneself of this it is only necessary to observe it attentively. When there is no more food for the young one in the egg and it has nothing on which to live, it makes violent movements, searches for food, and breaks the membranes. The mother, perceiving that the embryo is vigorously moving, smashes the shell. This occurs after 20 days. It is evident that this is how things happen for when the mother breaks the shell there is only an insignificant quantity of liquid in it. All has been consumed by the foetus. In just the same way, when the child has grown big and the mother cannot continue to provide him with enough nourishment, he becomes agitated, breaks through the membranes and incontinently passes out into the external world free from any bonds. In the same way among beasts and savage animals birth occurs at a time fixed for each species without overshooting it, for necessarily in each case there must be a point at which intra-uterine nourishment will become inadequate. Those which have least food for the foetus come quickest to birth and *vice versâ*. That is all that I had to say upon this subject.

The theory underlying this passage evidently is that the main food of the fowl embryo is the white and that the yolk is there purely for constructional purposes. Had the author not been strongly attached to this erroneous view he could not have failed to notice the unabsorbed yolk-sac which still protrudes from the abdomen of the hatching chick, and if he had given this fact a little more prominence he could hardly have come to enunciate the general theory of birth which appears in the above passage.[1] Moreover, had he been acquainted with the circulation of the maternal and foetal blood in viviparous animals, he could hardly have held that there was less food in a given amount of maternal blood at the end of development than at the beginning. But his attempted theory of birth was a worthy piece of scientific thinking, and we cannot yet be said to understand the principles governing incubation time.[2]

The treatises on food and on flesh περὶ τροφῆς and περὶ σαρκῶν (*ca.* 400 B.C.) contain points of embryological interest. Section 30 of the former contains some remarks on embryonic respiration, and Section 3 of the latter has a theory of the formation of nerves, bones, etc., by differences in composition of glutinous substances, fats, water, etc. Section 6 supports the view that the embryo is nourished *in utero* by sucking blood from the placenta, and the proof given is that its intestine contains the meconium at birth. Moreover, it is argued, if this were not so, how could the embryo know how to suck after it is born?

7. Aristotle's great Systematisation

After the Hippocratic writings nothing is of importance for our subject till Aristotle. It is true that in the *Timaeus* Plato deals with natural phenomena, eclectically adopting opinions from many previous writers and welding them into a not very harmonious or logical whole. But he has hardly any observations about the development of the embryo. The four elements—earth, fire, air and water—are, according to him, all bodies; and therefore have plane surfaces which are composed of triangles. Applying this semi-atomic hypothesis to the growth of the young animal, he says,

The frame of the entire creature when young has the triangles of each kind new and may be compared to the keel of a vessel that is just off the stocks; they are locked firmly together and yet the whole mass is soft and delicate, being freshly formed of marrow and nurtured on milk. Now when the triangles out of which meats and drinks are composed come in from without, and are comprehended in the body, being older and weaker than the triangles already there, the frame of the body gets the better of them and its newer

---

[1] In connection with the views of the Hippocratic embryologist on the exhaustion of nutriment as the cause of birth, it is of interest that modern research is pointing to a probable failure or inefficiency of the mammalian placenta towards the end of intra-uterine life. The well-known increase of erythrocytes, haemoglobin, blood-volume, etc., in the foetus at the end of pregnancy, together with a shift of the dissociation-curve of foetal blood, may be reactions adaptive to a relative anoxaemia caused by placental inefficiency, and comparable with those found at high altitude. See the monographs of Barcroft and the short survey of Needham (1933).

[2] Cf. Needham (1931) and Nice.

triangles cut them up and so the animal grows great, being nourished by a multitude of similar particles.

This is as near as Plato gets to embryological speculation. His description has a causal ring about it, which is in some contrast with the predominantly teleological tone of the rest of his writings; for instance, only a few pages earlier he has been speaking of the hair as having been arranged by God as "a shade in summer and a shelter in winter." It is also true that Plato may have said more about the embryo than appears in the dialogues. Plutarch mentions various speculations about sterility, and adds, "Plato directly pronounceth that the foetus is a living creature, for that it moveth and is fed within the bellie of the mother."[1]

But all this was only the slightest prelude to the work of Plato's pupil, Aristotle. Aristotle's main embryological book was that entitled περὶ ζῴων γενέσεως, On the Generation of Animals, but embryological data appear in περὶ ζῴων, The History of Animals, περὶ ζῴων μορίων, On the Parts of Animals, περὶ ἀναπνοῆς, On Respiration, and περὶ ζῴων κινήσεως, On the Motion of Animals. All these were written in the last three-quarters of the fourth century B.C.

With Aristotle, general or comparative biology came into its own. That almost inexhaustible profusion of living shapes which had not attracted the attention of the earlier Ionian and Italo-Sicilian philosophers, which had been passed over silently by Socrates and Plato, intent as ever upon ethical problems, but which had been for centuries the inspiration of the vase-painters and other craftsmen (ζωγράφοι), was now for the first time exhaustively studied and reduced to some sort of order. The Hippocratic school with their "Coan classification of animals," which Burckhardt has discussed, had indeed made a beginning, but no more. It was Aristotle who was the first curator of the animal world, and this comparative outlook colours his embryology, giving it, on the whole, a morphological rather than a physiological character.

The question of Aristotle's practical achievements in embryology is interesting, and has been discussed by Ogle.[2] There is no doubt that he diligently followed the advice of the author of the Hippocratic treatise on generation and opened fowl's eggs at different stages during their development, but he learnt much more than the unknown Hippocratic embryologist did from them. It is also clear that he dissected and examined all kinds of animal embryos, mammalian and cold-blooded. The uncertain point is whether he also dissected the human embryo. He refers in one place to an "aborted embryo," and as he was able to obtain

---

[1] On Plato and preformationism, see Praechter.
[2] And Montalenti.

easily all kinds of animal embryos without waiting for a case of abortion, it is likely that this was a human embryo. Ogle brings forward six or seven passages which all contain statements about human anatomy and physiology only to be explained on the assumption that he got his information from the foetus. So it is probable that his knowledge of biology was extended to man in this way, as would hardly have been the case if he had lived in later times, when the theologians of the Christian Church had come to severer conclusions about the sanctity of foetal as well as adult life.

The περὶ ζῴων γενέσεως, the first great compendium of embryology ever written, is not a very well-arranged work. There are a multitude of repetitions, and the order is haphazard, so that long digressions from the main argument are common. The work is divided into five books, of which the second is much the most important in the history of embryology, though the first has also great interest, and the third, fourth and fifth contain much embryological matter mixed up among points of generation and sexual physiology.

Book 1 begins with an introduction in which the relative significance of efficient and final causes is considered, and chapters 1 to 7 deal with the nature of maleness and femaleness, the nature and origin of semen, the manner of copulation in different animals and the forms of penis and testes found in them. Chapter 8 continues this, and describes the different forms of uterus in different animals, speaks of viviparity and oviparity, mentions the viviparous fishes (the selachians) and draws a distinction between perfect and imperfect eggs. Chapter 9 discusses the Cetacea; 10, eggs in general; and 11 returns to the differences between uteri. In chapter 12 the question is raised why all uteri are internal, and why all testes are not, and in chapter 13 the relations between the urinary and the genital systems are discussed. Copulation now receives attention again, in 14 with regard to Crustacea, in 15 with regard to Cephalopoda, and in 16 with regard to Insecta. After this point the argument lifts itself on to a more theoretical plane, and opens the question of pangenesis, into which it enters at length during the course of chapters 17 and 18, refuting eventually the widely held view that the semen takes its origin from all the parts of the body so as to be able to reproduce in the offspring the characteristics of the parent.[1] The nature of semen receives a long discussion; it is decided at last that it is a true secretion, and not a homogeneous natural part (a tissue), nor a heterogeneous natural part (an organ), nor an unnatural part such as a growth, nor mere nutriment, nor yet a waste product. It is here that the theory

[1] Special treatment of Aristotle's opinions on heredity will be found in Johannsen; Balss (1923); H. Meyer (1919); and Stiebitz.

is put forward that the semen supplies the "form" to the embryo and whatever the female produces supplies the matter fit for shaping. The obvious question has next to be answered, What is it that the female supplies? Aristotle concludes in chapters 19 and 20 that the female does not produce any semen, as earlier philosophers had held, but that the menstrual blood is the material from which the seminal fluid, in giving to it a form, will cause the complete embryo to be produced. This was not a new idea, but had already been suggested by the author of the Hippocratic περὶ γονῆς. What was quite new here was the idea that the semen supplied or determined nothing but the form. Chapters 21 and 22 are rather confused; they contain more arguments against pangenesis, and considerations upon the contrast between the active nature of the male and the passive nature of the female. Chapter 23, which closes the first book, compares animals to divided plants, for plants in Aristotle's view fertilise themselves.

Book II opens with a magnificent chapter on the embryological classification of animals, showing Aristotle, the systematist, at his best—his classification is reproduced in Chart I. But the chapter also includes a brilliant discussion of epigenesis or preformation, fresh development or simple unfolding of pre-existent structures, an antithesis which Aristotle was the first to perceive, and the subsequent history of which is almost synonymous with the history of embryology. The question in its acutest form was not settled until the eighteenth century, but since then it has become clear that there were elements of truth in the opinion which was the less true of the two. Chapter 2 is not so important, though it has some interesting chemical analogies; it compares semen to a foam, and suggests that it was this foam, like that of the sea, which gave birth to the goddess Aphrodite.[1] But chapter 3 returns to the high level of speculation and thought found in the opening part of the book, for it deals with the degree of aliveness which the embryo has during its passage through its developmental stages. Aristotle does not here anticipate the form of the recapitulation theory, but he certainly suggests the essence of it in perfectly clear terms. This chapter has also an interest for the history of theological embryology, for its description of the entry of the various souls into the embryo was afterwards made the basis for the legal rulings concerning abortion. This chapter also discusses embryogeny as a whole, as does the succeeding one. Chapter 5 is a digression into the problem of why fertilisation by the male is necessary, but it has also some curious speculations as to what extent the hen's egg is alive if it is infertile. The main thread is resumed in

---

[1] To the Greeks all natural foams possessed a generative virtue, and a Zeus Aphrios was worshipped at Pherae in Thrace.

CHART I

ARISTOTLE'S CLASSIFICATION OF ANIMALS ACCORDING TO EMBRYOLOGICAL CHARACTERISTICS

LIVING MATTER

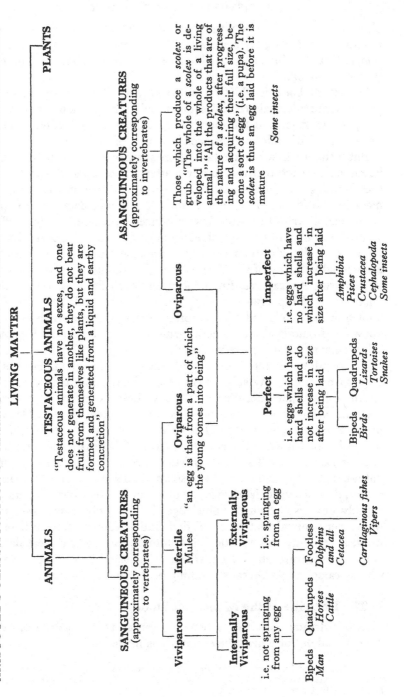

ANIMALS

PLANTS

TESTACEOUS ANIMALS

"Testaceous animals have no sexes, and one does not generate in another, they do not bear fruit from themselves like plants, but they are formed and generated from a liquid and earthy concretion"

ASANGUINEOUS CREATURES
(approximately corresponding to invertebrates)

Those which produce a *scolex* or grub. "The whole of a *scolex* is developed into the whole of a living animal." "All the products that are of the nature of a *scolex*, after progressing and acquiring their full size, become a sort of egg" (i.e. a pupa). The *scolex* is thus an egg laid before it is mature

Some insects

SANGUINEOUS CREATURES
(approximately corresponding to vertebrates)

Oviparous
"an egg is that from a part of which the young comes into being"

Oviparous

Infertile
Mules

Internally Viviparous
i.e. not springing from any egg

Bipeds
Man

Quadrupeds
Horses
Cattle

Externally Viviparous
i.e. springing from an egg

Footless
Dolphins and all Cetacea

Cartilaginous fishes
Vipers

Viviparous

Perfect
i.e. eggs which have hard shells and do not increase in size after being laid

Bipeds
Birds

Quadrupeds
Lizards
Tortoises
Snakes

Imperfect
i.e. eggs which have no hard shells and which increase in size after being laid

Amphibia
Pisces
Crustacea
Cephalopoda
Some insects

chapters 6 and 7, two very fine ones, in which embryogeny and foetal nutrition are thoroughly dealt with, but dropped again in the last section, chapter 8, which is devoted to an explanation of sterility. This ends the second book.

The third book is chiefly concerned with the application of the general embryological principles, described in the previous book, to the comparative field, and the fourth book contains a collection of minor items which Aristotle has not been able to speak of before.

But if the work as a whole tails off in a rather unsatisfactory manner, its merits are such that this hardly matters. The extraordinary thing is that building on nothing but the scraps of speculation that had been made by the Ionian philosophers, and the exiguous data of the Hippocratic school, Aristotle should have produced, apparently without effort, a text-book of embryology of essentially the same type as Graham Kerr's or Balfour's. It is even very possible that Aristotle was unacquainted with any of the Coan school; for, though he often mentions Democritus, Anaxagoras, Empedocles and even Polybus, yet he never once quotes Hippocrates, and this is especially odd, as Aristotle is known to have collected a large library. Perhaps Hippocrates was only known to Aristotle as an eminent medical man; if this is so, Aristotle's achievements are still more wonderful.

The depth of Aristotle's insight into the generation of animals has not been surpassed by any subsequent embryologist, and, considering the width of his other interests, cannot have been equalled. At the same time, his achievements must not be over-estimated. Charles Darwin's praise of him in his letter to Ogle (which is almost too well known to quote) is not without all reservations true.[1] There is something to be said for Lewes as well as Platt. Aristotle's conclusions were sometimes not warranted by the facts at his disposal, and some of his observations were quite incorrect. Moreover, he stood at the very entrance into an entirely unworked field of knowledge; he had only to examine, as it were, every animal that he could find, and set down the results of his work, for nobody had ever done it before. It was like the great days of nineteenth-century physiology, when, as the saying was, "a chance cut with a scalpel might reveal something of the first importance."

8. The Doctrine of the Menstrual Blood

As has already been said, Aristotle regarded the menstrual blood as the material out of which the embryo was made.

---

[1] "Linnaeus and Cuvier have been my two gods, though in very different ways, but they were mere schoolboys to old Aristotle," C. D. to W. O. 22/2/1882, from *Life and Letters*, ed. F. Darwin, 1888, vol. 3, p. 252.

That, then, the female does not contribute semen to generation [says Aristotle], but does contribute something, and that this is the matter of the catamenia, or that which is analogous to it in bloodless animals, is clear from what has been said, and also from a general and abstract survey of the question. For there must needs be that which generates and that from which it generates, even if these be one, still they must be distinct in form and their essence must be different; and in those animals that have these powers separate in two sexes the body and nature of the active and passive sex also differ. If, then, the male stands for the effective and active, and the female, considered as female, for the passive, it follows that what the female would contribute to the semen of the male would not be semen but material for the semen to work upon. This is just what we find to be the case, for the catamenia have in their nature an affinity to the primitive matter.[1]

Thus the male dynamic element (τὸ ἄρρεν ποιητικόν) gives a shape to the plastic female element (τὸ θῆλυ παθητικόν). Aristotle was right to the extent that the menstrual flow is associated with ovulation, but as he knew nothing of the mammalian ovum, and indeed, as is shown in his embryological classification, expressly denied that there was such a thing, his main menstruation theory is wrong. Yet it was not an illegitimate deduction from the facts before him.[2]

9. Denials of Maternity and Paternity

These views of Aristotle's about the contribution of the female to the embryo are in striking contrast with certain conceptions of a century before which were probably generally held in Greece. There is a most interesting passage relating to them in the *Eumenides* of Aeschylus, when, during the trial scene, Apollo, defending Orestes from the charge of matricide, brings forward a physiological argument. "The mother of what is called her child," Apollo is made to say, "is no parent of it, but nurse only of the young life that is sown in her (τροφὸς δὲ κύματος νεοσπόρου). The parent is the male, and she but a stranger, a friend, who, if fate spares his plant, preserves it till it puts forth."

There is evidence that this doctrine was of Egyptian origin, for Diodorus Siculus says, "The Egyptians hold the father alone to be the author of generation, and the mother only to provide a nidus and nourishment for the foetus."[3] Whether this was so or not, the influence

[1] 729ᵃ 22.
[2] The further (and long) history of this theory will be found principally on pp. 78, 145-6 and 237-8, below. For Aristotle, as for all other Greek authors, the menstrual blood was normally an excretion of impure material. Cf. the impurity of the woman producing it in folklore, both modern and ancient Greek (Licht, vol. 2, p. 77; Crawfurd). Biochemical investigations have tentatively traced the inhibitory and other biological effects of menstrual blood and the sweat of menstruating women to the presence of considerable amounts of the base choline.
[3] Loeb edn. p. 275.

of such a doctrine must have been tremendous. We know that the conception of the female sex as playing the part of farm-land, i.e. of woman as a field in which grain was sown, was widespread in antiquity; Hartland[1] and S. A. Cook[2] have collected examples of it from Vedic, Egyptian and Talmudic sources. A late echo of it is to be found in Lucretius, who refers to "Venus sowing the field of woman"—

atque in eost Venus ut muliebria conserat arva.[3]

Nor would resemblances between mothers and children suffice to kill this belief, for plants may differ slightly according to the soil in which they are planted. Such an idea would have been a natural concomitant of the practice—also widespread in antiquity—of putting captured males to death, and retaining the females as concubines. The conquerors would thus have had no fear of corrupting the race with alien blood. The whole matter affords an excellent illustration of the way in which an apparently academic theory may have the most intimate connections with social and political behaviour, and Aristotle, far from being remote from practical affairs as he examined his viviparous fishes and made marginal notes on his copy of Empedocles, is seen to be labouring at their very root.

There is a good deal more to be said about this Graeco-Egyptian doctrine, which we might term "the denial of physiological maternity." For its precise opposite is met with in anthropology—"the denial of physiological paternity." Just as the Egyptians claimed that the father alone produced the child, so the Melanesians claim that the child is produced solely by the mother.

Malinowsky, in his brilliant account of the sexual life of the Trobriand Islanders,[4] describes their belief that children originate only in Tuma, the spirit-world,[5] and that sexual intercourse has nothing whatever to do with pregnancy and childbirth. Of the fertilising power of semen, they have, according to him, no idea. Tuma is a kind of world of the unborn, reminiscent of Cooke's eighteenth-century theory (see p. 208) and of Origen's pre-existence (see p. 95 n). Menstrual blood is the substratum of the embryo, and souls come to inhabit it as it accumulates in individual bodies.

---

[1] Vol. i, p. 309.   [2] Vol. i, p. 537.
[3] IV, 1107. And another in Sophocles, *Antigone*, l. 569:
> *Ismene.* Wilt thou slay the betrothed of thine own son?
> *Creon.* Nay, there are other fields for him to plough.
> (ἀρώσιμοι γὰρ χάτέρων εἰσὶν γύαι).

[4] Ch. 7, sect. 3, pp. 147, 149, 153.
[5] Cf. the belief of the Australian Arunta in the origin of children from *ratappa* stones, described by Spencer & Gillen, vol. i, p. 363; and now by Ashley Montagu (1937). Vaughan has further explored the Greek parallels.

The Trobrianders' argument, when pressed, was twofold: (1) that women were often sterile, even when married and having frequent sexual intercourse, and (2) that unmarried girls, though permitted by custom to have sexual intercourse, invariably remained sterile until officially married. Nothing could be said against the first of these observations, but the second presented a sufficiently intriguing problem, not for the anthropologist only, but also for the biologist. Malinowsky was able to convince himself that contraceptives were not in common use, and the subject remained something of a mystery until Hartman discovered a high relative sterility of the adolescent organism in experimental colonies of apes. Puberty and maturity, as he points out, are neither synchronous nor synonymous. In Hartman's colony, the young females were mated at the first menses (wt. 3350 gm.) but not a single female conceived before attaining the weight of 4400 gm. Mirskaia & Crew, again, observed in the mouse that pregnancy followed first mating in only 24 per cent. of the cases, while the same mice were 90 per cent. fertile in later matings. In India (see p. 26), where cohabitation began from about 12 years onwards, returns from maternity hospitals placed the average first parturition at about 19 years (18.3–19.4, Clark). The same picture is given by Mondière for Cochin-China. Malinowsky's phenomena, says Hartman, are probably explained by the fact that the first menstruation (puberty) marks merely an early manifestation of a train of events (adolescence) which only after three or four years leads to ovulation and conception, the proof of maturity. This explanation is made more plausible by the fact that although childbirth before marriage was stated to be exceedingly rare among the Trobrianders, occasional cases occurred.[1]

Much interest attaches to the further problem, namely whether these two opposed theories of primitive man—the denial of physiological paternity and maternity respectively—could have had any connection with the patriarchal and matriarchal frameworks of human societies.[2]

Finally, the resemblance of the Graeco-Egyptian view to the consequences of extreme animalculism (see pp. 205–12 of the present work) should be noticed. On the whole, the eighteenth century refrained from drawing the logical consequences of animalculism as regards heredity, and sometimes saved the situation by falling back on the force of the mother's imagination (see p. 215), etc., but a remark of Good,[3] who

[1] Cf. the review on adolescent sterility by Ashley Montagu (1939).
[2] After proposing this connection, I learnt that the Oresteian legend had been made the basis of similar arguments by J. J. Bachofen in his *Mutterrecht u. Urreligion*, p. 174, by F. Engels in his *L'origine de la famille, de la propriété privée, et de l'état*, p. xvii, and by G. P. Thomson in *Aeschylus and Athens*, p. 287. Cf. Bachofen's *Ur-religion und antike Symbole*, pp. 114 ff.
[3] Lucretius translation and notes, vol. 2, pp. 196 ff.

wrote in 1805, unearthed by Cole,[1] is very illuminating. Speaking of the wide acceptance of the animalculist theory during the preceding fifty years, he says: "Every naturalist, and indeed every man who pretended to the smallest portion of medical science, was convinced that his children were no more related, in point of actual generation, to his own wife, than they were to his neighbour's."[2]

10. Formation, Recapitulation and Fermentation

The embryo, then, took its origin from the menstrual blood, on which, and in which, the seminal essence operated to produce it. But the perplexing question of the order of formation of the parts remained unsettled, though it had already been opened by earlier thinkers. What they had not done was to put the question, as it were, into the form of a motion; they had not grasped the existence of two main alternatives, one of which would have to be chosen before any further progress could be made. This is just what Aristotle did:

There is considerable difficulty in understanding how the plant is formed out of the seed or any animal out of the semen. Everything that comes into being or is made must (1) be made out of something, (2) be made by the agency of something, and (3) must become something. Now that out of which it is made is the material; this some animals have in its first form within themselves, taking it from the female parent, as all those which are not born alive but produced as a *scolex* or egg; others receive it for a long time from the mother by sucking, as the young of all those which are not only externally but also internally viviparous. Such is the material out of which things come into being, but we are now enquiring not out of what the parts of an animal are made, but by what agency. Either it is something external which makes them or else it is something existing in the seminal fluid and the semen; and this must either be soul or a part of a soul, or something containing soul.[3]

Aristotle concludes that there is no external shaping influence, but only something or other contained in the embryo itself. To this extent he was wrong, for the influence of the proper physico-chemical environment on

[1] *Early Theories*, p. 122.
[2] With this may be compared the curious passages in L. Sterne's *Tristram Shandy* which discuss the proposition that the mother is not of kin to her child (Book IV, chapter 29), and the long consideration which Boswell gave (vol. 2, p. 428 ff.) to the question of whether his family estate should be entailed for heirs general or male heirs only (1776). "I had," he tells us, "a zealous partiality for heirs male, however remote, which I maintained by arguments which appeared to me to have considerable weight. As, first, the opinion of some distinguished naturalists, that our species is transmitted through males only, the female being all along no more than a nidus, or nurse, as Mother Earth is to plants of every sort; which notion seems to be confirmed by that text of scripture—'He was yet in the loins of his Father when Melchizedek met him' (Heb. vii. 10)," etc., etc. In spite of the efforts of Lord Hailes and Dr Johnson, Boswell retained the partiality.
[3] 733[b] 23.

the growing embryo is as important as its physico-chemical internal constitution (later he modified his views on this). But now he goes on to deal with the main question, and says,[1]

> How then does it (the shaping influence) make the other parts? All the parts, as heart, lung, liver, eye and all the rest, come into being either together or in succession, as is said in the verse ascribed to Orpheus, for there he says that an animal comes into being in the same way as the knitting of a net. That the former is not the fact is plain even to the senses, for some of the parts are clearly visible as already existing in the embryo while others are not. That it is not because of their being too small that they are not visible is clear, for the lung is of greater size than the heart, and yet appears later than the heart in the original development.

This passage demonstrates that Aristotle had opened hen's eggs at different stages, and was well acquainted with the appearances presented there as early as the third day. He goes on to set forth a further alternative. Agreeing that a continuously new formation of parts takes place, and not merely an unfolding of parts already present in the semen or the menstrual blood, is this brought about by a chain of creations or by one original creation? In other words, does the heart come into being first, and then proceed to form the liver, and then the liver go on to form the lungs, or do they simply appear one after the other without such a creative inter-relationship? Aristotle argues against the former view on the ground that if one organ formed another, the second one would have to resemble the first in some way, which is not the case. His words on this subject cannot be condensed.[2]

> But neither can the (formative) agent be external and yet it must needs be one or other of the two. We must try then to solve this difficulty, for perhaps some one of the statements made (already) cannot be made without qualification, e.g. the statement that the parts cannot be made by what is external to the semen. For if in a certain sense they cannot, yet in another sense they can. [Thus Aristotle does some justice to the environment.] It is possible, then, that A should move B and B should move C, that, in fact, the case should be the same as with the automatic machines shown as curiosities. For the parts of such machines while at rest have a sort of potentiality of motion in them, and when any external force puts the first of them into motion, immediately the next is moved in actuality. As, then, in these automatic machines the external force moves the parts in a certain sense (not by touching any part at the moment but by having touched one previously), in like manner also that from which the semen comes, or in other words that which made the semen, sets up the movement in the embryo and makes the parts of it by having touched first something though not continuing to touch it. In a way it is the

[1] 734ᵃ 18.   [2] 734ᵇ 3.

innate motion that does this, as the act of building builds a house. Plainly, then, while there is something which makes the parts, this does not exist as a definite object, nor does it exist in the semen at the first as a complete part.

This idea of the setting in motion of a wound-up clock is substantially modern and underlies the physico-chemical analysis of the developing embryo. It is really striking to find Aristotle using the machine analogy in order to explain himself, for he, of all biologists, emphasised the final cause in natural operations. However, he soon returns to a more vital-istic attitude in the succeeding section.[1]

But how is each part formed? We must answer this by starting in the first instance from the principle that in all products of Nature or art, a thing is made by something actually existing out of that which is potentially the same as the finished product. Now the semen is of such a nature and has in it such a principle of motion, that when the motion is ceasing each of the parts comes into being and that as a part having life or soul. . . . And just as we should not say that an axe or other instrument or organ was made by the fire alone, so neither shall we say that foot or hand were made by fire alone. . . . While, then, we may allow that hardness and softness, stickiness and brittleness, and whatever other qualities are found in the parts that have life and soul, may be caused by mere heat and cold, yet when we come to the principle ($\lambda\acute{o}\gamma o\varsigma$) in virtue of which flesh is flesh and bone is bone, that is no longer so; what makes them is the movement set up by the male parent, who is in actuality what that out of which the offspring is made is in potentiality. That is what we find in the products of art; heat and cold may make the iron soft or hard, but what makes a sword is the movement of the tools employed, this movement con-taining the principle of the art. For the art is the starting-point and form of the product; only it exists in something else (i.e. potentially in the mind of the artist) whereas the movement of nature exists in the product itself, issuing from another nature (i.e. the parent) which has the form in actuality.

Thus Aristotle, evidently influenced by his doctrine of "form" and "matter," decided against preformation and pictured at one and the same time the unformed catamenia as containing a kind of clockwork mechanism which, once set in motion, would inevitably produce the finished embryo, and also as an inchoate substance on which the seminal essence should act like a swordmaker producing a sword according to the motions of a natural art.[2] These two ideas are not completely recon-

[1] 734[b] 20.
[2] Balss (1936, p. 60) interprets Aristotle as leaning more to the former of these two ideas than I did when I first wrote the above passage. If so, the conception of "A moving B, and B moving C" and the analogy of the "automatic machines shown as curiosities" give a remarkable vindication of Aristotle's insight; since modern embry-ology, with its theory of first-, second- and third-grade organisers, has found many facts of this kind. The neural system is induced by the primary dorsal lip organiser, and the lens of the eye in turn by the optic outgrowth of the neural system (see Needham, 1936; 1950). Many other cases of this succession of influences are known,

ciled in Aristotle, and a consideration of artificial fertilisation would have provided a test case, had he been able to know of the experiments of Delage and Loeb. For on his second theory, butyric acid would transmute a sea-urchin's egg into butyric acid and not into a sea-urchin; while, on his first theory, the egg would make the sea-urchin irrespective of what influence it was that swung the starting-handle.

Aristotle has a good deal to say about the theory of recapitulation, as it was afterwards to be called. He thought there was no doubt that a vegetative or nutritive soul[1] existed in the unfertilised material of the embryo,

for nobody would put down the unfertilised embryo as soulless or in every sense bereft of life (since both the semen and the embryo of an animal have every bit as much life as a plant) and it is productive up to a certain point. . . . As it develops it also acquires the sensitive soul[2] in virtue of which an animal is an animal. . . . For first of all such embryos seem to live the life of a plant, and it is clear that we must be guided by this in speaking of the sensitive and the rational soul.[3] All three kinds of soul, not only the nutritive, must be possessed potentially before they are possessed actually.[4]

These passages show very clearly the line of thought contained in the recapitulation theory, as do the following.[5] "An animal does not become at the same time an animal and a man or a horse or any other particular animal," i.e. the more general appears first and the more particular later. "The end is developed last, and the peculiar character of the species is the end of the generation in each individual," i.e. the embryo attains the point of being definitely not a plant before it attains that of being definitely not a mollusc but a horse or a man. Aristotle concludes that the different sorts of souls enter the embryo at different stages of development, just as the shape of the embryo gradually approximates to whatever adult shape it is destined to possess.[6] He did not think, how-

and it has been suggested as the explanation of the facts for which the recapitulation theory was fashioned (Needham, 1930).

Another argument used against preformation by Aristotle was that if the embryo was preformed either in the male or female contributions to generation, a double off-spring would always result. Balss (1936) points out the sharpsightedness of this criticism, which really did not receive an answer till the discovery of the reduction division of the chromosomes two thousand years later.

[1] The ψυχὴ θρεπτική.   [2] The ψυχὴ αἰσθητική.   [3] The ψυχὴ διανοητική.
[4] 736ª 33; cf. Schmidt.   [5] 736ᵇ 2.
[6] On Aristotle's doctrine of souls cf. Sir Thomas Browne's "Who admires not Regiomontanus his Fly beyond his Eagle, and wonders not more at the operation of *two* souls in those minute bodies, than but *one* in the trunk of a Cedar?" It has recently been shown that closely similar doctrines of a ladder or succession of souls or vital forces in ontogeny and phylogeny were current in Chinese thought through the ages (see Lu & Needham, and more fully in *Science and Civilisation in China*, vol. 2). The dating of the thinkers concerned makes any transmission of Greek ideas very improbable.

The recapitulation theory has an entertaining echo in sixteenth-century theological ever, that they were in-breathed from any source external to the embryo, but rather that they were internally generated each in due time.[1]

Aristotle continues to discuss the central problems of embryology, but now in a way which presents features of directly physico-chemical interest.[2]

When the material secreted by the female in the uterus has been fixed by the semen of the male (this acts in the same way as rennet acts upon milk, for rennet is a kind of milk containing vital heat, which brings into one mass and fixes the similar material, and the relation of the semen to the catamenia is the same, milk and the catamenia being of the same nature), when, I say, the more solid part comes together, the liquid is separated off from it, and as the earthy parts solidify membranes form all round it; this is both a necessary result and for a final cause, the former because the surface of the mass must solidify on heating as well as on cooling, the latter because the foetus must not be in a liquid but separated from it.

Later on, he also says,[3]

The reason is similar to that of the growth of yeast, for yeast also grows great from a small beginning as the more solid part liquefies and the liquid is aerated. This is effected in animals by the nature of the vital heat, in yeasts by the heat of the juice contained in them.

polemic, for the *Epistolae Obscurorum Virorum*, written on the Protestant side in German to ridicule, *inter alia*, Catholic scrupulosity, contains (p. 446) the following:

Letter xxvi. *Heinrich Schaufmaul to Mag. Ortwin Gratius.*

"I write to ask your reverence what opinion you hold concerning one who on a Friday . . . should eat an egg with a chicken in it. For you must know that we were lately sitting in an inn in the Campo dei Fiori, having our supper, and were eating eggs, when on opening one I saw that there was a young chicken within. This I showed to a comrade, whereupon quoth he to me, 'Eat it up speedily, ere the taverner see it, for if he mark it, you will have to pay . . . for a fowl. It is a rule of the house that once the landlord has put anything on the table, you must pay for it, he won't take it back.' . . . In a trice I gulped down the egg, chicken and all, and then I remembered that it was a Friday. So I said to my companion, 'You have made me commit a mortal sin in eating flesh on the sixth day of the week.' But he averred it was no mortal sin, nor even a venial one, seeing that such a chick is accounted an egg merely, until it is born. He told me, too, that it is just the same in the case of cheese, in which there are sometimes mites, as there are maggots in cherries, peas, or new beans; yet all these may be eaten on Fridays and even on Apostolic Vigils. But taverners are such rascals that they call them flesh, to get the more money. Thus I departed, and thought the matter over, and, by the Lord, Master Gratius, I am in a mighty quandary and know not what to do. . . . It seemeth to me that these young fowls in eggs are flesh, because their substance is formed and fashioned into the limbs and body of an animal, and possesseth a vital principle. It is different in the case of cheese-mites and such-like, because grubs are accounted fish, as I learnt from a physician who is skilled also in natural philosophy. Most earnestly do I entreat you to resolve the question I have propounded, for if you hold that the sin is mortal, then I would fain get shrift here before I return to Germany."

[1] See the careful study of Moraux.
[2] 739^b 22. On Aristotle's chemical ideas see von Lippmann.
[3] 755^a 18.

These remarkable passages contain the first reference to enzyme action ever made in a discussion in embryology. The solidification of the outer crust is of course Hippocratic, as we have already seen. The part about the amnios is unfortunate; for the facts are exactly contrary.

The heart is first differentiated [says Aristotle[1]], as is clear not only to the senses (for it is so) but on theoretical grounds. For whenever the young animal has been separated from both parents it must be able to manage itself, like a son who has set up house away from his father.

This is good observation. "The heart is the principle and origin of the embryo," says Aristotle.[2] This conception of *cor primum vivens, ultimum moriens* (a phrase never used by Aristotle himself) has henceforward a long and tortuous history, which has been described by Ebstein and others.

Aristotle goes on to describe the membranes of the mammalian foetus with its umbilical cord:[3] "The vessels join on to the uterus like the roots of plants and through them the embryo receives its nourishment. This is why the embryo remains in the uterus"; not, as Democritus thought, so that it might be moulded into the maternal shape. The embryo "straightway sends off the cord like a root to the uterus." He carefully notes, as if the conception of axial gradients was existing deep down in his mind, that the cephalic parts of the embryo are formed first.[4]

The greater become visible before the less even if some of them do not come into being before them. First the parts above the *hypozoma* [a term more or less corresponding to "diaphragm"] are differentiated and are superior in size; the part below is both smaller and less differentiated. This happens in all animals in which exists the distinction of upper and lower, except in the insects.

Aristotle gives as his explanation of this a teleological argument:[5]

This is why the parts about the head and especially the eyes appear largest in the embryo at an early stage, while the parts below the umbilicus, as the legs, are small; for the lower parts are for the sake of the upper and are neither parts of the end, nor able to form it.

Embryonic growth is thus described by Aristotle:[6]

The homogeneous parts (tissues) are formed by heat and cold, for some are put together and solidified by the one and some by the other. . . . The nutriment oozes through the blood-vessels and the passage in each of the parts, like water in unbaked pottery, and thus is formed the flesh or its analogues, being solidified by cold, which is why it is dissolved by fire. But all the particles given off which are too earthy, having but little moisture and heat,

[1] 740ᵃ 3.   [2] 740ᵃ 20.   [3] 740ᵃ 33.   [4] 741ᵇ 26.   [5] 742ᵇ 14.   [6] 743ᵃ 4.

cool as the moisture evaporates along with the heat, so they become hard and earthy in character, as nails, horns, hoofs and beaks, and therefore they are softened by fire but none of them is melted by it, while some of them, as egg-shells, are soluble in liquids. The sinews and bones are formed by the internal heat as the moisture dries, and hence the bones are insoluble by fire like pottery, for like it they have been as it were baked in an oven by the heat in the process of development. . . . The skin, again, is formed by the drying of the flesh, like the scum upon boiled substances; it is so formed not only because it is upon the outside, but also because what is glutinous, being unable to evaporate, remains on the surface.

Here is a splendid collection of mechanical processes, but Aristotle is careful to add:[1] "As we said, all these things must be understood to be formed in one sense of Necessity, but in another sense not of Necessity but for a Final Cause."

Concurrent growth and differentiation, the former being temporally sequent to the latter, he thus describes:[2]

The upper half of the body, then, is first marked out in the order of development; as time goes on the lower also reaches its full size in the *sanguinea*. All the parts are first marked out in their outlines and acquire later on their colour and softness or hardness, exactly as if Nature were a painter producing a work of art, for painters too first sketch in the animal with lines and only after that put in the colours.

Aristotle had some difficulty about the eyes; he noted that they were very disproportionately large in early bird embryos, but he seems to have thought that they shrank absolutely as well as relatively during further development. It takes him a great deal of ingenuity to invent a teleological explanation for this quite imaginary fact.

The food which the embryo derives from the mother, according to Aristotle, is of two distinct kinds, nutritious, formative or creative, τό θρεπτικόν, and that which is concerned with simple increase of size, τό εἰς μέγεθος ποιοῦν τὴν ἐπίδοσιν. This distinction is difficult to understand, and, though it would be attractive to interpret the former as vitamins and the latter as fats, proteins and carbohydrates, that would probably be putting too much of a strain on our belief in Aristotle's insight. He has much to say of the placenta, and ascribes to it its correct function. He combats the idea that foetal nutrition is maintained by uterine paps, alleging against it the fact that all embryos are enclosed in membranes. He discusses birds' eggs in great detail, referring to infertile or "wind-eggs" and to the action of heat during incubation. He considered that the embryo was formed from the white exclusively, and only got its nourishment from the yolk, which was a backward step

[1] 743[b] 16.   [2] 743[b] 17.

in view of what had already been said by the Hippocratic embryologist. He knew of the whiteness of the yolk when first formed in the oviduct and of the yellow colour of the layers of yolk added to it in its passage down that tube, but he held that the yellow colour was "sanguineous," and therefore hot, while the white was cold. He held also that the bird embryo always developed at the pointed end;[1] no doubt, as Platt has suggested, Aristotle belonged to Swift's class of "little-endians," and must have always opened them at that end, in which case he would find the embryo there, for the yolk always swims embryo uppermost. He knew also that the yolk liquefied during the first week of development, and that it grew larger, but he did not guess the right reasons for these phenomena. He knew the arrangements for embryonic development in the dolphins and ovoviviparous sharks.[2] He takes a strong line over spontaneous generation; "nothing," he says,[3] "comes into being by putrefying, but by concocting." And so in many other passages where detailed observation is joined with acute reasoning.

So far only the treatise on the generation of animals has been under consideration. But in the περὶ ζῴων, also, there are many embryological data, and it is strange that those detailed observations upon the developing fowl embryo, which demonstrate more than anything else Aristotle's wonderful powers of observation, are not contained in the *Generation of Animals* at all, but in the *History of Animals*. He takes animals one by one in order, and in each case deals with their generative peculiarities, such as their mode of hatching, their incubation period, their fertility, etc. For instance, he correctly relates how the embryos of cartilaginous fishes possess a yolk-sac like bird embryos, but no allantois. In his account of the fowl he is unusually precise.[4]

Most of the sixth book is occupied with the account of the generation of birds and fishes, and the seventh treats also very fully of that of man. But in both cases it is description that is given; the theoretical considerations are left to the book on generation, and for this reason the latter work is the more interesting. The *History of Animals* has a wonderful wealth of material in it, but at the same time includes many extravagant stories, such as those of the "kindly and gentle dolphin" and the equine Oedipus, so that the austerity of the book on generation charms us more.

[1] 754^b 10.
[2] The placentoid structure in *Mustelus laevis* was rediscovered by Johannes Müller in the nineteenth century; the full story is given by Haberling.
[3] 762^a 14. See on the question of spontaneous generation in antique authors (including Aristotle) von Lippmann and Rodemer. Later Rabbinic texts mention birds as originating from the slime of the sea (e.g. *Pesiqta Rabbathi*, ed. Friedmann, p. 61*a*). I owe this reference to Dr H. Loewe.
[4] 561^a.

Other treatises also mention embryology. The περὶ ζῴων μορίων, *On the Parts of Animals*, has a passage in which the appearance of the third-day chick embryo is described, and refers to observations on the lack of pigment and of distinct medullary canals in bones in foetal life. The small work entitled περὶ ἀναπνοῆς, *On Respiration*, also refers to the heart as the first organ to be formed, and so as the seat of the soul. But these minor sources contribute little to the progress of the science, and it is upon the great work *On the Generation of Animals* that Aristotle's well-deserved fame as an embryologist will always rest.[1]

11. The Aristotelian Balance-sheet

If I have devoted such ample space to an account of Aristotle's contributions to embryology, it is, firstly, because they are actually greater in number than those of any other individual embryologist, and secondly, because they had so profound an influence upon the following twenty centuries. Embryology from the third century B.C. to the seventeenth century A.D. is meaningless unless it is studied in the light of Aristotle.

His outstanding contributions to embryology may be put in the following way:

1. He carried to their logical conclusion the principles of the observation of facts suggested by the unknown Hippocratic embryologist, and added to them a discipline of classification and correlation of facts which gave embryology a quite new coherence.
2. He introduced the comparative method into embryology, and by studying a multitude of living forms was able to lay the foundation for future science of the various ways in which embryonic growth can take place. Thus he knew of oviparity, ovoviviparity, and viviparity, and one of his distinctions is substantially the same as that known to modern embryology between holoblastic and meroblastic yolks.
3. He distinguished between primary and secondary sexual characteristics.
4. He pushed back the origin of sex-determination to the very beginning of embryonic development.[2]
5. He associated the phenomena of regeneration with the embryonic state.
6. He realised that the previous speculations on the formation of

[1] Our knowledge of the numerous later translations of Aristotle's *On the Generation of Animals* into Arabic, Latin and other languages, is still imperfect, but Sarton's great work contains a good deal of information on this subject.
[2] Cf. the special study of this by Blersch.

the embryo could be absorbed into the definite antithesis of pre-formation and epigenesis, and he decided that the latter alternative was the true one.

7. He put forward a conception of the unfertilised egg as a complicated machine, the wheels of which would move and perform their appointed function in due course when once the master-lever had been released.

8. He foreshadowed the theory of recapitulation in his speculations on the order in which the souls came to inhabit the embryo during its growth, and in his observation that universal characteristics precede particular characteristics in embryogeny.

9. He foreshadowed axial gradient theory by his observations on the greater and more rapid development of the cephalic end in the embryo.

10. He allotted the correct functions to the placenta and the umbilical cord.

11. He gave a description of embryonic development involving comparison with the action of rennet and yeast, foreshadowing thus our knowledge of organic catalysts in embryogeny.

But there was another side to the picture. Aristotle made three big mistakes, and here I do not refer to any matters of detail, in which it would not have been humanly possible to be more than very often right, but rather to general notions, such as the eleven correct ones just noted. They were as follows:

1. He was incorrect in his view that the male supplies nothing tangible to the female in the process of fertilisation. To say that the semen gave the "form" to the inchoate "matter" of the menstrual blood was equivalent to saying that the seminal fluid carried nothing in it but simply an immaterial breath along with it. Aristotle could not, of course, envisage the existence of spermatozoa.

2. He was entirely wrong in his teaching about the *scolex*. The caterpillar is not, as he supposed, an egg laid too soon, but has already passed through the embryonic state.[1]

[1] The study of metamorphosis in animals would be worth following all through the ages since the changes undergone by the pupa so closely resemble the differentiation of embryos. The time was to come, in the seventeenth century (pp. 139, 183 below), when the study of insect morphogenesis and the embryology of mammals were to react strongly together. But first it was necessary to clear away a mass of erroneous mediaeval beliefs about non-existent metamorphoses. For example, there was the ancient myth of the generation of geese from barnacles, which naturally played a not unimportant part in moral theology. The best accounts of it are in von Lippmann (pp. 36 ff.) and in the monograph of Heron-Allen. The myth was subject, says Heron-Allen, to a number of smaller or larger variations, but, broadly speaking, it ran that

3. He was misled by some observations on castrated animals and so did not ascribe to the testis its true function.

12. Aristotle's Theory of Causation

Such mistakes as these, however, were not nearly so important as the solid ground gained by his correct answers. They were always open to experimental test, even though the authority of his name precluded it until the Renaissance. But there was one aspect of his embryological work which was to exercise an unfortunate influence on the subsequent progress of the science, namely, his insistence on teleological explanations. He was always seeking for final as well as efficient causes.[1] "The ancient Nature-philosophers did not see that the causes were numerous; they only saw the material and efficient causes and did not distinguish even these, while they made no enquiry at all into the formal and final causes." "Democritus," he says, "neglecting the final cause, reduces to Necessity all the operations of Nature. Now they are necessary it is true, but yet they are also for a final cause, and for the sake of what is best in each case."

Aristotle's theory of causation is best studied in the *Physica* (194^b 16 ff.). Santayana has applied it in an amusing passage to embryology.

Aristotle distinguished four principles in the understanding of Nature. The ignorant think that these are all, equally, forces producing change, and the cooperative sources of all natural things. Thus, if a chicken is hatched, they say that the Efficient Cause is the warmth of the brooding hen, yet this heat would not have hatched a chicken out of a stone, so that a second condition, which they call the Material Cause, must be invoked as well, namely, the nature of an egg; the essence of eggness being precisely a capacity to be hatched when warmed gently—because, as they wisely observe, boiling would drive away all potentiality of hatching. Yet, as they further remark, gentle heat-in-general joined with the essence-of-eggness would produce only

"the fruits (or leaves) of certain trees, falling into the sea (or on land) become Barnacles (or birds), or that the Barnacles themselves grow upon a tree (or upon a log, or upon ship's timbers), and when developed to a certain point, fall off and become geese (or ducks), in fact the Barnacle-goose or Brent-goose (*Branta bernicla*)." The barnacle itself is of course a sessile cirripede (crustacean), and retains on account of the age of the legend the name *Lepas anatifera*. Heron-Allen's conclusion is that the myth arose from the striking resemblance between the feathers of a bird and the plumose appendages of a cirripede. But its antiquity is rather unexpected; he was able to trace it back to the Mycenaean age, though it does not occur in Graeco-Roman literature.

One of the most extraordinary things about the barnacle-geese legend is that it has close parallels in Chinese zoological literature, also connecting birds and molluscs. The facts will be given in the author's *Science and Civilisation in China*, vol. 8.

[1] The exact meaning of the word "entelechy" in connection with the final cause, as used by Aristotle and revived by certain modern writers, especially Hans Driesch, is rather a vexed question. Balss (1936), Burchard and Ritter are to be consulted on the subject.

hatching-as-such and not the hatching of a chicken, so that a third influence, which they call the Final Cause, or the End-in-view, must operate as well, and this guiding influence is the divine idea of a perfect cock or a perfect hen presiding over the incubation and causing the mere eggness in the egg to assume the likeness of the animals from which it came. Nor, finally, do they find that these three influences are sufficient to produce here and now this particular chicken, but are compelled to add a fourth, a Formal Cause, namely, a particular yolk, a particular shell, and a particular farmyard, on which and in which the other three causes may work, and laboriously hatch an individual chicken, probably lame and ridiculous despite so many sponsors.

Santayana puts this description[1] into the mouth of Avicenna in his imaginary dialogue, and makes him go on to say,

Thus these learned babblers would put Nature together out of words, and would regard the four principles of interpretation as forces mutually supplementary combining to produce material things; as if perfection could be one of the sources of imperfection or as if the form which things happen to have could be one of the causes of their having it. Far differently do these four principles clarify the world when discretion conceives them as four rays shed by the light of an observing spirit.

It is essential for an understanding of the following centuries to realise that these Aristotelian conceptions went without serious contradiction,[2] and thus formed the framework for all the biological work that was done. Owing to its association with the idea of the plan of a divine being, the final cause tended in the Middle Ages to eclipse the others. In the seventeenth century this feeling is well shown in a remarkable passage which occurs in the *Religio Medici* of Sir Thomas Browne:

There is but one first cause, and four second causes of all things; some are without Efficient, as God; others without Matter, as Angels; some without Form, as the first matter; but every Essence, created or uncreated, hath its Final cause, and some positive End both of its Essence and Operation; this is the cause I grope after in the works of Nature; on this hangs the providence of God; to raise so beauteous a structure as the World and the Creatures thereof, was but his Art; but their sundry and divided operations, with their predestinated ends, are from the Treasure of his Wisdom. In the causes,

---

[1] Actually Santayana used much philosophical licence in his account. The best explanations of the Aristotelian causes I know of are in the brilliant introductions to A. L. Peck's editions of the *Generation of Animals* (1943) and the *Parts of Animals* (1937). The more usual interpretation would be that the yolk and white of the egg are the Material Cause, the sperm of the cock the Efficient Cause, the generic and specific nature of the animal (in this case a bird) the Formal Cause, and the end-in-view, the perfected adult cock or hen in the future, the Final Cause. Peck's introductions are worth very careful study.

[2] Cf. Dante, *Purgatorio*, canto 25 and the comments of del Gaudio. See further, pp. 94 ff. below.

nature, and affections of the Eclipses of the Sun and Moon there is most excellent speculation, but to profound farther, and to contemplate a reason why his providence hath so disposed and ordered their motions in that vast circle as to conjoyn and obscure each other, is a sweeter piece of Reason and a diviner point of Philosophy; therefore sometimes, and in some things, there appears to me as much Divinity in Galen his books *De Usu Partium*, as in Suarez' *Metaphysicks*: Had Aristotle been as curious in the enquiry of this cause as he was of the other, he had not left behind him an imperfect piece of Philosophy but an absolute tract of Divinity.

This was written in Harvey's time, and in Harvey's thought the four causes were still supreme; his *De Generatione Animalium* is deeply concerned with the unravelling of the causes which must collaborate in producing the finished embryo (see p. 140). But the end of their domination was at hand, and the exsuccous Lord Chancellor, whose writings Harvey thought so little of, was making an attack on one of Aristotle's causes which was destined to be peculiarly successful. It is needless to quote his immortal passages about the "impertinence," or irrelevance, of final causes in science, for they cannot but be familiar to all scientific men.[1] Bacon demonstrated that from a scientific point of view the final cause was a useless conception; recourse to it as an explanation of any phenomenon might be of value in metaphysics, but was pernicious in science, since it closed the way at once for further experiments. To say that embryonic development took the course it did because the process was drawn on by a pulling force, by the idea of the perfect adult animal, might be an explanation of interest to the metaphysician, but as it could lead to no fresh experiments, it was nothing but a nuisance to the man of science. Later on it became clear also that the final cause was irrelevant in science owing to its inexpressibility in terms of measurable entities. From these blows the final cause never recovered. In England the seventeenth century was the time of transition in these affairs, and in such books as Joseph Glanville's *Plus Ultra* and *Scepsis Scientifica*, for instance, or Thomas Sprat's *History of the Royal Society*, the stormy conflict between the "new or experimental philosophy" and the Aristotelian "school-philosophy" can easily be followed. Francis Gotch has given a delightful account of the evening of Aristotelianism, but it involved a stormy sunset, and the older ideas did not give way without a struggle. Harvey's work is perfectly representative of the period of transition, for, in his preface under the heading "Of the Method to be observed in the knowledge of Generation," he says, "Every inquisition is to be derived from its Causes, and *chiefly* from the Material and Efficient." As for the formal cause, Bacon ex-

---

[1] *De Augmentis Scientiarum*, Bk. III, ch. 4.

pressly excluded it from Physic, and it quietly disappeared as men saw that scientific laws depended on the repeatableness of phenomena, and that anything unique or individual stood outside the scope of science. Thus in the case of the developing egg, the formal and the final causes are scientifically meaningless, and if it were desired to express modern scientific discourse in Aristotelian terminology, the material and efficient causes would alone appear.

Aristotle alone was unharmed by Aristotelianism. A metaphysician as well as a scientific worker, he was able to use the concept of purposiveness as a heuristic aid, but he never *rested* upon it. The trouble was that he introduced it into the discussion at all. It is an interesting speculation to consider what would have happened if the first great biologist had not brought final causes into his teaching; perhaps the subsequent history of biology, and science as a whole, would have been very different. For final causes irresistibly led to the theological blind alleys into which men's thoughts were ushered and there left to grope till the end of the Middle Ages.

Perhaps Aristotle would not have made so many great discoveries if he had been more of a Democritus. For teleology is, like other varieties of common sense, useful from time to time; e.g. Harvey told Boyle that he was led to certain important considerations by meditating upon the final cause of the valves in the veins;[1] and every biologist acts in the same way at the present time. But the important thing is not to give the last word to teleology. And those attractive shady places which Aristotle, guided by his genius, quickly passes through on his perpetual journeys into the hot sunlight of research and speculation were so many traps for those who followed him. He himself knew how to change rapidly from metaphysician into physicist and back again, how to bow politely to the final cause and press on with the dissection; but the later Peripatetics had no knowledge of this art, nor had the Patristic doctors, nor the mediaeval Aristotelians; who all remained sleeping quietly in the shade of the will of God. He knew very well from the sea (to use Bacon's metaphor at last) the look of the Circë country of teleology, but

---

[1] The interview was related by Boyle in his "Disquisition about the Final Causes of Natural Things," 1688—"And I remember that when I asked our famous Harvey, in the only discourse I had with him (which was but a while before he dyed), What were the things that induc'd him to think of a Circulation of the Blood? He answer'd me, that when he took notice that the Valves in the Veins of so many several parts of the Body, were so Plac'd that they gave free passage to the Blood Towards the Heart, but oppos'd the passage of the venal blood the Contrary way: He was invited to imagine that so Provident a Cause as Nature had not so Plac'd so many Valves without Design; and no design seemed more probable, than that, since the Blood could not well, because of the interposing Valves, be sent by the Veins to the Linbs; it should be Sent through the Arteries, and return through the Veins, whose valves did not oppose its course that way."

he never visited it for long at a time, being an authentic Odysseus, unlike so many later heads, who, following the example of Plato, "anchored upon that shore" and, dropping their hooks to the sound of plain-song, there rode, never to hoist sail again.

13. The Hellenistic Age

Aristotle died in 322 B.C. From that year until 1534, the date of the birth of Volcher Coiter, first in time of the Renaissance embryologists, embryology has very little history.

The founder of the Stoic philosophy, Zeno of Citium, was born some twenty years before the death of Aristotle.

Pious and magnanimous as Stoicism was in the field of conduct [says Allbutt], creating or nourishing that elevation of mind which distinguished the nobler Roman of the Empire, yet in Rome, as in England, its natural science was of no account. The spirit of it was indeed rather alien than akin to science. The mind of the Porch which called itself "practical" was reluctant to all "speculation," natural science included.

The Stoics regarded the four qualities of cold, hot, wet and dry as ultimate, instead of the earth, fire, air and water of the Peripatetics and their predecessors. Plutarch, in his summary of philosophic opinions already mentioned, has some passages relating to their views on the development of the embryo.

The Stoicks say that the foetus is fed by the secundine and navell; whereupon it is that midwives presently knit up and tie the navell string fast, but open the infants mouth, to the end that it be acquainted with another kind of nourishment.

And elsewhere,

The Stoicks say that it is a part of the wombe and not an animall by itselfe. For like as fruits be parts of trees, which when they be ripe do fall, even so it is with an infant in the mother's wombe. . . . The Stoicks are of opinion that the most parts are formed all at once; but Aristotle saith the backbone and loines are first framed like as the keele in a ship.

But to which of Zeno's successors—Cleanthes, Chrysippus, Crates or the rest—these sayings are to be attributed is not known.

The Epicureans also had opinions on these subjects. They thought that the foetus *in utero* was fed by the amniotic liquid or the blood, and they also believed, in contradistinction to the Peripatetics, that both male and female supplied seed in generation, as is shown by the lines of Lucretius:

usque adeo magni refert, ut semina possint
seminibus commisceri genitaliter apta
crassaque conveniant liquidis et liquida crasso.[1]

But much more important than the teaching of these philosophers was the rise of what might be called the scientific faculty of the great University of Alexandria. That seat of learning, perhaps the most glorious, after Athens, of any in antiquity, and greater than its contemporary rival Pergamon, was important because all the traditions of earlier times were united in it like a bundle of strands coming together to form a rope. Democritean atomism, Peripatetic science and metaphysics, Coan biology, Coan and Cnidian medicine, above all, Athenian mathematics and astronomy, all were gathered in the μουσεῖον of Alexandria under the benevolent dynasty of the Ptolemies. The link between the Alexandrian biologists and the school of Aristotle was Strato of Lampsacus, who, though apparently not making any contribution to embryology himself, must have brought the knowledge of generation gained by Aristotle to Alexandria as he sailed south across the Mediterranean to be the tutor of Ptolemy Philadelphus. The link between Cos and Alexandria was Diocles of Carystus, who was the last of the Hippocratic school and also a pupil of Philistion of Locri. Diocles has a certain importance in the history of embryology; for Oribasius refers to him as the discoverer of the *punctum saliens* in the mammalian embryo, "on the ninth day a few points of blood, on the eighteenth beating of the heart, on the twenty-seventh traces of the spinal cord and head." He thus showed that the early development of chick and mammal was very alike. Plutarch also tells us that he occupied himself with the question of sterility. He described the human placenta, as well as embryos of twenty-seven and

---

[1] "A matter of great moment 'tis in truth,
    That seed may mingle readily with seed
    Suited for procreation, and that thick
    Should mix with fluid seed, with thick the thin."

IV, 1257. For the further history of this view, which might also be called Hippocratic, see pp. 80, 127, 150 and 217. It could still be defended in the seventeenth century, as by Kijper and Mauriceau.

This is perhaps the place to refer to the fact, perhaps more singular than important, that an association between small animals and the male seed was made in antiquity. In 1885 Ladelci figured a painted marble sarcophagus in the museum at Tarragona, on which are two human figures in Minoan (?) costume, one male, the other female, standing under two date-palms, of which one is fertile and the other not. From the breasts of the female there comes a stream of milk (as in the device of the University of Cambridge); and from the male a stream of seed, which, however, instead of falling naturally, curls around in a spiral (cf. the vortex theories satirised by Aristophanes in the *Clouds*). Within this spiral many little animals are drawn. There is, unfortunately, doubt about the authenticity of the sarcophagus, which might immediately be dismissed were it not for the story, found in several Greek authors, e.g. in the second century, Antoninus Liberalis, that the seed of Minos contained all sorts of noxious animals (snakes, scorpions and scolopendras). As a result all his lovers died until he was cured by Procris. Cf. A. B. Cook, vol. 2 pp. 2, 1211.

forty days, and he held that both male and female contribute seed in generation. Cnidian medicine influenced Alexandria through Chrysippus of Cnidus—not the Stoic—whose embryological doctrine seems to have been that the embryo had only a vegetative soul until birth or hatching.

All these influences were fruitful, for they produced the two greatest physiologists of ancient times—Herophilus of Chalcedon and Erasistratus of Chios. These two, who were contemporaries during the third century B.C., experimented much and wrote voluminously, but all except fragments of their writings have been lost, and can now only be pieced together out of the books of Galen, as has been done by Dobson. Allbutt has well described the differences between them, such as the predilection of Herophilus for the humoral pathology and pharmacy, and the greater interest taken by Erasistratus in atomistic speculations. "Herophilus," says Plutarch, "leaveth to unborne babes a mooving naturall, but not a respiration, of which motion the sinewes be the instrumentall cause, but afterwards they become perfect living animall creatures, when being come forth of the wombe, they take in breath from the aire."

Herophilus described the ovaries and the Fallopian tubes, but did not advance further than Aristotle towards correct sexual physiology in this respect. We gather that he made many dissections of embryos from the testimony of Tertullian, though this may not be worth much. Moreover, he called the outer membrane of the brain, chorion, after the membranes which surround the embryo. He gave a correct description of the umbilical cord, except that he assigned to it four vessels instead of three, carrying blood and breath to the embryo. The veins, he thought, communicated with the venae cavae, and the arteries with the great artery running along the spine. Herophilus also occupied himself much with obstetrical matters, and wrote a treatise on them, μαιωτικόν. Together with Erasistratus he denied that there were any diseases special to women other than those attendant on their special sexual functions, but the greatest contribution which he made to biology was the association of the brain with the intellect,[1] for even Aristotle had made the heart the seat of the mental individual.

Erasistratus did not study embryology as much as Herophilus, but a passage in Galen throws an interesting light on his notions of embryonic growth.

The heart is no larger at first than a millet seed, or, if you like, a bean. Ask yourself how it could grow large otherwise than by being distended and re-

[1] This was not absolutely new: Alcmaeon had held the same view (see Burnet).

CHART II

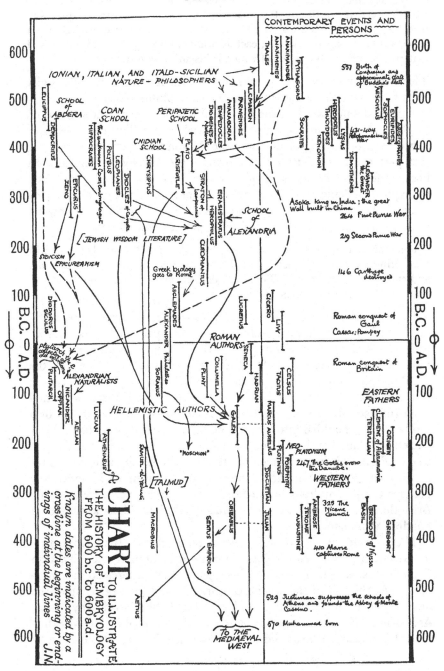

CONTEMPORARY EVENTS AND PERSONS

IONIAN, ITALIAN, AND ITALO-SICILIAN NATURE-PHILOSOPHERS

THALES · ANAXIMANDER · ANAXIMENES · PYTHAGORAS

557 Birth of Confucius and approximate date of Buddha's death.

SCHOOL of ABDERA · LEUCIPPUS · DEMOCRITUS

COAN SCHOOL · PERIPATETIC SCHOOL

ALCMAEON · PARMENIDES · ANAXAGORAS · DIOGENES of Apollonia · EMPEDOCLES · XENOPHON · SOCRATES

HERODOTUS · THUCYDIDES · LYSIAS · AESCHYLUS · SOPHOCLES · EURIPIDES · ARISTOPHANES

431-404 Peloponnesian War

The unknown Coan Embryologist · HIPPOCRATES · POLYBUS · LEOPHANES · DIOCLES of Carystus · CHRYSIPPUS · CNIDIAN SCHOOL

PLATO · ARISTOTLE · STRATON of Lampsacus · ERASISTRATUS · HEROPHILUS · CLEOPHANTUS

DEMOSTHENES · ALEXANDER the Great

ZENO · EPICURUS

SCHOOL of ALEXANDRIA

Asoka king in India; the great Wall built in China.

264 First Punic War

219 Second Punic War

[JEWISH WISDOM LITERATURE]

STOICISM · EPICUREANISM

Greek biology goes to Rome.

146 Carthage destroyed

ASCLEPIADES · ALEXANDER PHILALETHES

LUCRETIUS · CICERO · LIVY

Roman conquest of Gaul

Caesar; Pompey

DIODORUS SICULUS

ROMAN AUTHORS

SENECA · COLUMELLA · PLINY · CELSUS · TACITUS

Roman conquest of Britain

Plutarch i.e. the collection of Opinions · ALEXANDRIAN NATURALISTS · PLUTARCH · OPPIAN · NICANDER · AELIAN · LUCIAN · ATHENAEUS · SORANUS · GALEN · HADRIAN · MARCUS AURELIUS · DIOCLETIAN · JULIAN

EASTERN FATHERS

CLEMENT of Alexandria · TERTULLIAN · ORIGEN

HELLENISTIC AUTHORS

"MOSCHION"

NEO-PLATONISM · PLOTINUS · PORPHYRY

247 The Goths cross the Danube.

WESTERN FATHERS

SAMUEL-EL-YEHUDI · [TALMUD] · MACROBIUS · ORIBASIUS · SEXTUS EMPIRICUS · AETIUS

325 The Nicene Council

AMBROSE · JEROME · AUGUSTINE · BASIL · GREGORY of Nyssa · GREGORY

410 Alaric captures Rome

529 Justinian suppresses the schools of Athens and founds the Abbey of Monte Cassino.

570 Muhammad born

TO THE MEDIAEVAL WEST

A CHART TO ILLUSTRATE THE HISTORY OF EMBRYOLOGY FROM 600 B.C. to 600 A.D.

Known dates are indicated by a crossline at the beginning or endings of individual lines. J.N.

B.C. 0 A.D.

600 500 400 300 200 100 0 100 200 300 400 500 600

ceiving nutriment throughout its whole extent, just as we have shown above that the seed is nourished. But even this is unknown to Erasistratus, who makes so much of Nature's Art. He supposes that animals grow just like a sieve, a rope, a bag, or a basket, each of which grows by the addition to it of materials similar to those out of which it began to be made.

This is only one instance out of many in which Galen the teleologist finds fault with Erasistratus the mechanistic philosopher.

During the period when the biological school of Alexandria was at its height, that city became an important Jewish centre. Two centuries later it was to produce Philo, but now the Alexandrian Jews were writing that part of the modern Bible known as the Wisdom Literature. In books such as the *Wisdom of Solomon, Ecclesiasticus, Proverbs*, etc. the typical Hellenic exclusion of the action of gods in natural phenomena is clearly to be seen. There are two passages of embryological importance. Firstly, in the *Book of Job* (x. 10), Job is made to say,

Remember, I beseech thee, that thou hast fashioned me as clay; and wilt thou bring me into the dust again? Hast thou not poured me out as milk, and curdled me like cheese? Thou hast clothed me with skin and flesh, and knit me together with bones and sinews.

This comparison of embryogeny with the making of cheese is interesting in view of the fact that precisely the same comparison occurs in Aristotle's book *On the Generation of Animals*, as we have already seen.[1] Still more extraordinary, the only other embryological reference in the Wisdom Literature, which occurs in the *Wisdom of Solomon* (vii. 2), also copies an Aristotelian theory, namely, that the embryo is formed from (menstrual) blood. There the speaker says, "In the womb of a mother was I moulded into flesh in the time of ten months, being compacted with blood of the seed of man and the pleasure that accompanieth sleep." Perhaps it is no coincidence that both these citations can be referred back to Aristotle, and in the second case even to Hippocrates; perhaps the Alexandrian Jews of the third century B.C. were studying Aristotle as attentively as Philo Judaeus studied Plato a couple of hundred years later.

The Alexandrian school[2] was directly responsible for the introduction of Greek medicine and biology into Rome, through the physician Cleophantus, who seems to have been particularly interested in gynaecology. At the end of the second century B.C. and the beginning of the first, Rome received the first and greatest of her Greek physicians, Asclepiades of Parion, who brought atomism with him. He was thus the link between Epicurus and the methodistic school of physicians, and

[1] P. 50.   [2] See Meyerhof.

may have been a potent influence upon Lucretius. Again, Alexander Philalethes provides the link between Cleophantus and Soranus. Soranus lived in Rome from about A.D. 30 till just after the end of the first century, and so twenty years before the birth of Galen.

Of all the ancient writers on embryology Soranus is the one whose works were in later times most widely appropriated, mutilated, furbished up, quoted from rightly and wrongly, and generally upset. Allbutt, Barbour and Singer give accounts of the way in which this process went on, and the whole question has given rise to a considerable literature (see Lachs, Ilberg, Sudhoff, etc.). It lasted right into the Middle Ages, and was particularly vehement in the case of the treatise on gynaecology, περὶ γυναικείων παθῶν. This was translated into Latin under the name of Moschion, then back into Greek and finally back into Latin again. It is largely obstetrical, but it shows an advanced knowledge of embryology, and especially an accurate idea of the anatomy of the uterus. (See Plate III, facing page 66.)

Mention may here be made of a woman writer, Cleopatra, whose short treatise on obstetrics was often reprinted in the collective works of the Renaissance (Bauhin and Spach, q.v.). She appears to have been a sensible gynaecologist contemporary with Soranus and Galen (cf. the papers of Hurd-Mead). At the time of the first publication of the present work, my friend Dr R. W. Gerard brought to my notice a curious story, the origin of which he was unable to trace, that Cleopatra, the Ptolemaic queen, had investigated the process of foetal development by the dissection of slaves at known intervals of time from conception, following the precepts of Hippocrates with regard to hen's eggs.[1] The story is, it seems, Rabbinic (cf. Preuss, p. 451). R. Ismael (Nidd. III. 7) taught that the male foetus was complete in 41, the female in 81, days, and cited as his authority the results of the above Alexandrian experiment. Sceptics urged that copulation might have taken place before the experiment began, but supporters replied that an abortifacient was, of course, given. Sceptics begged leave to doubt the universal efficiency of these drugs. They also questioned whether intercourse between the slaves and the prison guards had been absolutely guarded against.

The whole subject is not as absurd as it seems at first sight, for it provides an example, in the Hellenistic or Patristic period, not common perhaps even in the Talmud, of a serious discussion on scientific method, and the planning of an experiment. It demonstrates how near men could come to the Baconian outlook. Other considerations, economic and theological, such as those referred to in the introduction to the present

---

[1] A similar story is found in Chinese legend concerning one of the early kings. Particulars will be found in the author's *Science and Civilisation in China*, vol. 8.

work, demonstrate how far men really were from it. It may also be proper to point out here that the Hellenistic, as opposed to the later mediaeval and post-mediaeval, arguments about "perfection-time" were related to a quite serious scientific problem, namely the respective part played by growth and differentiation in development. These concepts were clear in Aristotle's mind (see e.g. p. 52) and it was legitimate to investigate their speeds and end-points. The theological aspect of the subject was secondary.

Whether the story itself rests upon a confusion between Cleopatra the gynaecologist and Cleopatra the queen, or whether it arose entirely in R. Ismael's imagination, cannot at present be decided.

The other writers of this period are unimportant embryologically. Among the Greeks, Aelian wrote a *De natura animalium*, in which he spoke of eggs, but without adding anything to our knowledge of them. Nicander in his *Theriaca* refers to mammalian embryos, and alleges that they breathe and eat through the umbilical cord, and Oppian has a few unsystematic remarks about the embryos of various animals. Junius Columella's work on husbandry contains two chapters on eggs,[1] but he was not much interested in the theoretical aspect of development. In Aulus Gellius we have the cheese analogy appearing in conjunction with obscurantist views about the powers of the number seven.[2] It is not generally known that a clear statement of the preformationist or "Entfaltung" theory of embryogeny[3] occurs in Seneca's *Quaestiones Naturales*, where there is the following passage:[4]

In the seed are enclosed all the parts of the body of the man that shall be formed. The infant that is borne in his mother's wombe hath the rootes of the beard and hair that he shall weare one day. In this little masse likewise are all the lineaments of the bodie and all that which Posterity shall discover in him.

Perhaps this notion was derived by Seneca from the Homoeomereity of Anaxagoras, for a discussion of which in relation to embryology, see Cornford. "Hair cannot come out of not-hair, nor flesh out of not-flesh," said Anaxagoras.[5]

[1] Bk. VIII, ch. 5.   [2] Bk. III, ch. 10.
[3] See pp. 121, 167 and 213 ff.   [4] Bk. III, ch. 29.
[5] Nekrassov points out that another link in the obscure early chain of preformationist doctrine is to be found in St Augustine, as quoted expressly on the point by Vallisneri in 1739. But the strict statement of Homoeomereity may, as here, be diluted to a mysticism hardly distinguishable from Tennyson's "flower in the crannied wall." The best discussion of St Augustine's ideas is that of Meyer; he traces them back to the λόγος σπερματικός of the Stoics, who regarded these seeds of things as to some extent conscious. Meyer describes the views of Philo and of many Patristic writers, such as Justin Martyr, Clement of Alexandria, Origen and Gregory of Nyssa. He regards Augustine as linked to the Stoics by way of Seneca (v. the quotation given

PLATE III

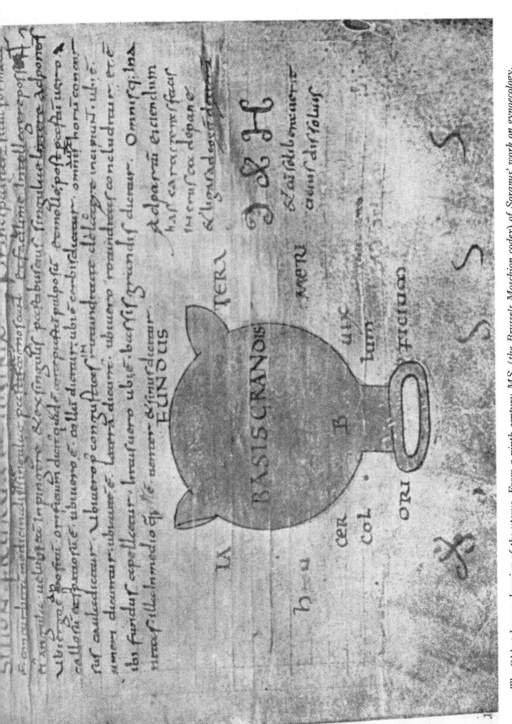

The Oldest known drawing of the uterus. From a ninth-century MS. (the Brussels Moschion codex) of Soranus' work on gynaecology.

The *Natural History* of Pliny, that "voluminous, industrious, un-philosophical, gullible, unsystematic old gossip," as Singer justly calls him, contains little of embryological importance, although he devotes many sections to eggs, and what there is comes straight from the fountain-head, Aristotle. As, for example,

All egs have within them in the mids of the yolk, a certain drop, as it were of bloud, which some thinke to be the heart of the chicken, imagining that to be the first that in everie bodie is formed and made; and certainlie a man shall see it within the verie egge to pant and leape. As for the chick, it taketh the corporall substance, and the bodie of it is made of the white waterish liquor in the egge, the yellow yolke serves for nourishment; whiles the chick is un-hatched and within the egge, the head is bigger than all the bodie besides; and the eies that be compact and thrust together be more than the verie head. As the chick within growes bigger, the white turneth into the middest, and is enclosed within the yolke. By the 20 day (if the eggs be stirred) ye shall heare the chicke to peepe within the verie shell; from that time forward it beginneth to plume and gather feathers; and in this manner it lies within the shell, the head resting on the right foot, and the same head under the right wing, and so the yolke by little and little decreaseth and faileth.

But the best way to illustrate Pliny's embryology is to copy out some of his index, as follows:

This last item exhibits Pliny at his worst. It is worth quoting, apart from any intrinsic value, for it shows to what depths embryological

above) and Cicero, who in the *De Natura Deorum* makes one of his characters outline the Stoic doctrine of seeds.

The devious connections between Greek atomism and seventeenth-century biological preformationism are now fairly clear (see Balss and also the note on the Kabbalah, p. 79). But otherwise excellent histories of atomism, such as that of Gregory, often jump direct from Epicurus to Gassendi, entirely neglecting the Stoic-Kabbalistic "seeds."

knowledge descended within four hundred years after Aristotle collected his specimens on the shores of the lagoon of Pyrrha, and talked with the fishermen of Mitylene.[1]

I will not overpasse one kind of eggs besides, which is in great name and request in France, and whereof the Greeke authors have not written a word; and this is the serpents egg, which the Latins call Anguinum. For in Summer time yerely, you shall see an infinit number of snakes gather round together into an heape, entangled and enwrapped one within another so artificially, as I am not able to expresse the manner thereof; by the means therefore, of the froth ór salivation which they yeeld from their mouths, and the humour that commeth from their bodies, there is engendred the egg aforesaid. The priests of France, called Druidae,[2] are of opinion, and so they deliver it, that these serpents when they have thus engendred this egg do cast it up on high into the aire by the force of their hissing, which being observed, there must be one ready to catch and receive it in the fall again (before it touch the ground) within the lappet of a coat of arms or souldiours cassocks. They affirme also that the party who carrieth this egg away, had need to be wel mounted upon a good horse and to ride away upon the spur, for that the foresaid serpents will pursue him still, and never give over until they meet with some great river betweene him and them, that may cut off and intercept their chace. They ad moreover and say that the only marke to know this egg whether it be right or no, is this, that it will swim aloft above the water even against the stream, yea though it were bound and enchased with a plate of gold.

But one must not be too severe upon Pliny, for he and his translator, Philemon Holland, provide unequalled entertainment.

To some extent the same applies to Plutarch of Chaeronea, who lived about the same time. Plutarch's writings, inspired as they were throughout by the desire to commend the ancient religion of Greece to a degenerate age, represent no milestone or turning-point in the history of embryology, yet there is a passage in the *Symposiaques, or Table-questions* which bears upon it. The third question of Book II is "Whether was before, the hen or egg?"

This long time [says Plutarch] I absteined from eating egges, by reason of a certaine dream I had, and the companie conceived an opinion or suspition of me that there were entred into my head the fantasies and superstitions of Orpheus or Pythagoras, and that I abhorred to eat an egge for that I believed it to be the principle and fountaine of generation.

He then makes the various characters in the dialogue speak to the motion, and one of them, Firmus, ends his speech thus,

[1] See d'Arcy Thompson.
[2] For further information about the serpents' eggs of the Druids, see Kendrick, p. 125; they were probably fossil echinoderms.

And now for that which remaineth (quoth he and therewith he laughed) I will sing unto those that be skilfull and of understanding one holy and sacred sentence taken out of the deepe secrets of Orpheus, which not onely importeth this much, that the egge was before the henne, but also attributeth and adjudgeth to it the right of eldership and priority of all things in the world, as for the rest, let them remaine unspoken of in silence (as Herodotus saith) for that they bee exceeding divine and mysticall, this onely will I speake by the way; that the world containing as it doth so many sorts and sundry kinds of living creatures, there is not in manner one, I dare well say, exempt from being engendred of an egge, for the egge bringeth forth birdes and foules that flie, fishes an infinit number that swimme, land creatures, as lizards, such as live both on land and water as crocodiles, those that bee two-footed, as the bird, such as are footlesse, as the serpent, and last of all, those that have many feet, as the unwinged locust. Not without great reason therefore it is consecrated to the sacred ceremonies and mysteries of Bacchus as representing that nature which produceth and comprehendeth in itselfe all things.

This emphatic passage looks at first sight as if it was a statement of the Harveian doctrine *omne vivum ex ovo*.[1] But the fact that no mammals are mentioned makes this improbable.[2] Firmus then sits down and Senecius opposes him with the well-worn argument that the perfect must precede the imperfect, laying stress also on the occurrence of spontaneous, i.e. eggless, generation, and on the fact that men could find no "row" in eels. Three hundred years later, Ambrosius Macrobius[3] handled the question again in his *Saturnalia*,[4] and the progress in embryological knowledge could be strikingly shown by the difference in treatment. It would be an interesting study to make a detailed comparison.

14. Galen and the Vital Faculties

Another fifty years brings us to Galen of Pergamos, second in greatness among ancient biologists, though in spite of his multitudinous writings he does not quite take this high rank in embryology. That knowledge of the development of the foetus was at this time specially associated with Peripatetic tradition appears from a remark of Lucian of Samosata, Galen's contemporary. In the satire called *The Auction of the Philosophies*, Hermes, the auctioneer, referring to the Peripatetic who is being sold, says, "He will tell you all about the shaping of the embryo in the womb." But Galen was now to weld together all the biological knowledge of antiquity into his voluminous works, and so transmit it to the Middle Ages.

[1] See on, p. 133 ff.
[2] Firmus was doubtless referring to the cosmic egg of Orphic speculation, see p. 27.
[3] See Whittaker, p. 56.   [4] Ch. 7.

Most of Galen's writing was done between A.D. 150 and 180. Out of the twenty volumes of Kühn's edition of 1829, less than one is concerned with embryology, a proportion considerably less than in the case of Aristotle. Galen's embryology is to be found in his περὶ φυσικῶν δυνά- μεων, *On the Natural Faculties*, which contains the theoretical part, and in his *On the Formation of the Foetus*, which contains the more anatomical part. There is also the probably spurious treatise εἰ ζῷον τὸ κατὰ γαστρός, *On the Question of whether the Embryo is an Animal*.[1]

It is important to realise at the outset that Galen was a vitalist and a teleologist of the extreme kind. He regarded the living being as owing all its characteristics to an indwelling *physis* or natural entity with whose "faculties" or powers it was the province of physiology to deal. The living organism according to him has a kind of artistic creative power, a τέχνη, which acts on the things around it by means of the faculties, δυνάμεις, by the aid of which each part attracts to itself what is useful and good for it, τὸ οἰκεῖον, and repels what is not, τὸ ἀλλότριον. These faculties, such as the "peptic faculty" in the stomach and the "sphygmic faculty" in the heart, are regarded by Galen as the causes of the specific functions or activity of the part in question. They are ultimate biological categories; for, although he admits the theoretical possibility of analys- ing them into simpler components, he never makes any attempt to do so, and evidently regards such an effort as doomed to failure, unlike Wilhelm Roux, whose "interim biological laws" were really conceived of as interim.

The effects of Nature [says Galen] while the animal is still being formed in the womb are all the different parts of the body, and after it has been born an effect in which all parts share is the progress of each to its full size and thereafter the maintenance of itself as long as possible.

Galen divides the effects of the faculties into three, genesis, growth and nutrition, and means by the first what we mean by embryogeny.

Genesis is not a simple activity of Nature, but is compounded of *alteration* and of *shaping*. That is to say, in order that bone, nerve, veins and all other tissues may come into existence, the underlying substance from which the animal springs must be altered; and in order that the substance so altered may acquire its appropriate shape and position, its cavities, outgrowths, and attachments, and so forth, it has to undergo a shaping or formative process. One would be justified in calling this substance which undergoes alteration the material of an animal, just as wood is the material of a ship and wax of an image.

[1] For an analysis of the views of Galen on heredity, see Balss (1934).

This is a very remarkable passage. Galen's words express quite modern views about growth and differentiation. They are also applicable to our current distinction between chemical and histological differentiation on the one hand, and morphogenesis on the other.

Galen then goes on to treat of embryogeny in more detail.

The seed having been cast into the womb or into the earth—for there is no difference—[he says (see p. 44)] then after a certain definite period a great number of parts become constituted in the substance which is being generated; these differ as regards moisture, dryness, coldness and warmth, and in all the other qualities which naturally derive therefrom [such as hardness, softness, viscosity, friability, lightness, heaviness, density, rarity, smoothness, roughness, thickness and thinness]. Now Nature constructs bone, cartilage, nerve, membrane, ligament, vein and so forth at the first stage of the animal's genesis, employing at this task a faculty which is, in general terms, generative and alterative, and, in more detail, warming, chilling, drying and moistening, or such as spring from the blending of these, for example, the bone-producing, nerve-producing and cartilage-producing, faculties (since for the sake of clearness these terms must be used as well). . . . Now the peculiar flesh of the liver is of a certain specific kind, also that of the spleen, that of the kidneys and that of the lungs, and that of the heart, so also the proper substance of the brain, stomach, oesophagus, intestines and uterus is a sensible element, of similar parts all through, simple and uncompounded. . . . Thus the special alterative faculties in each animal are of the same number as the elementary parts, and further, the activities must necessarily correspond each to one of the special parts, just as each part has its special use. . . . As for the actual substance of the coats of the stomach, intestine and uterus, each of these has been rendered what it is by a special alterative faculty of Nature; while the bringing of these together, the combination therewith of the structures that are inserted into them, etc., have all been determined by a faculty which we call the shaping or formative faculty; this faculty we also state to be artistic—nay, the best and highest art—doing everything for some purpose, so that there is nothing ineffective or superfluous, or capable of being better disposed.

Thus the alterative faculty takes the primitive unformed raw material and changes it into the different forms represented by the different tissues, while the formative faculty, acting teleologically from within, organises these building-stones, as it were, into the various temples which make up the Acropolis of the completed animal. Galen next goes on to speak of the faculty of growth. "Let us first mention," he says, "that this too is present in the foetus *in utero* as is also the nutritive faculty, but that at that stage these two faculties are, as it were, handmaids to those already mentioned, and do not possess in themselves supreme authority."

71

Later on, until full stature is reached, growth is predominant, and finally nutrition assumes the hegemony.

So much for Galen's embryological theory. But before leaving the treatise *On the Natural Faculties*, it may be noted that he ascribes a retentive faculty to the uterus as well as to the stomach, and explains birth as being due to a cessation of action on the part of the retentive faculty "when the object of the uterus has been fulfilled," and a coming into action of a hitherto quiescent propulsive faculty. This wholesale allotting of faculties can obviously be made to explain anything, and is eminently suited to a teleological account such as Galen's. It was not inconvenient as a framework within which all the biological knowledge of antiquity could be crystallised, but it was utterly pernicious to experimental science. Fifteen hundred years later it received what would have been the death-blow to any less virile theory, at the hands of Molière in his immortal *Malade Imaginaire*:

> *Bachelirius*. Mihi a docto doctore
> Demandatur causam et rationem quare
> Opium facit dormire
> A quoi respondeo
> Quia est in eo
> Virtus dormitiva
> Cujus est nature
> Sensus assoupire
>
> *Chorus*. Bene, bene, bene, bene respondere.
> Dignus, dignus est entrare
> In nostro docto corpore.
> Bene, bene, respondere.[1]

But to return to Galen. The book on the formation of the embryo opens with a historical account of the views of the Hippocratic writers with whom Galen was largely in agreement. It goes on to describe the anatomy of allantois, amnios, placenta and membranes with considerable accuracy. The embryonic life consists, it says, of four stages: (1) an unformed seminal stage, (2) a stage in which the *tria principia* (a concept here met with for the first time) are engendered, the heart, liver

---

[1] *Bachelor*. The learned doctor asks
The cause and reason deep
Why opium sends to sleep
To him I make reply affirmative
Because it has a virtue dormitive
And can our senses lull.

    Chorus. Hooray, hooray, an answer splendid!
Right worthy is a candidate who shows such knowledge
To enter the Physicians' learned College.

and brain, (3) a stage when all the other parts are mapped out and (4) a stage when all the other parts have become clearly visible. Parallel with this development, the embryo also rises from possessing the life of a plant to that of an animal, and the umbilicus is made the root in the analogy with a plant. The embryo is formed, firstly, from menstrual blood, and secondly, from blood brought by the umbilical cord, and the way in which it turns into the embryo is made clearer as follows: "If you cut open the vein of an animal and let the blood flow out into moderately hot water, the formation of a coagulum very like the substance of the liver will be seen to take place." And in effect this viscus, according to Galen, is formed before the heart.

Galen also taught that the embryo excreted its urine into the allantois. He was acquainted with foetal atrophy. He gave a fairly correct account of the junction of the umbilical veins with the branches of the portal vein, and the umbilical with the iliac arteries, of the *foramen ovale*, the *ductus Arantii* and the *ductus Botalli*.[1] He maintained that the embryo respired through the umbilical cord, and said that the blood passed in the embryo from the heart to the lungs and not *vice versa*. The belief that male foetuses were formed quicker than female ones he still entertained, explaining it as being due to the superior heat and dryness of the male germ. He also associated the male conception with the right side and the female with the left and asserted that the intra-uterine movements are sooner felt in the case of the male than in that of the female. Dry foods eaten by the mother, he thought, would lead to a more rapid development of the foetus than other kinds.

In this account of the Galenic embryology I have drawn not only upon the book on the formation of the foetus, but also upon his ὑπόμνημα, *Commentary on Hippocrates*, his περὶ αἰτίων συμπτωμάτων, *On the Causes of Symptoms*, and his book περὶ χρείας τῶν μορίων, *On the Use of Parts*. It is this latter work that had the greatest influence on the ages which followed Galen's life. In the course of seventeen books, he tries to demonstrate the value and teleological significance of every structure and function in the human and animal body, and to show that, being perfectly adapted to its end, it could not possibly be other in shape or nature than what it is. At the conclusion of this massive work with all its extraordinary ingenuity and labour, he says,

Such then and so great being the value of the argument now completed, this section makes it all plain and clear like a good epode, I say an epode, but not in the sense of one who uses enchantments (ἐπῳδαῖς) but as in the melic poets whom some call lyric, there is as well as strophe and antistrophe, an

---

[1] Whether Galen knew of the *ductus venosus* Franklin considers doubtful.

epode, which, so it is said, they used to sing standing before the altar as a hymn to the Gods. To this then I compare this final section and therefore I have called it by that name.

This is one of the half-dozen most striking paragraphs in the history of biology; worthy to rank with the remarks of Hippocrates on the "sacred disease."[1] Galen, as he wrote the words, must have thought of the altar of Dionysus in the Athenian or Pergamene theatre, made of marble and hung about with a garland, but they were equally applicable to the altar of a basilica of the Christian Church with the bishop and his priests celebrating the liturgy at it. What could be more charged with significance than this? At the end of the antique epoch the biology of all the schools—Crotona, Acragas, Cos, Cnidus, Athens, Alexandria, Rome— is welded together and as it were deposited at the entrance into the sanctuary of Christendom. It was the turning-point, in Spengler's terminology, between Apollinian civilisation and Faustian culture. Galen's words are the more extraordinary, for he himself can hardly have foreseen that the long line of experimentalists which had arisen in the sixth century B.C. would come to an end with him. But so it was to be, and thenceforward experimental research and biological speculation were alike to cease, except for a few stray mutations, born out of due time, until in 1453 the city of Byzantium should burst like a ripe pod and distributing her scholars all over the West help to bring all the fruits of the Renaissance, as if by a fertilising process, into being.

[1] "As regards the disease called sacred" (epilepsy) "it appears to me to be no more divine than any other disease, but to have a natural cause from which it originates even as do other diseases. Men regard its nature as divine from ignorance and wonder, since it is a peculiar condition and not easily understood. Yet if it be reckoned divine merely because it is wonderful, then instead of one there should be many sacred diseases. . . . The sacred disease arises like all other diseases from things which enter and quit the body, such as cold, the sun, and the winds, which are never at rest and are always changing. Such things are divine or not, as you wish, for the distinction makes no difference, and there is no need to make the division anywhere in nature, for all things are alike divine and all things are alike human."

CHAPTER II

EMBRYOLOGY FROM GALEN TO THE RENAISSANCE

1. Patristic Speculation

WE are now at the beginning of the second century A.D. The next thousand years can be passed over in as short a time as it has taken to describe the embryology of Galen alone. The Patristic writers, who on the whole were careful to base their psychology on the physiology of the ancients, had little to say about the developing embryo. Most of their interest in it was, as would naturally be expected, theological; Tertullian,[1] for instance, held that the soul was present fully in the embryo throughout its intra-uterine life, thus denying that kind of psychological recapitulation which had been suggested by Aristotle. "Reply," he says in his *De Anima*, "O ye Mothers, and say whether you do not feel the movements of the child within you. How then can it have no soul?" These views were not held by other Fathers, of whom St Augustine of Hippo (*De Immortalitate et de Quantitate Animae*) may serve as a representative, for he thought that the embryo was "besouled" in the second month and "besexed" in the fourth. These various opinions were duly reflected in the law, and abortion, which had even been recommended theoretically by Plato and defended practically by Lysias[2] in the fourth or fifth century B.C., now became equivalent to homicide and punishable by death. This fact leads Singer and Jones to the view that the Hippocratic oath is late, perhaps early Christian. The late Roman law, which, according to Spangenberg,[3] regarded the foetus as not *Homo*, not even *Infans*, but only a *Spes animantis*, was gradually replaced by a stern condemnation of all pre-natal infanticide. "And we pay no attention," said the Bishops of the Quinisext Council, held at Byzantium in 692,

---

[1] Obstructionist organicism can count Tertullian on its side. Writing in A.D. 200 he said: "Herophilus, the physician, or rather butcher, dissected 600 persons that he might scrutinise nature; he hated man that he might gain knowledge. I know not whether he explored clearly all the internal parts of man, for death changes them from their state when alive, and death in his hands was not simply death, *but led to error from the very process of cutting up.*"
[2] On the status of abortion in Classical Greece, see Moissides.
[3] Consult also Goeckel and Morache.

75

"to the subtle distinction as to whether the foetus is formed or unformed." Other authorities, following St Augustine, took a more liberal
view, and the canon law as finally crystallised recognised first the
fortieth day for males and the eightieth day for females as the moment
of animation,[1] but later the fortieth day for both sexes. The *embryo
informatus* thus had no soul, the *embryo formatus* had, and as a corollary
could be baptised. St Thomas Aquinas was of opinion that embryos
dying *in utero* might possibly be saved: but Fulgentius denied it.[2] As
for the ancient belief that male embryos were formed twice as quickly
as female ones, it lingered on until Goelicke took the trouble to disprove
it experimentally in 1723.

Clement of Alexandria, in his book λόγος προτρεπτικὸς πρὸς
"Ελληνας, has some remarks to make on embryology, but adds nothing
to the knowledge previously gained. He adopts the Peripatetic view
that generation results from the combination of semen with menstrual
blood, and he uses the Aristotelian illustration of rennet coagulating
milk. Lactantius of Nicomedia, who lived about the date of the Nicene
Council (A.D. 325), perpetuated the deeply rooted association of male
with right and female with left in his book *On the Work of God, De
opificio Dei*. He also maintained that the head was formed before the
heart in embryogeny, and seems to have opened hen's eggs systematically at different stages, so that to this extent he was a better embryologist
than Galen.

The inherent formative power of the egg has been translated by
biologists of every period into the language of their time. Just as Driesch
sought to acclimatise it to the unfavourable environment of a post-
Cartesian world, so St Gregory of Nyssa, about A.D. 370, clothed it in
Patristic terminology, and produced a theological variety of neo-vital-
ism. His most important biological works, the περὶ κατασκευῆς
ἀνθρώπου, *On the Making of Man* and περὶ ψυχῆς, *On the Soul*, contained such passages as these:

The thing so implanted by the male in the female is fashioned into the
different varieties of limbs and interior organs, not by the importation of any
other power from without, but by the power which resides in it transforming
it.

And elsewhere:

For just as a man when perfectly developed has a soul of a specific nature,
so at the fount and origin of his life he shows in himself that conformation of
soul which is suitable for his need in preparing for itself its peculiarly fit

[1] See the discussion of Cleopatra (p. 65).
[2] *De Fide*, ch. 27. See Coulton, and p. 205 below.

dwelling-place by means of the matter implanted in the maternal body; for we do not suppose it possible that the soul is adapted to a strange building, any more than it is possible that a certain seal should agree with a different impression made in wax.

Thus the soul makes its body as if it were a gem making a stamp upon some soft substance, and acting during development from within. "No unsouled thing," says Gregory, "has the power to move and grow."

Late Latin writers, other than the theologians, do not say much about it. There is a passage in Ausonius, however, which describes the development of the foetus (*Eclog. de Rat. puerp.*), but it is almost wholly astrological. Elsewhere he says:

> juris idem tribus est, quod ter tribus; omnia in istis;
> forma hominis coepti, plenique exactio partu,
> quique novem novies fati tenet ultima finis.[1]
>
> *Idyll* II (Gryphus ternarii numeri), 4–6.

But this is probably a late echo of the Pythagoreans rather than an early prelude to Leonardo da Vinci and the mâthematisation of nature.

2. Contributions of Jewish Thinkers

That great mass of Jewish writings known as the Talmud, which grew up between the second and sixth centuries A.D., also contains some references to embryology, and certain Jewish physicians, such as Samuel ha-Yehudi, of the second century, are said to have devoted special attention to it. The embryo was called *peri habbetṭen* (fruit of the body), פרי הבטן. It grew through various definite stages:

(1) *golem* (formless, rolled-up thing), גולם, 0–1.5 months.

(2) *shefir meruqqām* (embroidered foetus), שפיר מרקם.

(3) *'ubbar* (something carried), עובר, 1.5–4 months.

(4) *walad* (child), ולד, 4–7 months.

(5) *walad shel qayāmā* (viable child), ולד של קיימא, 7–9 months.

(6) *ben she-kallu khadāshāw* (child whose months have been completed), בן שכלו חדשיו.

The ideas of the Talmudic writers on the life led by the embryo *in utero* are well represented by the remark, "It floateth like a nutshell on the waters and moveth hither and thither at every touch".

ואמר רבי אלעזר למה ולד דומה במעי אמו לאגוז מונח בספל של מים אדם
בותן אצבעו עליו שוקע לכאן ולכאן.

[1] The power of 3, in 3 times 3 lies too,
Thus 9 rules human form and human birth,
And 9 times 9 the end of human life.

And the classical passage,[1]

Rabbi Simlai lectured: the babe in its mother's womb is like a rolled-up scroll, with folded arms lying closely pressed together, its elbows resting on its hips, its heels against its buttocks, its head between its knees. Its mouth is closed, its navel open. It eats its mother's food and sips its mother's drink: but it doth not excrete for fear of hurting.

דרש רבי שמלאי למה הולד דומה במעי אמו לפנקס שמקופל ומונח ידיו על שתי צדדיו שתי אציליו על ב׳ ארכבותיו וב׳ עקביו על ב׳ עגבותיו וראשו מונח לו בין ברכיו ופיו סתום וטבורו פתוח ואוכל ממה שאמו אוכלת ושותה ממה שאמו שותה ואינו מוציא רעי שמא יהרוג את אמו.

It was thought, moreover, that the bones and tendons, the nails, the marrow in the head and the white of the eye, were derived from the father, "who sows the white," but the skin, flesh, blood, hair, and the dark part of the eye from the mother, "who sows the red." This is evidently in direct descent from Aristotle through Galen, and may be compared with the following passage[2] from the latter writer's *Commentary on Hippocrates*:

We teach that some parts of the body are formed from the semen and the flesh alone from blood. But because the amount of semen which is injected into the uterus is small, growth and increment must come for the most part from the blood.

It might thus appear that, just as the Jews of Alexandria were reading Aristotle in the third century B.C., and incorporating him into the Wisdom Literature,[3] so those of the third century A.D. were reading Galen and incorporating him into the Talmud. As for God, he contributed the life, the soul, the expression of the face, and the functions of the different parts. This participation of three factors in generation—male, female, and God—is exceedingly ancient, as may be read in Robertson-Smith. Some Talmudic writers held that development began with the head, agreeing with Lactantius, and others that it began at the navel, agreeing with Alcmaeon. Weber has given an

---

[1] Nidd. 30 b.
[2] Ten centuries later it was still worth while for Harvey to have a hit at this opinion. "In the interim," he says (1653, p. 116), "we cannot chuse but smile at that fond and fictitious Division of the Parts, into Spermatical and Sanguineous; as if any part were immediately framed of the semen, and were not all of one extract and original." Anthropology may throw light on the ultimate origin of some of these curious ideas. Thus Mr Bateson informs me that the natives of New Guinea make a distinction between the red flesh provided by the mother, and the white bone provided by the father. They can hardly have learned this from Galen. Similarly, the natives of Lesu, according to Powdermaker, hold the "Aristotelian" view that the menstrual blood is the material from which the foetus is formed.
[3] See p. 64.

account of the Talmudic beliefs about the infusion of the soul into the embryo.[1] They do not seem to have embodied any new or striking idea.

Although the Talmud contained certain references of embryological interest, the first Hebrew treatise on biology was not composed till the tenth century, when Asaph Judaeus or Asaph ha-Yehudi wrote on embryology about A.D. 950. His MSS. are exceedingly rare, but, according to the descriptions of Gottheil, Steinschneider, Simon and Venetianer, they contain several sections on embryonic life. For further details on the whole subject of Jewish embryology, see Macht, and especially Preuss.

As is well known, the general view of the world in the Kabbalah is that of the emanation doctrines of neo-Platonism. The world is full of Ideas or Daemons which are the spiritual representatives of all living things. A thing has life if it works according to certain aims. Living things are *nizzuzoth* (sparks): a conception which may be connected with the *synderesis* of the mediaeval mystical authors such as Dionysius the Pseudo-areopagite. But according to the emanation theory these sparks are not simply situated in the world side by side. They are contained (inserted, *eingeschachtelt*) in other things, which can again split into endless other sparks (monads). In this sense all men are contained in the body of Adam Protoplastes, and the human frame is the microcosm or imitation in little of the macrocosm. Both can be divided into an infinite number of parts or limbs, each having a spiritual representative, which is evidently identical with the *archaeus insitus* of van Helmont. But the spiritual representative does not enter the body from outside. It builds the body by splitting itself into an infinite number of new limbs or sparks, and in this monistic view of matter and spirit there are all stages from the non-corporeal through the finest corporeal essences to the grossest materials (the ladder of emanations). Such a view occurs in Leibniz[2] (see Feilchenfeld and Cassirer[3]) and Spinoza as well as van Helmont, but was of course contrary to that of Descartes and Stahl.

In the *Kabbalah Denudata* there is no embryology as such.[4] The *Sefer Yesirah* or *Book of Creation*, translated into German by Lazarus Goldschmidt, does contain embryological ideas, but they are only mystical

[1] *Jüdäische Theologie*, p. 225.
[2] In Leibniz' thought "each part of the organism can be considered as a garden of plants or a whole pond of fishes, but even each branch, each limb, of the organism, each drop of its fluids, is itself such a pond or garden." Here and in similar passages of van Helmont there are important aspects of the history of the concept of the relation between the whole and its parts in biology and pathology. Life is the process of development of certain preformed things, and each monad mirrors all the others like the nodes of Indra's Net. There can be little doubt that Leibniz was influenced considerably by neo-Confucian and Buddhist ideas (cf. *Science and Civilisation in China*, vol. 2, pp. 496 ff.).
[3] Pp. 46, 405.   [4] Cf. Vol. 2, pt. II, tractate III, pneum. 2.

and allegorical pictures of the work of creation, without scientific value.

But from the Kabbalistic ideas already mentioned there resulted a speculative embryology dominated by the suggestion of a general pre-formationism. The monad of Leibniz has no windows. The Kabbalah stresses the differences between individual persons rather than their likeness. Their fate, talents, personal gifts, etc., are determined according to the virtues of the parents and their thoughts in the moment of conception. The nature of the soul determines the sex. The individual personality is marked by the particular name which is bestowed upon the soul in heaven before the creation of the body. For the development of the human body itself there is required (as in van Helmont's view) the seed, a portion of matter with a spiritual Archaeus, the *aura vitalis*, in it, corresponding to the Aristotelian *anima vegetativa*. The world is full of such seeds, because all things, including diseases, owe their existence to development from seeds. As the classical examples of diseases in the writings of Paracelsus and van Helmont are the plague and other infections, the seeds were probably thought of much as our micro-organisms are. Imagination of a disease leads to its contraction, the Archaeus of the body generating the disease from its pre-existing seed. All generation is imagination of an idea. The picture imagined by the generating individual is the middle term between God and the World, corresponding to the Logos, God's Son, or Christ, who is the *causa exemplaris et formalis*, the representative of God's *sapientia* in each living thing. This seventeenth-century doctrine of seeds links up the *logos spermatikos* of the Stoics, the Kabbalah, the preformation theory in embryology, and the "bacteriology" of Athanasius Kircher.[1]

But the Matter and the *aura vitalis* alone are not sufficient to create life, in spite of the fact that they can develop parts of the body such as *molae*, or the whole body as in stillborn infants. The *lumen formale et vitale*, an entity of the subtlest corporeality and greatest activity, like light, immediately proceeding from God, is required. This light is the beginning of life—the Hebrew *or*, אוֹר, means light as well as beginning.

All this speculative embryology has been somewhat overlooked, and should make us hesitate, as W. Pagel says, in accepting the view of Bilikiewicz that the Baroque period was wholly dominated by the developing mechanism of Descartes. Its relation to "light-mysticism" led to one development of extraordinary interest, namely the work of Marcus Marci of Kronland, a Bohemian. His *Idearum Operatricium Idea*, published in 1635, was a mixture of purely scientific contributions to optics (see Hoppe; Rosenfeld), and speculative theories about embry-

[1] For further discussion of preformationism and seeds, see p. 66 of the present work.

ology. Thus he explained the production of manifold complexity from the seed in generation by an analogy with lenses, which will produce complicated beams from a simple light-source. The formative force radiates from the geometrical centre of the foetal body, creating complexity but losing nothing of its own power. Monsters originate from accidental doubling of the radiating centre, or from abnormal reflections or refractions at the periphery (cf. mirror-image reduplications, accessory organisers, *situs inversus viscerum*, etc.).

Marcus Marci thus links together the following trends of thought: (1) the old Aristotelian theory of seed and blood, (2) the new rationalistic mathematical attitude to generation as e.g. in Gassendi and Descartes, (3) the new experimental approach, in his contributions to optics, (4) the cabbalistic mysticism of light as the fountain and origin of things. Finally (5) by his brilliant guess of centres of radiant energy, he anticipates much of modern embryology (field theories, fate of part as function of position, etc.). Pagel and Baumann give an elaborate discussion of his opinions.

The only parallel to this occurs, it seems, in a quarter far removed from Marci at Prague, but equally devoid of influence on contemporaries, namely the *De Motu Animalium* of Borelli, the founder of the iatro-mathematical school (p. 153). Chiarugi gives an account of the chapter on generation.[1] Its interest is that Borelli compares the semen to a magnet arranging iron particles in a field of force. There is really little difference between this conception and the "individuation field" of modern embryologists. In Harvey, too, a reference to the magnetic field can be found. In the discourse on Conception (1653, p. 539) he says:

The Woman or Female doth seem, after the spermatical contact in coition, to be affected in the same manner, and to be rendered prolifical, by no sensible corporeal Agent; as the Iron touched by the Loadstone is presently indowed with the virtue of the Loadstone, and doth draw other iron-bodies unto it.

In the eighteenth century, of course, traces of this are easier to find. Thus from Bourguet, one of the saner ovistic preformationists (see p. 207), may be quoted (1789):

Le Méchanisme Organique [which works in generation] n'est autre chose que la Combinaison du Mouvement d'une infinité de Molécules éthériennes, aériennes, aqueuses, oléagineuses, salines, terrestres, etc., accommodées à des systèmes particuliers, déterminés dès le commencement par la Sagesse

---

[1] Pt. II ch. 14, in vol. 2, pp. 378 ff.

suprême, et unis chacun à une Activité ou Monade singulière et dominante, à laquelle *celles qui entrent dans son système sont subordonnées*"[1]

The ideas of Parsons (1752) are also relevant; they will be found discussed on p. 192 below.

3. Embryology among the Arabs

Arabic science, so justly famed for its successes in certain fields such as optics and astronomy, was not of great help to embryology. My friend Professor Reuben Levy has collected for me the following embryological excerpts from the Koran:

XXXIII (12 ff.) We created man of a choice extract of clay, then we placed him as semen in a sure place, then we created (?) the semen into clotted blood, then we formed the clotted blood into a morsel of flesh, then we created the morsel into bones, and we covered the bones with flesh, then we produced out of it a new creature.

XXIV (44) God created every beast out of water.

XXXV (12) God created you from earth, then from a clot, then he made you pairs.

LXXV (36) Does man think that he shall be neglected?

(37) Was he not a clot of emitted seed?

(38) Then he was congealed blood, then God created him and fashioned him.

(39) And made of him the pair, male and female.

LXXVI (3) Verily, we created man from a clot of mixtures.

A seventh-century echo of Aristotle and the *Āyur-veda*.

The treatises of the Brethren of Sincerity (*Rasā'il Ikhwān al-Ṣafā'*), an anonymous group who wished to popularise science in the late tenth century at Basra in Iraq, contain a few references to generation, again Aristotelian, mentioning the cheese analogy, but mostly astrological. Abū'l-Ḥasan 'Alī ibn Sahl ibn Rabban al-Ṭabarī, a Muslím physician who flourished under the Caliphate of al-Mutawakkil about A.D. 850, wrote a book called *The Paradise of Wisdom*, in which an entire part was devoted to embryology, all the more interesting as it is a mixture of Greek and ancient Indian knowledge. Browne gives a description of it. Ibn Rabban's contemporary, Thābit ibn Qurra, is also said to have written on embryology. The great Avicenna, or, to give him his proper name, Abū 'Alī al-Ḥasan ibn 'Abdallāh ibn Sīnā, who lived from 980 to 1037, devoted certain chapters of his *Canon Medicinae* to the development of the foetus, but added nothing to Galen. His contemporaries, Abū'l-Qāsim Maslama ibn Aḥmad al-Majrīṭī and 'Arīb ibn Sa'īd al-Kātib, a Spanish Muslím, wrote treatises on the generation of animals, but neither has survived.

---

[1] Italics mine. I am indebted to my friend Dr W. Pagel for most of the foregoing information concerning the Kabbalah.

4. Alchemy and Embryology

What was alchemy doing all this time? It was engaged on many curious pursuits, but among them the interpretation of embryonic development was not one. Alchemical texts before the tenth century do make reference to eggs from time to time, but it is safe to say never with any trace of an interest in the development of the embryo out of them (cf. Berthelot's collection[1]). It is not until after the time of Paracelsus that the notion of applying chemical methods to eggs or embryos arises at all.

Although somewhat out of chronological order, a word may be said here concerning Paracelsus. Though deserving of little remark by the embryologist, his recipe for making a homunculus cannot be passed over. It occurs in his *Treatise concerning the Nature of Things*, Book I, concerning the generation of natural things, p. 124. Human semen is allowed to putrefy in a cucurbite for forty days "with the highest putrefaction of the *venter equinus*" till it moves and is agitated; it is then fed cautiously and prudently with the arcanum of human blood for forty weeks. The *venter equinus* may have meant an apparatus for maintaining a temperature of about blood heat by the use of fermenting horse-dung. Paracelsus also wrote a *Liber de generatione hominis* which only exists in fragmentary form. His view that "putrefaction is the first initiative of generation" (p. 120) may stand in some relation with the cheese analogy.[2]

It is of interest that this doctrine is embedded in the Hebrew Liturgy (p. 190), where in chapter 3 of the *Ethics of the Fathers* we find

Aqabya, the son of Mahalalel, said, reflect upon three things . . . whence thou camest, whither thou art going, and before whom thou wilt in future have to give account and reckoning. Whence thou camest—from a *putrefying drop* (מאין באת מטפה סרוחה), etc., etc.

The date of Aboth is uncertain; it is first cited by name in A.D. 299 but is certainly much older (30 B.C.–A.D. 120). The particular author in question here, Aqabya ben Mahalalel, was one of the earliest Tannaim (Rabbis of the Mishnah), since he has no title, probably a contemporary of Hillel, and therefore about the end of the first century B.C. The doctrine of generation implying putrefaction is doubtless connected with the doctrine of spontaneous generation, the history of which has been so well written by von Lippmann, but the origin of both is still very obscure.

---

[1] E.g. vol. 2, pp. 56 ff.
[2] Pp. 50, 85 of the present book; see also Cole, p. 1.

5. The Visions of St Hildegard

Not long after the death of Avicenna, St Hildegard was born. She lived from 1098 to 1180, and was abbess successively of Disibodenberg and Bingen in the Rhineland. Her treatises on the world, which are an extraordinary medley of theological, mystical, scientific and philosophical speculation, have been brilliantly described by Singer, and though in her books, *Liber Scivias* and *Liber Divinorum Operum simplicis hominis*, there is little of embryological interest, yet she does give an account of development and especially of the entry of the soul into the foetus.[1]

This is seen in an illustration (Plate IV, opposite) from the Wiesbaden Codex B of the *Liber Scivias*. The soul is here shown passing down from heaven into the body of the pregnant woman and so to the embryo within her. The divine wisdom is represented by a square object with its angles pointing to the four corners of the earth in symbol of stability. From it a long tube-like process descends into the mother's womb and down it the soul passes as a bright object, "spherical" or "shapeless," illuminating the whole body. The scene shows the mother in the foreground lying down; inside her there are traces of the foetal membranes; behind this ten persons are grouped, each carrying a vessel, into one of which a fiend pours some noxious substance from the left-hand corner. St Hildegard describes and expounds the scene as follows:[2]

Behold, I saw upon earth men carrying milk in earthen vessels and making cheeses therefrom. Some was of the thick kind from which firm cheese is made, some of the thinner sort from which more porous cheese is made, and some was mixed with corruption and of the sort from which bitter cheese is made. And I saw the likeness of a woman having a complete human form within her womb. And then by a secret disposition of the most high craftsman, a fiery sphere having none of the lineaments of a human body possessed the heart of the form and reached the brain and transfused itself through all the members. . . . And I saw that many circling eddies possessed the sphere and brought it earthward, but with ever-renewed force it returned upwards and wailed aloud, asking, "I, wanderer that I am, where am I?" "In death's shadow." "And where go I?" "In the way of sinners." "And what is my hope?" "That of all wanderers." . . . As for those whom thou hast seen carrying milk in earthen vessels, they are in the world, men and women alike, having in their bodies the seed of mankind from which are procreated the various kinds of human beings. Part is thickened because the seed in its

---

[1] It is thought that the book of the neo-Platonist Porphyrius may have been among her sources, as it deals expressly with the animation of the embryo (see Ueberweg & Praechter, p. 598). On her pathology, see Schulz. Cf. Liebeschütz, pp. 65 ff.
[2] Translation by Singer.

PLATE IV

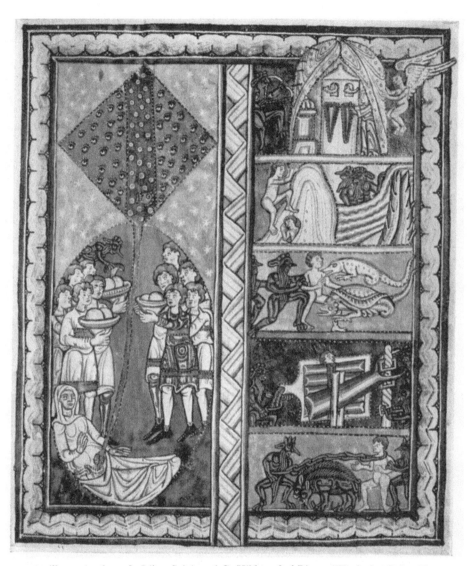

An illustration from the Liber Scivias *of St Hildegard of Bingen (Wiesbaden Codex B), showing the descent of the soul into the embryo (c. AD. 1150) (after Charles Singer).*

strength is well and truly concocted and this produces forceful men to whom are allotted gifts, both spiritual and carnal. . . . And some had cheeses less firmly curdled, for in their feebleness they have seed imperfectly tempered and they raise offspring mostly stupid, feeble and useless. . . . And some was mixed with corruption . . . for the seed in that brew cannot be rightly raised, it is invalid, and makes misshapen men who are bitter distressed and oppressed of heart so that they may not lift their gaze to higher things. . . . And often in forgetfulness of God and by the mocking devil a *mistio* is made of the man and the woman and the thing born therefrom is deformed, for parents who have sinned against me return to me crucified in their children.

We have already traced the wanderings of the cheese-analogy, which, beginning fresh with Aristotle, was taken to Alexandria, incorporated itself in the Wisdom Literature, and so found its way to the Arabic of 'Alī ibn al-'Abbās al-Majūsī, or Haly-Abbas, as he was known in the West, a Persian.[1] His *Liber Totius* appeared in Latin in 1523, but had been translated much earlier, at Monte Cassino between 1070 and 1085, by Constantine the African, who called it *Liber de Humana Natura*, and gave it out to be his own work. Thus St Hildegard obtained it, and worked it up into one of her visions. At this point embryology touched, perhaps, its low-water mark. But a great man was at hand, destined to carry on the Aristotelian tradition and to add to it much of originality, the Dominican Albertus of Cologne. Before speaking of him, however, a word must be said about that very queer character Michael Scot (1178–1234), who, according to Gunther,[2] "appeared in Oxford in 1230 and experimented with the artificial incubation of eggs, having got an Egyptian to teach him how to incubate ostrich eggs by the heat of the Apulian sun." That "muddle-headed old magician," as Singer severely calls him, was not the man to profit by it, but the point is interesting, especially as an Egyptian is mentioned. Haskins, in his curious studies of the scientific atmosphere of the court of the Emperor Frederick II of Sicily, has shown Scot, newly arrived from his alchemical studies in Spain, assisting that learned and unorthodox monarch in his artificial incubation experiments.

One should remember that about the same time as Hildegard, some progress was being made in gynaecology and obstetrics at the School of Salerno (cf. Bayon, 1940). A not uncommon mediaeval manuscript, *De Passionibus Mulierum*, is usually ascribed to Trotula of Salerno, a matron (cf. Hurd-Mead, 1930). It recommends support of the perinaeum in childbirth and primary suture of lacerations. The text contains

[1] His name means "the Magian"; one of the three greatest physicians of the Eastern Caliphate, he died in A.D. 994.
[2] Vol. 3, p. 151.

many references to Muslim and Hebrew physicians, speaks of numerous drugs from Arabic pharmacopoeias, and avoids magical formulae. There is a tradition that the "mulieres Salernitanae" taught obstetrics there, and the name of one woman professor from somewhat later at Naples has come down to us, Costanza Calenda of Salerno, who lectured at some period between 1326 and 1382.

6. Albertus Magnus; the Re-awakening of Scientific Embryology

Albertus Magnus of Cologne and Bollstadt was born in 1206, and died in 1280, six years after his favourite disciple, St Thomas Aquinas. The greater part of his life was spent in study and teaching in one or other of the houses of the Dominican friars, to which he belonged, though for a time he was Bishop of Regensburg. Albert resembles Aristotle in many points, but principally because he produced biological work with, as it were, no antecedents. Just as Aristotle's contributions to embryology were preceded by no more than the diffuse speculations of the Ionian nature-philosophers, so Albert's came immediately after the dead period represented by the visions of St Hildegard. In many ways, Albert's position was much less conducive to good work than Aristotle's.

Albert follows Aristotle closely throughout his biological writings,[1] quoting him word for word in large amounts, but the significant thing is that he does not follow him slavishly. He resembled Aristotle in paying much attention to the phenomena of generation, as a rough computation shows; Aristotle devoting 37 per cent. of his biological writings to this subject, and Albert 31 per cent., to which Galen's 7 per cent. may with interest be compared. Albert is extremely inferior to Aristotle, however, in point of arrangement, for Aristotle, although some of his books, such as the *De Generatione Animalium*, are sufficiently confused and repetitive, does yet succeed in infusing a clarity and incisiveness into his style. Albert, on the other hand, allows his argument to wander through his twenty-six books *De Animalibus* in the most complex convolutions, so that the sections on generation and embryology are found indiscriminately in the first, sixth, ninth, fifteenth, sixteenth and seventeenth. In Book I he gives a kind of summary or skeleton of his views on the embryo. These follow Aristotle fairly closely; thus he accepts the Aristotelian classification of animals according to their manner of generation, and thinks still that caterpillars are immature eggs; he derives the embryo from the white, not the yolk, and he explains why soft-shelled eggs, being imperfect, are of one colour only. But there are new observations; for instance, he describes an *ovum in ovo*, which he has seen, calling it a *natura peccatis*, and he speaks

[1] See Balss.

86

definitely of the seed of the woman, thus departing from Peripatetic opinion, and adopting the Epicurean view. The female seed, he thinks, suffers coagulation like cheese by the male seed, and to these two humidities there must be added a third, namely the menstrual blood (corresponding to the yolk in the case of the bird).

When these three humidities therefore have been brought into one place, all the similar members except the blood and fat are formed from the two humidities of which one generates actively but the other passively. But the blood which is attracted for the nutriment of the embryo is double in virtue and double in substance. For a certain part of the blood is united with the sperm in such a way that it takes on some of the virtue of the seed, because a certain part of the spermatic humour remains in it, and from this are begotten the teeth and for this reason they grow again if they are pulled out at an age near the time of sperm-making and do not grow again at an age remoter from this, at which the virtue of the first generating principle has vanished from the blood. But another part of the blood is of twofold or threefold substance and from the thick part of the blood itself is generated the flesh. And this flows in and flows out and grows again if rubbed away. From the watery part of the same blood or of the nutritive humour are generated the fat and oil and this flows in and out more easily than the flesh itself, but other parts of the blood are its refuse and impurities and are not attracted to the generation of any part of the animal, but having been collected until birth are expelled with the embryo from the uterus in the foetal membranes, like the remnants in the hen's egg after the chick has hatched. There is a similar virtue in the liver and heart of animals, which organs after the animals are born form the flesh and fat from food in accordance with its twofold substance, and expel the refuse as we said before.

In the sixth book Albert contradicts Aristotle's opinion that the male chick develops out of the sharp-ended egg, and one hopes that he is going to say there is no relationship between egg-shape and sex; but no, he goes on to say that the Aristotelian statement rested on a textual error (in which he was quite wrong), so that really Aristotle agreed with Avicenna in saying that the males always develop from the more spherical eggs because the sphere is the most perfect of figures in solid geometry. These errors had a most persistent life; Horace has a passage in which they appear—

> longa quibus facies ovis erit, illa memento
> ut suci melioris, et ut magis alma rotundis
> ponere: namque marem cohibent callosa vitellum.[1]

[1] "When you would feast upon eggs, make choice of the long ones; they are whiter and sweeter and more nourishing than the round, for being hard they contain the yolk of the male." Book II, sat. 4, l. 12.

They were finally abolished by two naturalists, Günther and Bühle, who took the trouble to disprove them experimentally in the eighteenth century. Albertus refers here to artificial incubation:

For the alterative and maturative heat of the egg is in the egg itself and the warmth which the bird provides is altogether external (*extrinsecus est ammini-culans*) since in certain hot countries the eggs of fowls are put under the surface of the earth and come to completion of their own accord, as in Egypt, for the Egyptians hatch them out by placing them under dung in the sunlight.

Next he speaks of monsters and of the modes of corruption of eggs, which he divides into four: (1) decomposition of white, (2) decomposition of yolk, (3) bursting of the yolk-membrane, (4) *antiquitas ovi*.

And from the second cause it sometimes happens that in the corruption of the humours certain igneous parts are carried blazing to the shell of the egg and distribute themselves over it so that it shines in the dark like rotten wood; as happened in the case of that egg[1] which Avicenna said he saw in the city called Kanetrizine in the country of the Corascenes.

Albert is inclined to think that astrological influences may have an effect on foetal life, but he treats the suggestion with considerable scepticism, although he believes that thunder and lightning kill the embryos of fowls (a popular belief to which Féré tried not long ago to give a scientific foundation), and he regards the embryo of the crow as especially susceptible, though on what grounds he does not say.

The fourth chapter of the first tractate of the sixth book contains Albert's description of development of the chick, and is extremely interesting. He makes two principal mistakes: (*a*) he describes a quite non-existent fissure in the shell by which the chick may emerge, (*b*) he maintains that the yolk ascends after a day or two into the sharp end of the egg, adducing as the reason that there is found there more heat and formative force than elsewhere. On the other hand, he correctly describes (*a*) the pulsating drop of blood on the third day, and (*b*) he identifies it with the heart with its *systolen et dyastolen* sending out the "formative virtue" to all the parts of the growing body. He notices (*c*) that the differentiation of the chick at first proceeds rapidly and later more slowly. But the most notable characteristic of Albert's embryology is the way in which he is hampered by his inability to invent a technical terminology. Singer has studied the way in which anatomical terms, such as "syrach," etc., came into use, but whatever the causes were which produced them, they did not operate much in

[1] See on this subject Zäch.

Albert's mind. He represents the point beyond which embryology could not advance, until it had created a new set of terms. This is well illustrated by the following passage:

But from the drop of blood out of which the heart is formed, there proceed two vein-like and pulsatile passages, and there is in them a purer blood which forms the chief organs such as the liver and lungs, and these though very small at first grow and extend at last to the outer membranes which hold the whole material of the egg together. There they ramify in many divisions, but the greater of them appears on the membrane which holds the white of the egg within it [the allantois]. The albumen, at first quite white, is changed owing to the power of the vein almost to a pale yellow-green tint (*palearem colorem*). Then the path of which we spoke proceeds to a place in which the head of the embryo is found carrying thither the virtue and purer material from which are formed the head, and the brain, which is the marrow of the head. In the formation of the head also are found the eyes and because they are of an aqueous humidity which is with difficulty used up by the first heat they are very large, swelling out and bulging from the chick's head. A short time afterwards, however, they settle down a little and lose their swelling owing to the digestive action of the heat—and all this is brought about by the action of the formative virtue carried along the passage which is directed to the head, but before arriving there is separated and ramified by the great vein of the albumen-membrane, as may be clearly seen by anyone who breaks an egg at this time and notes the head appearing in the wet part of the egg and at the top of the other members. For what appears first in the making of a foetus are the upper parts because they are nobler and more spiritual, being compacted of the subtler part of the egg wherein the formative virtue is stronger. When this has happened one of the aforementioned two passages which spring from the heart branches into two, one of them going to the spiritual part which contains the heart and dividing there in it carrying to it the pulse and subtle blood from which the lungs and other spiritual parts are formed, and the other going through the diaphragm (*dyafracma*) to enclose within it at the other end the yolk of the egg, around which it forms the liver and stomach. It is accordingly said to take the place of the umbilicus in other animals and through it food is drawn in to supply the flesh for the chick's body, for the principle of generation of the radical members of the chick comes from the albumen but the food from which is made the flesh filling up all the hollows is from the yolk.

After ten days, Albert goes on to say, all the constituent organs are mapped out and the head is greater then than the rest of the body put together. He observes that the yolk liquefies early in development (see Fig. 7) and that slimy concretions are present in the allantoic fluid later on (uric acid). But the passage quoted demonstrates that before further progress could be made some better name must be found than

89

"the interior membrane to which the first vessel proceeds" for a given structure.

Albert, however, was accomplishing a good work. One of his best amplifications of Aristotle was his description of the relationship between yolk and embryo in fishes. Just as his words about the chick demonstrate that he must have opened hen's eggs at different stages during incubation, so his words about fish eggs show that he must have dissected and examined them also. In Book VI, tractate II, chapter I, he says,

> Between the mode of development (*anathomiam generationis*) of birds' and fishes' eggs there is this difference; during the development of the fish the second of the two veins which extend from the heart does not exist. For we do not find the vein which extends to the outer covering of the eggs of birds (which some wrongly call the umbilicus because it carries the blood to the outside parts) but we do find the vein which corresponds to the yolk vein of birds, for this vein imbibes the nourishment by which the limbs increase.[1] Therefore the generation of the fish embryo begins from the sharp end of the egg like that of birds, and channels extend from the heart to the head and eyes and first in them appear the upper parts. As the growth of the young fish proceeds the yolk decreases in amount being incorporated into the members and it disappears entirely when development is complete. The beating of the heart, which some call panting, is transmitted through the pulsating veins to the lower part of the belly carrying life to the inferior members. While the young fish are small and not yet fully developed they have veins of great length which take the place of the umbilicus, but as they grow these shorten till they contract into the body by the heart as has been said about birds. The young fish are enclosed in a covering just like the embryos of birds, which resembles the *dura mater* and beneath it another containing the foetus and nothing else, while between the two there is the moisture rejected during the creation of the embryo.

Albert also described ovoviviparous fishes but it is more difficult in that case to tell whether he had himself seen and dissected them. He notes also the prodigality of nature in producing so many marine eggs only destined to be eaten.

In Books IX and XV he treats of the Galenic views on generation and insists again that there is a seed provided by the female. In Book XVI he gives his opinions about the animation of the embryo, quoting the views of the ancients as given in Plutarch, e.g. Alexander the Peripatetic, Empedocles, Anaxagoras, Theodorus and Theophrastus, the Peripatetics, Socrates, Plato, the Stoics, Avicenna and Aristotle, "who saw the truth," but, and it is interesting to notice it, never the Christian Fathers,

---

[1] I.e. there is a yolk-sac but no allantois.

whose writings must have been well known to him. In discussing the
Aristotelian views he compares the menstrual blood to the marble and
the semen to the man with a chisel in his hand.

On the question of epigenesis and preformation, he follows Aristotle
almost word for word, using the same analogies, such as the "dead eye"
and the sleeping mathematician. Here his scholasticism comes out
clearly, for in rejecting altogether the theory that one part being formed
then forms the next part, he says, not that *A* would have to be in some
way like *B*, but is not, as Aristotle had, but simply *Generans et genera-
tum, est simul esset et non esset, quod omnino est impossibile*—a high-
handed and very unscientific manner of settling the question. In con-
formity with his theology and in contradistinction from Aristotle he
makes the vegetative and sensitive souls arrive automatically into the
embryo but the rational soul only by a direct act of God.

His mammalian embryology presents some points of interest. He
follows Hippocrates ("Ypocras") in an account of the co-operation of
heat and cold in member-formation, and he holds very enlightened
views about foetal nutrition.

It appears therefore that the embryo hangs from the cord and that the cord
is joined with the vein and that the vein extends through the uterus and has
blood running through it to the foetus like water through a canal. Round the
embryo there are membranes and webs as we have seen. But those who think
that the embryo is fed by little bits of flesh through the cord are wrong and
lie, because if this were the case with man it would happen also with other
animals and that it does not do so anybody can find out by investigation (*per
anathomyam*).

Finally, it is typical that in Book XVII Albert repeats what he has
already said in Book VI about the generation of the hen out of the egg all
over again with slight changes, but he adds the significant biochemical
remark that "eggs grow into embryos because their wetness is like the
wetness of yeast." The importance of Albert in the history of embryology is clear. With him the new spirit of investigation leapt up into
being, and, though there were many years yet to pass before Harvey,
the modern as opposed to the ancient period of embryology had
begun.

7. *Aristotle's Masterpiece*

Albert's writings were often copied and printed in the next few centuries, and even as late as 1601 *De Secretis Mulierum*, an epitome of his
books on generation, was published. In some sense, it still is, as it forms

the backbone of the little book *Aristotle's Masterpiece*, of which thousands of copies are sold in England every year. The copy of the *De Secretis* in the Caius College Library has, written across the title-page in faded ink, "*Simulacra sanctitas, duplex iniquitas, Nathan Emgross, Nov. 20. 1613.*" But in spite of Mr Emgross, Albertus, rightly called Magnus, has had the happy fate of being beatified both by the Church and by science.

The exact relations between Albertus' *De Secretis Mulierum* and the innumerable compendia of popular booklets on generation which appeared in the following centuries, often under the title *Aristotle's Masterpiece*, are complicated and would fittingly provide the subject for a serious historical research. This would be of great interest, since it is probably correct to say that these booklets, reprinted and modified a hundredfold, formed, and still form to-day, the main source of instruction on sexual and embryological matters for the working-class populations of Western Europe. I give in the bibliography a small selection of titles of these publications, which shade off into such modifications as those of Alletz, who improved upon Albertus Magnus by cutting out all the teaching on generation and substituting a collection of recipes. The bibliography of the *De Secretis* has been approached in a preliminary way by Ferckel, whose full paper on the subject was unfortunately only listed, not printed, in the Sudhoff-Festschrift.[1]

One of the sources of *Aristotle's Masterpiece* is undoubtedly Fortunius Licetus, *De Monstrorum Natura*. The illustrations of 1616 are still being reproduced to-day. The whole subject has lately been reviewed by d'Arcy Power.

This is perhaps the place to mention a curious mediaeval superstition, namely that the development of the human foetus might be unduly prolonged. The *proles lunatica* was a rare kind of embryo which waxed and waned with the phases of the moon, thus making no progress. In the collected miracles of King Henry VI of England (Grosjean) there is mentioned a pregnancy of twenty-eight months' duration, which was terminated at the intercession of the saint so that the woman produced a child "without deformity or monstrosity, such as oft-times befalleth in such cases as this." We may be forgiven for thinking twice about the probable origin of such a tale, since, as may be seen from the comprehensive review of Hamlett, the normal hibernation of embryos in many mammals is well known; to say nothing of the diapause of the silkworm.

[1] *Archiv f. d. Gesch. d. Med.* 1923.

8. Scholastic Ideas on Generation

Thomas of Aquino (1227–1274) incorporated the Aristotelian theories of embryology into his *Summa Theologica* especially under the head *De propagatione hominis quantum ad corpus*.[1] There are some striking passages, such as

> The generative power of the female is imperfect compared to that of the male; for just as in the crafts, the inferior workman prepares the material and the more skilled operator shapes it, so likewise the female generative virtue provides the substance but the active male virtue makes it into the finished product.

St Thomas' theory of embryonic animation was complicated.[2] He had a notion that the foetus was first endowed with a vegetative soul, which in due course perished, at which moment the embryo came into the possession of a sensitive soul, which died in its turn, only to be replaced by a rational soul provided directly by God. This led him into great difficulties, for if this scheme were true, it was difficult to say that man generated man at all; on the contrary he could hardly be said to generate more than a sensitive soul which died before birth, and on this view what was to happen to original sin? As Harris has put it,[3] Plato had said that the intellect was the man, using the body as a boatman uses a boat. Averroes[4] had said precisely the opposite, namely that the essence of humanity was in the body, and that the intellect was something extrinsic, not limited to the individual, but common to the race. Aristotle had taken the middle position, and given a soul to plants and animals, but, in doing so, he had made it into a vital rather than a psychological principle. The task of combining this ψυχή with the *anima* of the Fathers was what scholastic philosophy had before it. No wonder that St Thomas' account of embryonic animation was open to criticism. An echo of it appears in a poem of Jalāl al-Dīn al-Rūmī (1207–1273), the greatest of the Persian Sufi poets, and an exact contemporary of St Thomas Aquinas:

> I died from mineral and plant became;
> Died from the plant, and took a sentient frame;
> Died from the beast, and donned a human dress;
> When by my dying did I e'er grow less?

---

[1] See pt. I, qu. lxxvi, art. 3; qu. cxix, art. 2; cxviii, arts. 1 and 2; pt. III, qu. xxxii, art. 4; qu. xxxiii, art 1.   Cf. Lecky, *History of Rationalism*, vol. 1, p. 360, n. 2.
[2] See the special studies by Mitterer and Barbado.
[3] *Duns Scotus*, vol. 2, pp. 254 ff.
[4] Muḥammad ibn Aḥmad ibn Rushd of Cordova, A.D. 1126–1198, one of the greatest of Muslim philosophers.

Duns Scotus (1266–1308) objected to St Thomas' theory on the grounds already mentioned, and he himself abandoned the vegetative and sensitive souls altogether in his *De Rerum Principio*. This solution was no better than that of St Thomas, for agreeing with the latter as Duns did that the rational soul was not an ordinary form "educed" from the "potentiality" of the material, but rather an *ad hoc* creation of God injected by divine power into the embryo at the appropriate moment, it was difficult to see how the spiritual effects of Adam's fall could be transmitted to the men of each generation. It was as if only acquired characteristics were inherited. But the further course of embryological theology need not be pursued here; it runs in every century parallel with true scientific embryology, and it is not my purpose to do more than take a glance at its progress from time to time.

In the *Speculum Naturale*, which was written about 1250, by Vincent of Beauvais, the embryology of Constantine the African appears again;[1] and the embryology of Aristotle, Galen and the scholastics is to be found in Dante Alighieri (1265–1321), who dealt with the subject in his *Convivio*,[2] and especially in the *Divina Commedia*.[3] In Canto xxv of the *Purgatorio*, Statius (the personification of human philosophy enlightened by divine revelation) is made to speak to the poet thus:

If thy mind, my son, gives due heed to my words and takes them home, they will elucidate the question thou dost ask. Perfect blood which is in no case drawn from the thirsty veins, but which remains behind like food that is removed from table, receives in the heart informing power for all the members of the human body, like the other blood which courses through the veins in order to be converted into those members. After being digested a second time it descends to the part whereof it is more seemly to keep silence than to speak, and thence it afterwards drops into the natural receptacle (the uterus) upon another's blood; there the one blood and the other mingle. One is appointed to be passive, the other to be active according to the perfect place whence it proceeds (the heart). And being united with it, it begins to operate, first by coagulating it, and then by vivifying that to which it has given consistency, so that there may be material for it to work upon (*e poi avviva, Ciò che per sua materia fe' constare*). The active power having become a [vegetative] soul like that of a plant—only differing from it in this, that the former is in progress while the latter has reached its goal—thereafter works so much that it moves and feels like a sea-fungus and as the next stage it takes in hand to provide with organs the faculties which spring from it. At this point, my son, the power which proceeds from the heart of the begetter is expanded and

[1] See esp. Bks. xvi and xxxi.
[2] Tractate iv, ch. 21.
[3] *Purgatorio*, canto 25. A commentary on Dante's view of generation has been given by del Gaudio.

developed, that power in which Nature is intent on forming all the members, but how from being an animal it becomes a child, thou seest not yet, moreover this is so difficult a point that formerly it led astray one more wise than thou [Averroes], so that in his teaching he separated the active "intellect" from the soul because he could not see any organ definitely appropriated by it. Open thy heart to the truth and know that as soon as the brain of the foetus is perfectly organised, the Prime Mover, rejoicing in this display of skill on the part of Nature, turns towards it and infuses into it a new spirit replete with power which subsumes into its own essence the active elements which it finds already there, and so forms one single soul which lives and feels and is conscious of its own existence. And that thou mayst find my saying less strange, bethink thee how the heat of the sun passing into the juice which the grape distils, makes wine.

Having said this, Statius, with Virgil and Dante, passes on to the seventh ledge in Purgatory. It is interesting to see how Dante emphasises the dynamic teleological side of Aristotle and practically speaks of the soul enfleshing itself and arranging organs for its faculties. The reference to Averroes is explained by the fact that Averroes was a traducianist, and held that all the soul was generated by man at the same time as the body, whereas both St Thomas and Dante, as Creationists, held that each fresh soul was a special creation of God inserted by him into the brain of the embryo.[1]

The activity of Dante's contemporary, Mondino de Luzzi (1270–1326), brings us to the more practical aspects of embryology at this period. Mondino is the most outstanding figure among the Bolognese anatomists in what is really the first period of the revival of biology. After him, as we shall see, biology languished for a couple of centuries

---

[1] A concise account of these controversies is given by Shedd. According to him the views of the primitive Church ran in three directions, though not with equal strength, nor to an equal extent, Pre-existence, Creationism and Traducianism. Pre-existence, associated mainly with the names of Origen, Cyril of Alexandria and Nemesius of Emesa, taught that all finite spirits (human souls) were created at the beginning, before the creation of matter. They simply took up their residence in the blood-seed coagula "in rotation" as these were made ready. This view did not outlast the fourth century—Jerome says it is a *stulta persuasio* to believe that "souls were created of old by God and kept in a treasury." Creationism, dominant among the Eastern Fathers, taught that at some point during development, a new soul is created *de nihilo* by God, and infused into the embryo. The body, on the other hand, derives from Adam by propagation. For the souls, an infinite number of creative acts are necessary; for the bodies, only one. Traducianism, dominant among the Western Fathers, taught that both souls and bodies derived from Adam, so that in generation, both parts of man are derived from his parents. This was Tertullian's view, and it was more or less implicitly adopted by Augustine.

In the Middle Ages, Creationism prevailed over Traducianism because the latter doctrine seemed to conflict with orthodoxy on immortality. At the Reformation, with the revival of Augustinianism, Traducianism also returned to favour. It is obvious that these changes affected the outlook of the theological embryologists. "A very worthy Subject of philosophical Enquiry," remarked Sir John Hill, "because impossible to be determined."

until the advent of such men as Ulysses Aldrovandus in the sixteenth century, and Singer has shown that this was probably due to the fact that anatomy professors did not dissect in person. *A fortiori* embryotomy was infrequent.

But Mondino's *Anothomia*, published in 1316, contained statements about the organs of generation which were rather important.[1] He retains the notion of the seven-celled uterus, which had been introduced by Michael Scot, but he adopts a reasonable compromise between the opinions of Galen and Aristotle on the physiology of embryo formation. The distance between him and Leonardo da Vinci (1452–1519) would, however, be estimated rather at five or six centuries than at the century and a quarter that it actually was.

9. The Insights of Leonardo da Vinci

Among the artists of the Renaissance Leonardo was not alone in his anatomical interests, for Michaelangelo, Raphael, Dürer, Mantegna and Verrocchio all made dissections in order to increase their knowledge of the human body. But he penetrated more curiously into biology than they did, and he will always remain one of the greatest of biologists, for he first introduced the quantitative outlook. In this he was some four hundred years ahead of his time.

Leonardo's embryology is contained in the third volume of his notebooks, *Quaderni d'Anatomia*, published in facsimile by the admirable labours of three Norwegian scholars, Vangensten, Fohnahn and Hopstock, in 1911.[2] His notebooks are a remarkable and, indeed, charming miscellany of anatomical drawings, physiological diagrams, architectural and mechanical sketches and notes such as "Shirts, hose and shoes," "Go and see Messer Andreas," "get coal," "the supreme fool (is the) necromancer and enchanter."

His dissections of the pregnant uterus and its membranes are beautifully depicted, as can be seen from the figures which are here reproduced Plate V). He was acquainted with amnios and chorion, and he knew that the umbilical cord was composed only of vessels, though he seems to have thought the human placenta was cotyledonous. There is one drawing which the editors suppose to represent the developing hen's egg, but I do not feel that this ascription is likely. Indeed, Leonardo worked with eggs much less than with mammalian embryos, though there are references to the former. "See how birds are nourished in their eggs," he says in one place, to remind himself, perhaps, of possible

[1] Weindler reproduces the obstetrical illustrations of this period.
[2] See also the book of McMurrich on Leonardo.

PLATE V

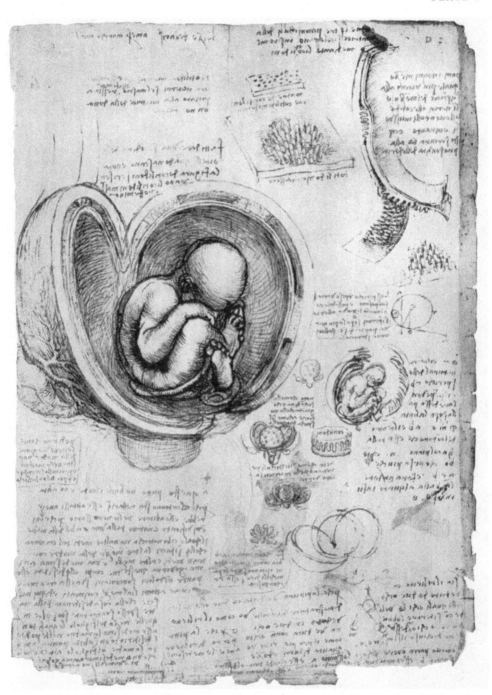

A page from Leonardo da Vinci's anatomical notebooks
(Quaderni d'Anatomia) c. *A.D. 1490.*

experiments, and, elsewhere, "Chickens are hatched by means of the ovens of the fireplace." Again, "Ask the wife of Biagino Crivelli (was she the Lucrezia Crivelli, whose portrait Leonardo painted?) how the capon rears and hatches the eggs of the hen when he is inebriated," a subject recently reopened by Lienhart. "You must first dissect the hatched egg before you show the difference between the human liver in foetus and adult." Leonardo perpetuates a persistent error in the note, "Eggs which have a round form produce males, those which have a long form produce females."

Concerning the mammalian foetus, he says,

The veins of the child do not ramify in the substance of the uterus of its mother but in the placenta which takes the place of a shirt in the interior of the uterus which it coats and to which it is connected but not united by means of the cotyledons.

Thus in one sentence Leonardo falls into a mistake in saying that the human placenta is cotyledonous, but at the same time asserts a fact which it took all the ingenuity of the seventeenth century to prove to be true, namely, that the foetal circulation is not continuous with that of the mother, for the placenta is only connected to the uterine wall and not united with it. Leonardo goes on to say,

The child lies in the uterus surrounded with water, because heavy things weigh less in water than in the air and the less so the more viscous and greasy the water is. And then such water distributes its own weight with the weight of the creature over the whole body and sides of the uterus.

The tendency towards quantitative and mathematical explanations is apparent at once.

Further notes are, "Note how the foetus breathes and how it is nourished through the umbilical cord and why one soul governs two bodies, as you see the mother desiring food and the child remaining marked (by a given amount of growth) because of it. Avicenna pretends that the soul generates the soul and the body the body. *Per errata.*" The child, says Leonardo, secretes urine while still *in utero*, and has excrement in its intestines; at four months it has chyle in its stomach, made perhaps from menstrual blood. But it has no voice *in utero*, "when women say that the foetus is heard to weep sometimes within the uterus, this is rather the sound of some flatus. . . ." Nor does it breathe there (on this point Leonardo contradicts himself). "The child does not respire within the body of its mother because it lies in water and he who breathes in water is immediately drowned." "Breathing is not necessary to the embryo because it is vivified and nourished by the life and food of the mother." Nor does the embryonic heart beat. To us the statement that there is no respiration in the uterus is obviously false, but we mean by the word tissue respiration, whereas in Leonardo's time pulmonary respiration was intended; he was therefore perfectly right in denying that the embryo breathed, as certain anatomists before him had asserted.

His only reference to the soul runs thus:

Nature places in the bodies of animals the soul, the composer of the body, i.e. the soul of the mother, which first composes, in the womb, the shape of man and in due time awakens the soul which shall be the inhabitant thereof, which first remains asleep and under the tutelage of the soul of the mother which through the umbilical vein nourishes and vivifies it.

This is not very revolutionary. But Leonardo was the first embryologist to make any quantitative observations on embryonic growth; he defined, for instance, the length of a full-grown embryo as one braccio and the adult as three times that.

The child grows daily far more when in the body of its mother than when it is outside of the body, and this teaches us why in the first year when it finds itself outside the body of the mother, or, rather, in the first 9 months, it does not double the size of the 9 months when it found itself within the mother's body. Nor in 18 months has it doubled the size it was 9 months after it was born, and thus in every 9 months diminishing the quantity of such increase till it has come to its greatest height.

Here Leonardo touches on one of the most modern quantitative aspects of embryology, and one almost expects to see him exemplify his words with a graph until one remembers with a shock that he lived two centuries before Descartes and five before Minot (see Fig. 5). His numerical data may also have included figures about the relative sizes of the parts, and the germ of the line of research so successfully pursued by Scammon and Calkins in our own times may be found in the note, "The liver is relatively much larger in the foetus than in the grown man." Other quantitative notes concern the length of the embryonic intestines, as in the laconic "20 braccia of bowels" and the statement that "the length of the umbilical cord always equals the length of the foetal body in man though not in animals."[1]

He said little about heredity, but in one place he mentions a case of sexual intercourse between an Italian woman and an Ethiopian, the outcome of which assured him that blackness was not due to the direct action of the sun and that the "seed of the female was as potent as that of the male in generation." Finally, the best instance of the wideness of

[1] Leonardo would have enjoyed Fog's statistical study of 8000 umbilical cords (1930).

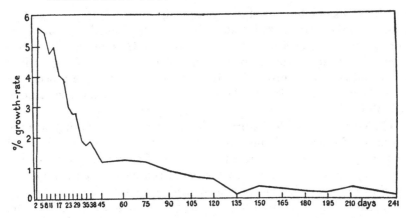

Fig. 5. Decline of the percentage growth-rate with increasing age in human males (from Minot).

his thought appears in the note, "All seeds have an umbilical cord which breaks when the seed is mature. And similarly they have matrix and secundines as the herbs and all the seeds which grow in shells show." We have met this idea before in Hippocrates of Cos, and we shall find it again in Nathaniel Highmore.

It is no coincidence that pictures of weights and cogs and pulleys stand side by side in Leonardo's notes with anatomical drawings of the embryo. As Hopstock says, "Leonardo arrives at the conclusion that there is but one natural law which governs the world, Necessity. Necessity is Nature's master and guardian, it is Necessity that makes the eternal laws." If Aristotle is the father of embryology regarded as a branch of natural history, Leonardo is the father of embryology regarded as an exact science.

10. The Macro-iconographers of the Sixteenth Century

After such a man, the writings of his contemporaries, such as the mythical Johannes de Ketham, Alessandro Achillini and Gabriele de Gerbi appear beyond description inferior.[1] De Ketham's embryology has been described by Ferckel. De Gerbi included in his *Liber Anatomiae corporis humani et singulorum membrorum illius* a section entitled *De Generatione Embryonis*, but there is nothing to be said about it except that it is a verbose compilation of the views of Aristotle and Galen taken from Avicenna. The work of Nolanus in 1532 presents

[1] Cf. Weindler's *Geschichte d. gynäkologisch-anatomische Abbildung*. The contemporary productions of Levinus Lemnius (described by Cole) and by Petrus Candidus are without value.

99

certain points of interest, but it is of little importance. Petrus Crescentius in his work on husbandry of 1548 mentions artificial incubation in ovens, but rather as a lost art. About this time also Hieronymus Dandinus Cesenas, a Jesuit, wrote a treatise on Galen's division of organs into white and red, those proceeding from the semen and those proceeding from the blood: it is cited by Aldrovandus, but I have not been able to consult it.

The most remarkable feature of the first half of the century was the encyclopaedic group of zoologists which now arose. Thus Belon and Rondelet, whose well-illustrated catalogues of animals were appearing from 1550 onwards, did a good service to comparative embryology in figuring the ovoviviparous selachians and viviparous Cetacea. Gesner belongs to this group.[1] All of them reproduce thin versions of Aristotle, when they speak of generation as such, and this is what differentiates them from Ulysses Aldrovandus, of whom I shall presently speak. Fig. 6 A and B shows Rondelet's picture of a viviparous dolphin and an ovoviviparous selachian.[2]

But the end of the twilight period was now at hand, for, within twenty-five years after the death of de Gerbi in 1505, four great embryologists were born as well as the greatest anatomist of any age, Andreas Vesalius (1514), of whom I shall say no more, for he had no opportunities for dissecting human embryos, and took hardly any interest in foetal development. But in 1522 Ulysses Aldrovandus was born, and in the following year Gabriel Fallopius, in 1530 Julius Caesar Arantius and in 1534 Volcher Coiter. Only three more years bring us to the birth of Andreas Laurentius and of Hieronymus Fabricius ab Aquapendente, the teacher of William Harvey.[3]

The senior member of this group, Ulysses Aldrovandus, was the first biologist since Aristotle to open the eggs of hens regularly during their incubation period, and to describe in detail the appearances which he found there. In his *Ornithologia*, published at Bologna in 1599, he set out to describe all the known kinds of birds, discussing in turn not only their zoological and physiological characteristics, but also their significance as presages and for augury, their mystical meaning, their use as allegories and for eating, and finally all the legends respecting them.[4] *Generositas, Temperantia, Liberalitas, aquilae* one finds. Beginning with

[1] *Historia*, Pt. III, p. 432.
[2] Oppenheimer has given us a special study of Guillaume Rondelet.
[3] Since this book was first written, I have had the good fortune to visit many of the scenes peopled by these great Italians, to find the little town of Aquapendente on the road to Rome, and to come upon the house of Aldrovandus unexpectedly during a stroll through a quiet street in Bologna.
[4] Vol. 2, pp. 183 ff.

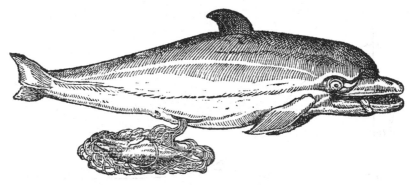

A. A (viviparous) dolphin.

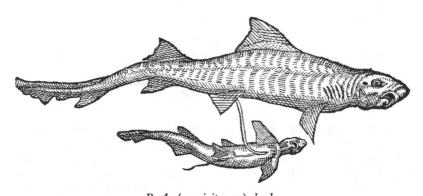

B. An (ovoviviparous) shark.
Fig. 6. Illustrations from Rondelet's "De piscibus marinis" of 1554.

the eagle, he proceeds to the vulture, the owl, the bat (the only vivi-parous bird!), the ostrich, the harpy (!), the parrot, the crow and so to the fowl. Side by side with a reference to the famous poem of Pruden-tius (*Multi sunt Presbyteri*, translated by J. M. Neale) about the steeple-cock, we find an excellent account of the generation of the chick in the egg. The book is sumptuously illustrated, but unfortunately there is only one picture of embryological interest, namely, a chick in the act of hatching.

In Aldrovandus' embryology there is much discussion of Aristotle and Galen, but traces of an independent spirit abound. Pliny's view that the heart was formed in the white is "exploded," and Aldrovandus says that it is formed on the yolk-membrane. He refutes the opinion of Galen also that the liver is first formed, in connection with which he says,

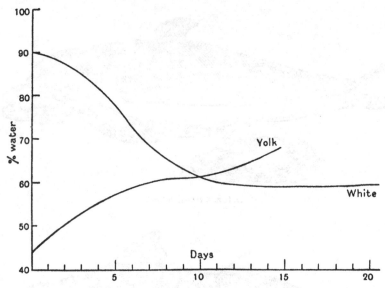

Fig. 7. *Water content of yolk and white during the development of the chick embryo.*

In order that I might bring to an end this controversy between the philosophers and the physicians I followed with the keenest curiosity and diligence the incubation of 22 hen's eggs, opening one each day; thus I found Aristotle's doctrine to be the truest. And because apart from the fact that these matters are most worthy of being looked into they provide also the greatest pleasure and entertainment, I have thought it well to describe them as clearly and briefly as possible.

Aldrovandus also contradicts Albertus, and propounds a new theory, namely, that the *spiritualia* (the organs in the thorax) are formed from the seed of the cock (*ex maris semine sunt*). This seed he affirms to be present in the egg, and he identifies it with the chalazae, thus anticipating Fabricius ab Aquapendente, but not going quite so far, and explicitly opposing Gaza, who had said not long before that the chalazae were simply congealed water. Aldrovandus' admiration for Aristotle is extreme, and, though he differs from him about the chalazae, he defends the Aristotelian opinion that the chick was made from the white but nourished from the yolk. His argument for this is new, however; it is that, during incubation, the latter liquefies but the former hardens[1]; now in all digestion liquefaction takes place, and in all growth hardening,

[1] During incubation the egg-white loses water and the yolk, up to a certain point, gains it, see Fig. 7.

102

therefore, etc. This argument is a great deal more cogent than most of those which were current between 1550 and 1650. He goes out of his way to castigate Albertus for saying that the yolk moves up into the sharp point of the egg, for experience assures him that it does not, "as I have observed by cutting open an egg after one day's incubation." A striking instance of his powers of observation was his description of the "egg-tooth" of embryonic birds, a discovery made anew in the nineteenth century by Yarrell and Rosenstadt. The chick was perfect in form, according to him, on the tenth day.

The peculiarity of Aldrovandus lies in the fact that he incorporated so many elements into one book, and was able to produce a collection of chapters in which good scientific observation sat at the closest quarters with literary allusion and semi-theological homily. So well-proportioned a mixture as the *Ornithologia* is not often found. As a final instance three consecutive paragraphs may be mentioned, in the first of which he discusses Plutarch's arid problem about the priority of egg or hen, next he makes some very reasonable remarks about teratology, suggesting that monsters come from yolks which are physico-chemically abnormal in some way, while in the third he expresses strong scepticism concerning the tale that the basilisk is sometimes hatched out from a hen's egg— *Ego ne jurantibus quidem crediderim,* he says. This last notion is found in the fourteenth-century poem of Prudentius alluded to above, and appears again in the *Miscellaneous Exercitations* of Caspar Bartholinus the younger,[1] whose second chapter is devoted to showing "That the basilisk hatcheth not from the egg of the hen," a conclusion which has been amply confirmed in the light of subsequent experience.[2]

Aldrovandus' disciple Volcher Coiter the Frisian,[3] as he described himself, did not suffer from the prevailing vice of the age, verbosity. His *Externarum et Internarum principalium Humani Corporis partium tabulae et exercitationes,* which appeared at Nuremberg in 1573—a beautifully printed book—contained a brief section entitled *De ovorum gallinaceorum generationis primo exordio progressuque et pulli gallinacei creationis ordine.* His Latin style betrays his German origin, for the constructions are Teutonic, though the meaning is always perfectly clear. Coiter says,

[1] See Petersen.

[2] Bartholinus gives a bibliography of this curious legend, on which see also Robin, pp. 84 ff. In an interesting paper L. J. Cole has considered the historical aspects of sex-reversal in fowls; the tendency of hens, especially old ones, to develop male characteristics, even to the extent of crowing. Hence the origin of "cock's eggs," sought by sorcerers as ingredients of magical preparations. Cases of the actual trial and condemnation of cocks for laying eggs are on record, e.g. at Basel in 1474. The question has wide-reaching implications, as is shown in the author's *Science and Civilisation in China,* vol. 2, pp. 574 ff.

[3] See Plate VI, facing page 104.

In the year 1564 in the month of May at Bologna, being instigated by that excellent professor of philosophy outstanding in varied sciences and arts, Doctor Ulysses Aldrovandus and by other doctors and students, I ordered 2 broody fowls to be brought and under each of them I caused 23 eggs to be placed and in the company of these persons I opened one every day so that we could see firstly the origin of the veins and secondly what organ is first formed in the animal.

What follows is practically a repetition of the facts available in Aristotle, but described with much greater clearness than either Aristotle or Aldrovandus had been able to bring to the matter. On the third day, he saw the *globulus sanguineus* which *in vitello manifeste pulsabat*, and so solved his first problem. He decides that the first organ to be formed is the heart, and quotes Lactantius' experiments. He explains the large size of the eye as due to the fact that the most complicated part of the body needs the longest time for its manufacture. He correctly describes the various membranes, and the *faeces subviridies* in the intestines at hatching. Once he contradicts Aristotle, maintaining that on the tenth day the body as a whole is larger than the head, and once he contradicts Albertus, denying that any yolk can be found in the stomach at hatching. He concludes his tractate by a succinct and clear account of the opinions of Aristotle and Hippocrates about embryonic development. His importance is that he drew the attention of scientific thinkers to the problems arising out of the hen's egg, and assisted in the formation of that iconographic phase in embryology which was later to find its climax in the plates of Fabricius, and its close in Harvey's *Exercitations*.

Gabriel Fallopius, who belongs to this time, must be mentioned as the discoverer of the organs which bear his name, but his services to embryology were only indirect. A. Benedictus, who was now growing old, and Caesar Cremonius, who was still young, may be remembered as the principal upholders of pure Aristotelianism. Realdus Columbus also wrote on the embryo. B. Telesius, in his *De Natura Rerum* of 1565, studied the hen's egg and suggested that the parts of animals were formed by the pressure of the uterus acting as a mould: he was thus the middle term between Galen and Buffon.

Julius Caesar Arantius has already been referred to. His *De Humano Foetu* was an important book, but, though it appeared in 1564, just at the time when the macro-iconographic school was at its height, it dealt with a rather different field and cannot be considered as a constituent of that group. He begins by relating that a pregnant woman was killed by an accident at Bologna a couple of years before, so that he had an opportunity of testing whether the opinions about certain points in generation, which he had formed on *a priori* grounds during the previous

PLATE VI

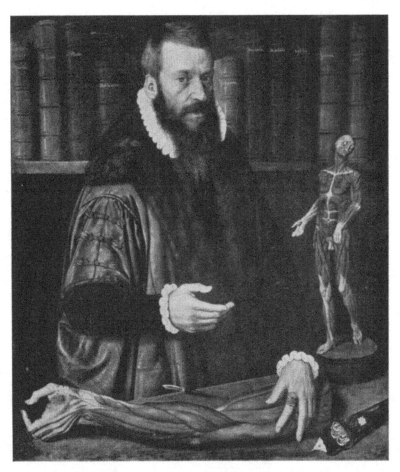

Volcher Coiter the Frisian, aet. 41 (painted in 1575 by an unknown master;
now in the Städtische Bibliothek, Nuremberg).

fifteen years, were true or not. In the first place, he found on dissection that the placenta was not cotyledonous, and he spoke thus of its formation:

> Blood flows out from the spongy substance of the uterus and this blood growing in bulk forms a soft and fungous-like mass of flesh, rather like the substance of the spleen, which adheres to the surface of the uterus and transmits to the foetus in proportion as it grows the nourishment for it which reaches the uterus in the form of blood and spirits.

Then, going on to discuss the functions of the *jecor uteri*, as he calls the placenta,[1] he devotes a chapter to *De vasorum umbilicalium origine*, and contradicting Hippocrates, Galen, Erasistratus, and Aetius, says that the maternal and foetal blood-vessels do not pass into each other by a free passage.

> This is repugnant to sense, and as may be seen by ocular inspection, these vessels do not reach the inner membrane of the uterus, for the substance of the placenta is placed between their ramifications and the proper substance of the womb.

He was thus the first to maintain that the maternal and foetal circulations are separate, but he naturally did not, and could not, speak of circulations, since he lived before Harvey. Nor could he have proved his point satisfactorily with the means then at his command, and, as we shall see, it was to take another century before the proof was given. Apart from this valuable contribution to embryology, Arantius gave some admirable anatomical descriptions of the foetal membranes.

Hieronymus Fabricius ab Aquapendente, the pupil of Fallopius, has always been given an important place in the history of embryology by those who have written on him.[2] As one comes upon him in the process of tracing out that history itself, however, he does not take such a high place. With the statement, for instance, that "Fabricius carried embryology far beyond where Coiter had left it and elevated it at one bound into an independent science" I find that I cannot agree. Embryologists who called themselves that and nothing else did not appear till the end of the eighteenth century, and it seems to me doubtful whether the anatomical advances in embryology made by Fabricius are not counterbalanced by the erroneous theories which he invented at the same time.

---

[1] Not until the discovery by Claude Bernard in 1858 that the glycogenic function of the liver is undertaken for the foetus by the placenta, could the justness of this intuition be assessed at its true value.

[2] We are now in possession of the sumptuous facsimile edition of Fabricius' embryological works, edited with a brilliant and exhaustive commentary by my friend Dr Howard B. Adelmann of Cornell University (1942).

His *De Formatione Ovi et Pulli Pennatorum*, and his *De Formato Foetu* of 1604 show much more scholasticism and sheer argumentativeness than is to be found in Coiter, and are remarkable for their bulk. Fabricius seems to have had a genius for exsuccous and formal discussions. He spends much time, for example, in taking up the problem of whether the yolk of the hen's egg is more earthy than the white, and looking at it from all possible angles. He disagrees at last with Aristotle and decides that the white is the more earthy. Bones, he says, are white, but also very earthy. The albumen is colder, stickier and heavier than the yolk: *sequitur, terrestrius esse*. In addition, he introduced a number of grave errors and misleading theories into embryology, so that subsequently Harvey had to spend a large part of his time refuting them. Fabricius was, indeed, a good comparative anatomist, and it is upon that ground that he deserves praise: his plates, some of which are reproduced herewith (Fig. 8), were far better than anything before and for a long time afterwards. He dissected embryos of man, rabbit, guinea-pig, mouse, dog, cat, sheep, pig, horse, ox, goat, deer, dogfish and viper, a comparative study which had certainly never been made previously.

In his first tractate he begins by dealing with a question not unlike that of how the sardines got into the tin, i.e. how the contents get into the hard-shelled egg. He rejects Aristotle's idea that the egg is formed in the oviduct by a kind of umbilicus, and ascribes its growth there to transudation through the blood-vessels. He marks a definite advance upon Aristotle when he says that silkworms and other insects are born into their larval state from an egg, though he still terms the chrysalis an egg, and therefore holds that they are generated twice. Then follows his discussion of what part of the egg the chick comes from. The chalazae, he says, are not semen, for the semen is not present at all in the fertilised egg. His argument sounds peculiar when he says that both the white and yolk of the egg are the food of the embryo, for neither of them is absent at the end of incubation, therefore neither of them is its material. Hippocrates had said, *ex luteo gigni, ex albo nutriri*; Aristotle had said, *ex albo fieri, ex luteo nutriri*. The latter was the view generally held in the sixteenth century, as may be gathered from Ambrosius Calepinus' dictionary; Scaliger's *Commentary on Aristotle* and the treatise on the soul by Joannes Philoponus.[1]

Fabricius now says both nourish, neither makes. This distinction between food and building-materials seems to us unnecessary, but it had a great influence on later thought. Fabricius devotes much time to proving, as he thinks, that yolk and white are of the same nature, and

---

[1] Bk. I, ch. 2.

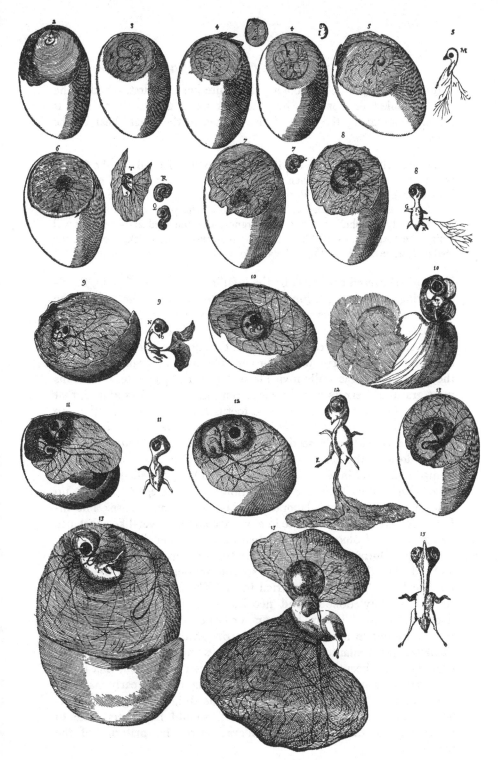

Fig. 8. Illustrations from Fabricius ab Aquapendente's "De Formatione Ovi et Pulli," 1604.

adduces the fact that "in cooking the white hardens first, whether the egg be boiled or poached, but the yolk hardens also if the heat is more," comparing the heat of the kitchen to the innate heat of the chick.

But you will say [he goes on] if the albumen and the yolk are the food of the chick in the egg, what then must we decide the material of the chick to be, since we have already said that the semen is not present in the eggs. You will find this material from an enumeration of the parts of the egg—there remains only the shell, the two membranes, and the chalazae—nobody will assign the membranes or the shell as the material of the chick, therefore the chalazae alone are the fitting substance out of which it can be made.

Having discovered this truth by the infallible processes of logic, Fabricius brings all kinds of arguments forward to support it; he adduces the three nodes in the chalazae as the precursors of brain, heart and liver; tadpoles, he thinks, resemble significantly the chalazae, being "armless legless spines." The eyes are transparent, so are the chalazae, therefore the latter must give rise to the former. The liver is formed as soon as the heart but is practically invisible as it does not palpitate. One of his most gratuitous errors was the suggestion, now newly introduced, that the heart (and other organs) of the foetus has no proper function, no *munus publicum*, but beats only in order to preserve its own life. Then there is a considerable section called *De Ovorum Utilitatibus*, which almost does for the hen's egg what Galen's *De Usu Partium* did for the human body, and in which such questions as Why the shell is hard and porous? and Why there are any membranes in the egg? are taken up and answered with an elaborate display of common sense. The influence of Galen is perceptible in a passage about a liver-like substance being formed if blood is freshly shed into hot water, in the usual terminology of formative faculties, and in the division of fleshes into white and red, though the former is not specifically derived from the semen nor the latter from the menstrual blood. The human placenta is described as cotyledonous, and needless confusion is caused by the doctrine that the "liquors, humours, or rather, excrements, around the foetus, are two in number, sweat and urine, the former in the amnios, the latter in the allantois." But the drawings and illustrations of Fabricius' work are beautiful and accurate, so much so, indeed, that it will long remain a mystery how the man who figured the early stages of the development of the chick as Fabricius did, showing the bloodvessels radiating from the minute heart, should have been able to propound the thesis that the chalazae were the material of the embryo.

The other biologist to whom Harvey was most indebted was Andreas Laurentius of Montpellier, whose *Historia Anatomica* (printed with his other works in 1628) contained a whole book (VII) devoted to embryology, but which presents us with nothing except a commentary on Hippocrates and Aristotle. The only evidences of life are furnished by two polemics, one of which was against Simon Petreus of Paris, who had propounded some new views about the foetal circulation. Laurentius gave also a table showing the changes which occur in the heart and lungs of the foetus at birth.

It was about this time that the embryological observations of that many-sided genius, Hieronymus Cardanus, began to attract attention. His main thesis was that the limbs of the embryo were alone derived from the yolk, while the rest of the body came from the white. This was a well-meant attempt to mediate between the two traditions headed respectively by Aristotle and Hippocrates, but the arguments in support of it were not remarkable even for ingenuity. Constantinus Varolius treated of the formation of the embryo in a book which appeared in 1591, but very inadequately.[1] He had certainly opened hen's eggs, and describes the fourth-day embryo as *forma minimi faseoli*. But nearly every one of his marginal headings begins with the word *Cur*, and this tells its own story, for the didactic style rarely hides genuine works of research. Johannes Fernelius, a rather earlier worker, in his *De Hominis Procreatione* followed Aristotle and Galen in nearly all particulars, and made no real contribution to embryology.[2]

11. The Movement to Rationalise Obstetrics

On its practical obstetrical side the sixteenth century produced some remarkable compilations of ancient gynaecological writings. The first of these was that of Caspar Wolf, which was published at Zürich in 1566, and, after having been enlarged by Caspar Bauhin in 1586, subsequently formed the backbone of the most important and famous one, namely that of Israel Spach (Strassburg, 1597). Although these composite text-books represented no real embryological progress, they yet showed that great interest in development was alive, an interest which, though doubtless utilitarian in its origin, could hardly fail to lead to advances of a theoretical nature. (See Fig. 9.)

The obstetrical literature intended for midwives is also of great

[1] *Resolutio*, Bk. IV, chs. 3 and 5.
[2] This was a section of his *Universa Medicinae* (*Physiologiae*, ch. 7). But Jean Fernel will always be remembered as the first man to use the term Physiology for a distinguishable branch of science. It was this that led one of the greatest physiologists of our own time, Sir Charles Sherrington, to make so notable a study of him.

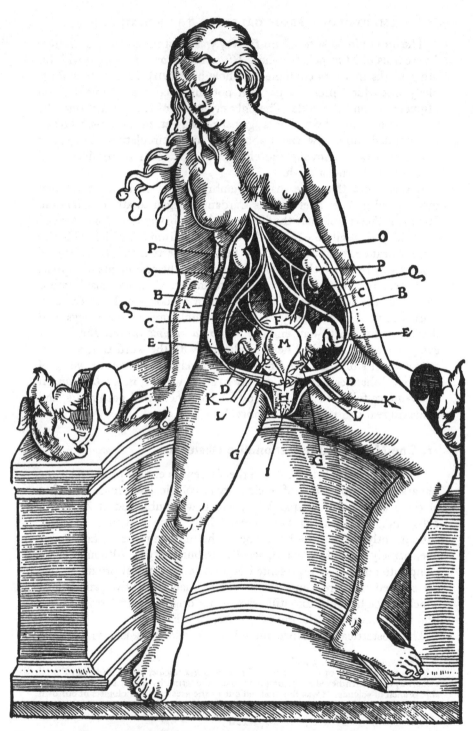

Fig. 9. Illustration from Walther Ryff's "Anatomia" of 1541. One of the nineteen woodcut plates by the great artist Hans Baldung Grien.

interest. It was about this time that the first popular guides to their subject began to appear, founded not upon mere superstition and the remnants of ancient knowledge derived in roundabout fashion through Syriac and Arabic, but either upon a careful study of Galen and Aristotle, or upon the results of dissections and living speculation. The principal representative of the former class is that of Jacob Rueff, which appeared in 1554 and was called *De Conceptu et Generatione Hominis*. Although written in Latin, it was soon translated into the vernacular languages. Its importance lies in its illustrations, which I reproduce in Fig. 10. I think they show very clearly what the general ideas were at this period about mammalian embryology, and thus afford us a precious insight into what was in the minds of such writers as Riolanus the elder, Mercurialis, Saxonia, Rondeletius, Venusti, Holler and Vallesius. There are many points which their expositions of foetal growth and development leave vague, and without Rueff it would be difficult or impossible to picture in what manner they imagined it to go on. Rueff's text follows Galen and Aristotle with fidelity, as does theirs—with the exception of a few minor ideas not quite consonant with this.

In (*a*) of Fig. 10 Rueff portrays the mixture of semen and menstrual blood in the womb, or, as he loosely refers to it, of both seeds, coagulating into a pink egg-shaped mass surrounded with a fine pellicle. (*b*) shows the same mass in the uterus and wrapped round with the three coats, amnion, chorion and allantois[1]—a lamentable but interesting misrepresentation of the facts. Then in (*c*) it is shown that upon the surface of the yolk-like mass of semen and blood appear "three tiny white points not unlike coagulated milk," these being the first origins of the liver, the heart and the brain. Next (*d*) shows the first bloodvessels springing from the heart, four in number, and distributing themselves over the surface of the mass. It is plain that Rueff must either have opened hen's eggs himself and seen the early growth of the blastoderm or have been told about it by some observer such as Coiter or Aldrovandus. He could not have copied his pseudo-blastoderm pictures from their works, for in 1554 none of them had appeared, and, as far as I know, there were no similar illustrations in existence at that time.

After this point the pictures grow even more fanciful, and, in (*e*), the first outline of the cranium is seen taking shape in the upper part of the "egg." In (*f*) the blood-vessels have suddenly assumed the outline of a human being, and in (*g*) the finished product is seen. Rueff gives what seems to be a mnemonic in hexameters:

[1] On the elusive human allantois see Meyer (1954).

iniectum semen, sex primis certe diebus
est quasi lac: reliquisque novem sit sanguis; at inde
consolidat duodena dies; bis nona deinceps
effigiat; tempusque sequens producit ad ortum
talis enim praedicto tempore figura consit.[1]

Rueff gives some excellent diagrams of the foetus *in utero* with relation to the rest of the body, and the various positions which are familiar to obstetricians. His teratology is less happy, for he attributes the production of monsters to the direct action of God, though he does venture upon a few speculations concerning "corrupt seed." But his principal significance for this history is that in his picture of the yolk-like mass of mixed semen and blood, with the pseudo-blastoderm upon it, he throws a brilliant light on the Aristotelian conceptions of his time.

These beliefs lasted far on into the eighteenth century (see p. 183). Thus as late as 1683 we find, in the English translation of Mauriceau's midwifery:

Hippocrates relates a story of a Woman, which at six days end cast forth, with a noise, at once, out of her Womb, the seeds she had conceived, resembling a raw Egg, without a shell, having only the small skin over it; or, to the abortive Eggs which have no shell: which membrane was on the outside a little covered with red.

Rueff's book was subsequently translated into English, and had many editions as *The Expert Midwife.*

The principal representative of the second class of popular books of this period is that of Euch. Rhodion, Rösslin, or Rösslein, which was translated into English, and published as his own work, by Thomas Raynold, "physition," in 1545, under the title of *The Byrth of Mankynde otherwyse named The Woman's Book.*[2] It was the first book in the English language to contain copper engravings. They were variants of the traditional Soranus-Moschion figures. The Rösslein-Raynold book pays less attention to Galenic theory than does that of Rueff, and includes much better drawings of actual dissections. Another famous obstetrical book was that of Scipio Mercurius; for further information on Renaissance midwifery see Spencer and Miller.

The minor embryologists of the sixteenth century included among them Ambroise Paré, the founder of modern surgery. His teaching on generation involved nothing original, and seems to have been Galenism

[1] "After the semen has been injected, for the first 6 days it is like milk, by the ninth there is nothing but blood, and on the twelfth all is consolidated, then successively for twice 9 days (the embryo) is shaped, after which for the rest of the time it develops that aspect which it is destined to have by the appointed time."

[2] For details consult d'Arcy Power, and Ballantyne (1907).

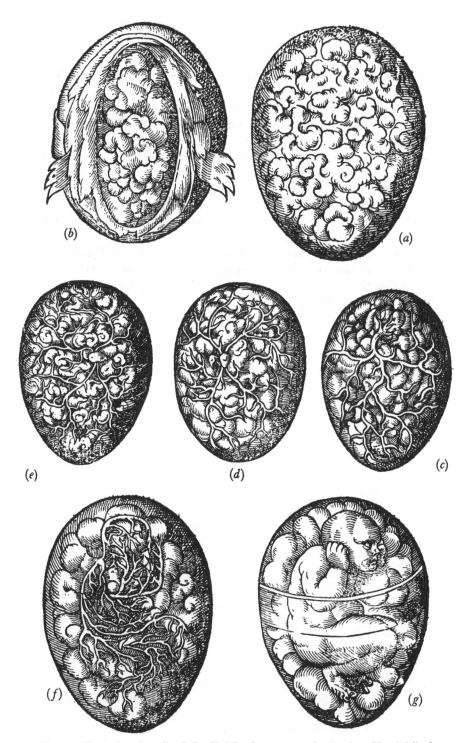

Fig. 10. Illustrations from Jacob Rueff's "De Conceptu et Generatione Hominis" of 1554 (arranged by Singer), showing the Aristotelian coagulum of blood and seed in the uterus.

interpreted by an intelligent, well-balanced, unspeculative mind. The three-bubble theory appears in him very clearly; thus, we read, "The seed boileth and fermenteth in the womb, and swelleth into three bubbles or bladders"—the brain, the liver and the heart. Paré's illustrations are copied wholesale from Vesalius and Rueff, without acknowledgment. The last authors to take the three-bubble theory seriously were Robert Fludd in 1617 and A. Deusingius, who wrote in 1665, after Harvey. Others who deserve a mention, but no more, were Severinus Pinaeus, L. Bonaciolus and Felix Platter. None of them made any advance, and the illustrations of the former's *De Virginitatibus notis Graviditate et Partu* were almost ludicrous.

Hieronymus Capivaccius, F. Licetus, J. Costaeus and V. Cardelinus, who wrote in 1608, were the last true supporters of the ancient theories, such as that the male embryo was twice as hot and developed twice as quickly as the female.

CHAPTER III

EMBRYOLOGY IN THE SEVENTEENTH CENTURY[1]

1. The Opening Years

A GOOD deal has been written on the history of biology in the seventeenth and eighteenth centuries by those who apply the distinction between the "Baroque" and "Rococo" periods. Since the art-styles from which these names are derived had relatively little influence in England, it is natural for English writers and readers to experience some hesitation in accepting at any rate all their applications to the history of science. Sigerist's essay on the position of Harvey may form a suitable introduction to this point of view, and the treatise of Bilikiewicz divides all the embryology of these centuries quite sharply into Baroque and Rococo.

Doubtless there is something to be said for such a division. Thus Harvey is said to stand as the typical Baroque biologist, since his outlook was "dynamic"; he studied the movement of the blood and the morphological movement in space-time of the developing embryo. With him embryology stepped from the confines of pure anatomy. Yet it seems to be overlooked that Hippocrates, Aristotle, Coiter and Aldrovandus (to say nothing of the Cleopatra legend, cf. p. 65) all employed the method of comparing morphological change against time in development.[2] Another characteristic of the Baroque period was its political absolutism, mirrored, it is suggested, in the absolutist claims for reason's supremacy which provided the basis for the wilder assertions of preformationism. But also in the hands of men like Gassendi, Descartes and Leibniz, this thorough-going rationalism gave rise to the *a priori* mathematical attitude to biological phenomena, exemplified in Descartes' own contribution to embryology (p. 155). Finally, it involved a preference for mechanistic as opposed to vitalistic interpretations, e.g. the Epicureanism of Highmore.

[1] Cf. the interesting recent résumé of H. Fischer.
[2] On the significance of the time-concept for seventeenth-century biology the obscure but interesting essays of d'Irsay should be consulted. Pagel has given us a brilliant study of J. B. van Helmont's tractate *De Tempore* on biological time (part of the *Ortus Medicinae*).

The Rococo period, it is said, brought in new movements towards freedom in the political sphere, and this took the form in science of a return to empiricism, so that the biological observations of Redi and Wolff were as much connected with the romantic movement as the philosophical speculations of Rousseau. In the Encyclopaedists, the connection between empiricism in science and political freedom is particularly well seen. But when it is suggested that the new eminence of the female sex in the Rococo period, unimaginable to previous ages, was connected with the temporary triumph of ovism,[1] the reader may question whether the Spenglerian method is not being carried too far.

Æmilius Parisanus, a Venetian, now dealt with embryology in the fourth, fifth and sixth books of his *De Subtilitate*. They were entitled as follows:

(4) Of the principles and first instruments of the soul and of innate heat, (5) Of the material of the embryo and of its efficient cause, (6) Of the part of the animal body which is first made, and of the mode and order of procreation.

Parisanus is very wordy, but he has the merit of giving many quotations from the lesser known authors, and providing (as a rule) accurate references. He held that the spleen was formed in all development before the heart, and that neither heart nor lungs moved *in utero*. With regard to the controversy over the function of white and yolk, he was in agreement with Fabricius, but he firmly opposed the view that the chalazae were the first material of the chick, rather, it must be confessed, because of the opinion of Aristotle than from personal conviction. Nevertheless, his own observations were noteworthy, and he will always be remembered for his opinion that the heart of the chick begins to beat some time before any red blood appears in it.

Parisanus was the last of the macro-iconographic group of sixteenth-century embryologists. Their labours established the fundamental morphological facts about the developing embryo; the first great step in the history of embryology. But there were numerous errors in their work, and Harvey, who occupies a terminal or boundary position, was destined to correct them. He marks the transition from the static to the dynamic conception of embryology, from the study of the embryo as a

[1] Bilikiewicz, p. 73. "Die Frau habe heute nicht nur das Recht, dass ihre Schönheit und Weiblichkeit in Dithyramben besungen werde; wenn sie den Platz auf dem Throne einnehmen oder über Throne verfugen könne, oder wenn sie im allgemein-gesellschaftlichen Leben mit der wachsenden Gleichberechtigung immer verant-wortlichere Rollen übernehmen könne, so habe sie auch das Recht, auf dem Gebiete der Embryologie dem männlichen Geschlechte in die Augen zu schauen als ein Wesen, das dieselben Rechte auf Freiheit habe. Der Ovismus liess diese Standarte wehen."

changing succession of shapes, to the study of it as a causally governed organisation of an initial physical complexity, in a word, from Coiter and Fabricius to Descartes and Mayow. Iconography did not die: on the contrary, the improvement of the microscope gave it new life, and the micro-iconographic school emerged with its principal glory, Malpighi.

Harvey sums up the work of the macro-iconographic period in the historical introduction contained in Ex. No. XIV of his *De Generatione Animalium*.[1] I give it in full in the beautiful seventeenth-century English into which Harvey's Latin was translated under his guidance by the physician Martin Llewellyn.

We have already discovered the Formation, and Generation of the Egge; it remains that we now deliver our Observations, concerning the Procreation of the Chicken out of the Egge. An undertaking equally difficult, usefull, and pleasant as the former. For Nature's Rudiments and Attempts are involved in obscurity and deep night, and so perplext with subtilties, that they delude the most piercing wit, as well as the sharpest eye. Nor can we easier discover the secret recesses, and dark principles of Generation than the method of the fabrick and composure of the whole world. In this reciprocal interchange of Generation and Corruption consists the Æternity and Duration of mortal creatures. And as the Rising and Setting of the Sun, doth by continued revolutions complete and perfect Time; so doth the alternative vicissitude of Individuums, by a constant repetition of the same species, perpetuate the continuance of fading things.

Those Authors which have delivered any thing touching this subject, do for the most part tread a several path, for having their Judgements prepossessed with their own private opinions, they proceed to erect and fashion principles proportionable to them.

Aristotle of old, and Hieronymus Fabricius of late, have written so accurately concerning the Formation and Generation of the Foetus out of the Egge, that they seem to have left little to the industry of Posterity. And yet Ulysses Aldrovandus hath undertaken the description of the Pullulation or Formation of the chicken out of the Egge, out of his own Observations; wherein he seems rather to have directed and guided his thoughts by the Authority of Aristotle, than by his own experience.

For Volcherus Coiter, living at Bononia at the same time did by the advice of the said Aldrovandus (whom he calls Tutor) dayly employ himself in the opening of Egges sat upon by the Hen, and hath discovered many things truer than Aldrovandus himself, of which he also could not be ignorant. Likewise Æmilius Parisanus (a Venetian Doctor) despising other mens opinions hath fancied A new procreation of the Chicken out of the Egge.

But because somethings, (according to our experience) and those of great

---

[1] P. 77 of the English edition (1653).

moment and consequence, are much otherwise than hath been yet delivered, I shall declare to you what dayly progress is made in the egge, and what parts are altered, especially about the first dayes of Incubation; at which time all things are most intricate, confused, and hard to observe, and about which authors do chiefly stickle for their own observations, which they accommodate rather to their own preconceived perswasions (which they have entertained concerning the Material and Efficient Causes of the generation of Animals) than to truth herself.

Aldrovandus, partaking of the same error with Aristotle, saith (which none but a blind man can subscribe to) that the Yolk doth in the first dayes, arise to the Acute Angle of the Egge; and thinks the Grandines to be the Seed of the Cock; and that the Pullus is framed out of them, but nourished as well by the yolk as the white; which is clean contrary to Aristotle's opinion, who conceived the Grandines to conduce nothing to the fecundity of the egge. Volcherus Coiter delivers truer things, and more consonant to Autopsie, yet his three Globuli are meer fables. Nor did he rightly consider the principle from whence the Foetus is derived in the Egg. Hieronymus Fabricius indeed contends, that the Grandines are not the seed of the cock, and yet he will have the body of the Chicken to be framed out of them (as out of its first matter) being made fruitful by the seed of the cock. He likewise saw the Original of the Chicken in the Egge; namely the Macula, or Cicatricula annexed to the membrane of the Yolke, but conceived it to be onely a Relique of the stalk broken off, and an infirmity of blemish onely of the Egge, and not a principle part of it. Parisanus hath plentifully confuted Fabricius his opinion concerning the Chalazae or Grandines, and yet himself is evidently at a loss in some certaine circles and points of the Principle parts of the Foetus (namely the Liver and the Heart) and seems to have observed a Principium or first Principle of the Foetus, but not to have known which it was, in that he saith, that the Punctum Album in the Middle of the Circles is the Cocks Seed out of which the Chicken is made. So that it comes to pass that while each of them desire to reduce the manner of the Formation of the Chicken out of the Egge to their own opinions they are all wide from the mark.

Before discussing how Harvey put them right, however, there are a number of other matters to be mentioned. Parisanus' work was published in 1623, and twenty-five years were to elapse before Harvey's *Exercitations* were to be put before the learned world by George Ent. In that time not a few events of importance for the history of embryology took place.

It will be convenient to speak first of Adrianus Spigelius, whose *De Formato Foetu* appeared in 1631. In this book the plates of the gravid uterus which had been prepared some years before for Julius Casserius were now published. They had more influence than Spigelius' text, perhaps, in contributing to the permanent fame of his book.

He gives for the most part straightforward anatomical descriptions, but he returns to the notion of a cotyledonous placenta in man, and he combats Arantius' opinions about the placenta. Arantius had said that the function of the *jecor uteri* was to purify the blood-supply to the foetus, a thoroughly modern idea, but Spigelius opposes this on two grounds, firstly, because the foetus has its own organs for purifying blood, and secondly, because, if Arantius was right, the placenta would always be as red as blood, but this is not the case in such animals as the sheep. Spigelius himself thought that the placenta was for the purpose of preventing severe loss of blood at birth, as would be the case if the embryo was joined to the mother with only one big vessel and not a great many little ones.

However, Spigelius upholds the view, taken by Rufus of Ephesus and by Vesalius, that the allantois contains the foetal urine, which has to be separated from the amniotic liquid in which the embryo is, because it would corrode the embryonic skin (*ne cuti tenellae aliquod damnum urinae acrimonia inferret*). The first discussion of the *vernix caseosa*, or *sordes*, as he calls it, appears in Spigelius, who, however, hazards no guess as to its nature. He is happy in his refutation of Laurentius, who had affirmed that the foetal heart did not beat *in utero*, and he shows some advance on all previous writers save Arantius in declaring that the umbilical vessels take vital spirits away from the foetal heart, not exclusively to it. He gave, moreover, the first denial of the presence of a nerve in the umbilical cord, and also made the first observation of the occurrence of milk in foetal breasts at birth.[1] Finally, he abolished at last the notion that the meconium in the foetal intestines argued eating *in utero* on the part of the embryo.

Riolanus the younger,[2] the correspondent and almost exactly the contemporary of Harvey, was professor in Paris and published his *Anthropographia* in 1618. As he was a keen advocate of the ancient views, his section on the formation of the foetus has little importance. Yet it contains the first known instance of the use of the lens in embryology, the germ of that powerful instrument which was to lead in due course to so many discoveries. "In aborted embryos," said Riolanus, "the structure is damaged and can often not be properly seen, even when you make use of lenses (*conspicilia*) which make objects so much bigger and more complicated than they ordinarily seem."

The *De Formatrice Foetus* of Thomas Fienus, professor at Louvain and a friend of Gassendi, published in 1620, is interesting because it is the middle term between Aristotle and Driesch. As the title-page in-

---

[1] The endocrinological aspects of the so-called "sorcerer's milk" have been studied by Halban and it has been analysed by Tschassovnikov.
[2] See Donley.

forms us, he sets out to demonstrate that the rational soul is infused into the human embryo on the third day after conception. This by itself would not be very attractive, but the most cursory inspection shows that Fienus' interests were not at all theological. He divides the book up into seven main questions. (1) What is the efficient cause of embryogeny? He concludes that it is neither God, nor Intelligence, nor *anima mundi* (influence of neo-Platonism here as on Galileo). (2) Is it in the uterus or in the seed? In the latter, says Fienus, adding a list of authorities who agree with this view—Haly-Abbas, Gaietanus, Zonzinas, Turisanus, Fernelius, Vallesius, de Peramato, Saxonia, Carrerius, Zegarra, Mercurialis, Massaria, and Archangelus, "*solus Fabio Pacio utero imprudenter adscribit*" (!). (3) Is it heat? Fienus nearly decided that it was, but gave his opinion against it, saying, "the process (of development) is so divine and wonderful that it would be ridiculous to ascribe it to heat, a mere naked and simple quality." After weighing various other alternatives in questions (4), (5) and (6), he asks whether it is *anima seminis post conceptum adveniens* (7), and concludes that it is. It is here that he becomes really interesting, for he quotes with approval certain writers, e.g. Alexander Aphrodisias (*organicum corpus esse organicum ab anima et anima prae-existere organizationi*), Themistius (*anima fabricatur architecturaque sibi domicilium et accommodatum instrumentum*) and Marsilio Ficino in his commentary on Plato's *Timaeus* (*priusquam adultum sit corpus, anima tota in illius fabrica occupatur*), and then maintains with them that the soul is the principle which organises the body from within, arranging an organ for each of its faculties and preparing its own residence, not merely consenting to be breathed into a physical being which has already organised itself. "The conformation of the foetus is a vital, not a natural, action," he says. He develops this idea in the remainder of the book; according to him, the seed first coagulates the menstrual blood into an amorphous cake, taking three days to do so, after which the rational (not vegetative or sensitive) soul (or entelechy), which has entered the uterus with the seed, finding a suitable mass of shapeless material, enters into it and begins to give it a shape. Fienus was attacked by several writers, and published a defence of his views.

Later writers on the same subject included Fidelis, Teichmeyer, Albertus, de Reies, Torreblanca and de Mendoza.[1] The Spanish influence here is perhaps significant. Hieronymus Florentinus, who adopted the same standpoint as Fienus in 1658, was forced to recant it.[2]

[1] Vol. 4, pp. 389 ff.
[2] I do not know why; but Fienus' vitalistic standpoint was certainly very repugnant to the Cartesian mechanical genius of the succeeding fifty years (cf. Bilikiewicz), as Digby's writings show.

In 1625 Joseph de Aromatari, of Assisi, included in his epistle on plants the first definite statement of the preformationist theory since Seneca, but he did not develop the idea.[1] He had noted that in bulbs and some seeds the rudiments of many parts of the adult plant can be seen even without glass or microscope, and this led him to suggest that probably in all animals as well as plants a similar thing was true. "And as for the eggs of fowls," he said, "I think the embryo is already roughly sketched out in the egg before being formed at all by the hen (*quod attinet ad ova gallinarum, existimamus quidem pullum in ovo delineatum esse, antequam foveatur a gallina*)." This suggestion did not begin to bear its malignant fruits till the time of Swammerdam. In his *De Rabia Contagiosa*, too, Joseph de Aromatari wrote against spontaneous generation, asserting that all animals arise from eggs (Bigelow). Here the logical connection between preformationism and belief in spontaneous generation appears, as also in its converse later, e.g. when, in the thought of J. T. Needham, epigenesis and spontaneous generation go side by side (see on, pp. 211 and 218).

Johannes Sinibaldi's *Geneanthropia* might be mentioned as belonging to this time. It was a compilation of facts relating to the generation of man, but it expressly excluded from its field any discussion of the embryo. It is no more important for our subject than the queer *Ovi Encomium* of Erycius Puteanus, another of Gassendi's friends.

2. Developmental Determinism and Transplantation; Digby, Highmore and Tagliacozzi

Much more significant was the controversy between Sir Kenelm Digby[2] and Nathaniel Highmore. In 1644, Sir Kenelm, whose intriguing personality will be sufficiently familiar to anyone even slightly acquainted with seventeenth-century England (biographic details in John Aubrey and in Bligh), published a work with the following title:*Two treatises, in the one of which, The Nature of Bodies, in the other, The Nature of Man's Soule is looked into, in way of discovery of the Immortality of Reasonable Soules.* It was inscribed in a charming dedication to his son, and consisted, in brief, in a survey of the whole realms of metaphysics, physics and biology from a very individual point of view.

One of Sir Kenelm's principal objects in writing apparently was to attack the old terminology of "qualities" in physics and "faculties" in biology. To say, as contemporary reasoning did, that bodies were red or blue because they possessed a quality of redness or blueness which

---

[1] See pp. 66, 163 and 213.   [2] See Plate VII, facing page 122.

caused them to appear red or blue to us, or again, to say that the heart beat because it was informed by a sphygmic faculty, or, to take the famous example, that opium sent people to sleep because it contained in it a dormitive virtue, appeared mere nonsense and word-spinning to Digby, "the last refuge of ignorant men, who not knowing what to say, and yet presuming to say something, do often fall upon such expressions."

Digby, like Galileo and Hobbes, wished to explain all phenomena by reference to two "virtues" only, those of rarity and density, "working by means of locall Motion." Chapters twenty-three, twenty-four and twenty-five contain his opinions and experiments in embryology. He begins by opening the question of epigenesis or preformation, practically for the first time since Albert the Great. "Our main question shall be," he says, "whether they be framed entirely at once, or successively, one part after another? And if this latter way, which part first?" He declares for epigenesis, but after a manner of his own, refuting "the opinion of those who hold that everything containeth formally all things."[1]

Why should not the parts be made in generation [he asks] of a matter like to that which maketh them in nutrition? If they be augmented by one kind of juyce that after severall changes turneth at the length into flesh and bone; and into every sort of mixed body or similar part whereof the sensitive creature is compounded, and that joyneth itself to what it findeth there already made, why should not the same juyce with the same progresse of heat and moisture, and other due temperaments, be converted at the first into flesh and bone though none be formerly there to joyn it self unto?

He gave a clearly deterministic account of development.

Take a bean, or any other seed and put it in the earth, and let water fall upon it; can it then choose but that the bean must swell? The bean swelling, can it choose but break the skin? The skin broken, can it choose (by reason of the heat that is in it) but push out more matter, and do that action which we may call germinating? Can these germs choose but pierce the earth in small strings, as they are able to make their way?... Thus by drawing the thrid carefully along through your fingers, and staying at every knot to examine how it is tyed; you see that this difficult progresse of the generation of living creatures is obvious enough to be comprehended and the steps of it set down; if one would but take the paines and afford the time that is necessary to note diligently all the circumstances in every change of it.... Now if all this orderly succession of mutations be necessarily made in a bean, by force of sundry circumstances and externall accidents; why may it not be conceived that the

[1] On this panspermatic view, see pp. 66 and 79.

PLATE VII

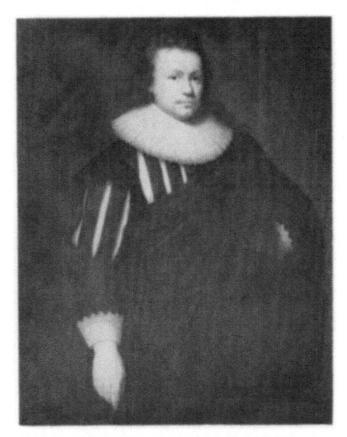

Sir Kenelm Digby (from the painting by Cornelius Jansen, at Althorp. Copyright: Earl Spenser).

like is also done in sensible creatures, but in a more perfect manner, they being perfecter substances? Surely the progresse we have set down is much more reasonable than to conceive that in the seed of the male there is already in act, the substance of flesh, bone, sinews, and veins, and the rest of those severall similar parts which are found in the body of an animall, and that they are but extended to their due magnitude by the humidity drawn from the mother, without receiving any substantial mutation from what they were originally in the seed. Let us then confidently conclude, that all generation is made of a fitting, but remote, homogeneall compounded substance upon which outward Agents, working in the due course of Nature, do change it into another substance, quite different from the first, and do make it lesse homogeneall than the first was. And other circumstances and agents do change this second into a third, that third, into a fourth; and so onwards, by successive mutations that still make every new thing become lesse homogeneall than the former was, according to the nature of heat, mingling more and more different bodies together, untill that substance bee produced which we consider the period of all these mutations.

This passage is indeed admirable, and well expresses the most modern conception of embryonic development, that of the ovum as a physico-chemical system, containing within itself only to a slight and varying degree any localisation answering to the localisation of the adult, and ready to change itself, once the appropriate stimulus has been received, into the completed embryo by the actions and reactions of its own constituents on the one hand and the influence of the fitting factors of the environment upon the other. Digby has not received his due in the past; he stands to embryology as an exact science, much in the same relationship as Bacon to science as a whole.

Generation is not made [he says] by aggregation of like parts to pre-supposed like ones; nor by a specifical worker within; but by the compounding of a seminary matter with the juice which accrueth to it from without and with the steams of circumstant bodies, which by an ordinary course of nature are regularly imbibed in it by degrees and which at every degree doe change it into a different thing. . . .[1] Therefore to satisfie ourselves herein, it were well we made our remarks in some creatures that might be continually in our power to observe in them the course of nature every day and hour. Sir John Heydon, the Lieutenant of his Majesties Ordnance (that generous and knowing Gentleman, and consummate Souldier both in theory and practice), was the first that instructed me how to do this, by means of a furnace so made as to imitate the warmth of a sitting hen. In which you may lay severall eggs to

[1] Digby would have appreciated the demonstration of modern biology that the eggs of many animals contain insufficient water and salts for the embryos produced from them, so that absorption from the environment has to take place (see Needham, 1931, p. 317).

hatch, and by breaking them at severall ages you may distinctly observe every hourly mutation in them if you please.

Sir Kenelm then goes on to describe the events that take place in the incubating egg, which he does very accurately, though briefly. In Vivipara, he says, the like experiments have been made, and the like conclusions come to by "that learned and exact searcher into nature, Doctor Harvey"—these he must have learnt of by word of mouth, for Harvey's book had not at that time been published. As regards heredity, he adopts a pure theory of pangenesis, and has more to say about it than any other writer of his time. He is sure that the heart is first formed both in Ovipara and Vivipara, "whose motion and manner of working evidently appears in the twinckling of the first red spot (which is the first change) in the egge."

Sir Kenelm Digby not only anticipated the outlook of the physico-chemical embryologist, but he also foreshadowed with considerable acumen Wilhelm Roux's definition of interim embryological laws.

Out of our short survey of which (anserable to our weak talents, and slender experience) I perswade myself it appeareth evidently enough that to effect this worke of generation there needeth not to be supposed a forming virtue or *Vis Formatrix* of an unknown power and operation, as those that consider things suddenly and in grosse do use to put. Yet in discourse, for conveniency and shortnesse of expression we shall not quite banish that terme from all commerce with us; so that what we mean by it be rightly understood, which is the complex assemblement, or chain of all the causes, that concur to produce this effect, as they are set on foot to this end by the great Architect and Moderatour of them, God Almighty, whose instrument Nature is: that is, the same thing, or rather the same things so ordered as we have declared, but expressed and comprized under another name.

Thus Sir Kenelm admits that it is allowable to speak of the "complex assemblement" of causes, as if it were one formative virtue, and this corresponds to Roux's "secondary components" or interim embryological laws. But that the portmanteau generalisations can be resolved into ultimate physico-chemical processes, Digby both believes and spends two entire chapters in trying to show. Digby has been one of the two seventeenth-century Englishmen most under-estimated in the history of biology, but his place is in reality a very high one. How far he was in advance of his time may be gauged from the work of his contemporary Sperlingen, whose book of 1641 was thoroughly scholastic and retrograde.

His *Treatise on Bodies* evoked several answers. Undoubtedly the most interesting from the progressive side was that of Nathaniel Highmore,[1] who will always be well remembered in embryological history. Highmore's *The History of Generation* came out in 1651, so that Harvey must have known of it, and it is one of the puzzles of this period why Harvey made no mention of it in his work, especially as J. D. Horst in a letter to Harvey refers to Highmore as his pupil. Harvey replying in 1655 said he had not seen Highmore for seven years. Highmore's title-page expressly states that his book is an answer to the opinions of Sir Kenelm Digby. But before discussing in what the answer consisted, we may look at the plate which is bound in immediately after the dedication (to Robert Boyle). It is interesting in that it shows again the idea initiated by Leonardo, namely that all growing things, plants as well as animals, have an umbilical cord. But the drawings of the chick embryos and eggs are more quaint than accurate (Fig. 11).

Highmore first describes the Aristotelian doctrine of form and matter, and then censures both it and the extensions of it with their "qualities," etc., much as Digby himself had done.

Some of our later philosophers have showed us that those forms wch they thought and taught to bee but potentially in the matter, are there actually subsisting, though till they have acquired fitting organs they manifest not themselves. And that the effects which were done before their manifestation (as the forming and fashioning of the parts wherein they are to operate) can rise from nothing else than from the Soul itselfe. This likewise I shall leave to the Readers enquiry, and shall follow that other way of introducing Forms, and Generation of creatures (as well animals as vegetables) which gives Fortune and Chance the preheminency in that work.

He then describes Sir Kenelm's opinions, quoting from him in detail, and dissents from them mainly on the ground that they do not sufficiently account for embryogeny, as it were, from a technical point of view. That they subvert the "antique principals of philosophy" does not worry Highmore, but in his view their detailed mechanisms do not explain the facts, a much more serious drawback. Highmore is himself by way of being an atomist, and it is because embryology was first treated by him from an atomistic standpoint that he derives his importance.

The blood, that all parts may be irrigated with its benigne moisture, is forc'd by several channels to run through every region and part of the body; by which meanes every part out of that stream selects those atomes which they finde to be cognate to themselves. Amongst which the Testicles abstract some spiritual atomes belonging to every part, which had they not here been anticipated, should have been attracted to those parts, to which properly they

[1] Physician at Sherborne in Dorset, see Fig. 12.

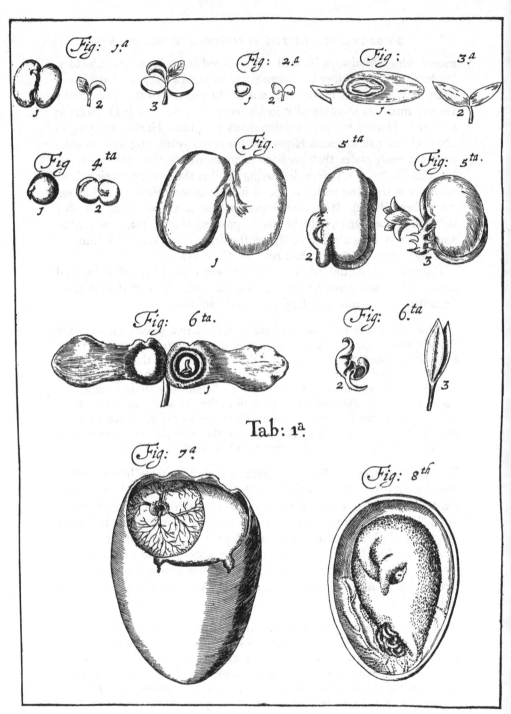

Fig. *11. Illustration from Nathaniel Highmore's "History of Generation,"* 1651.

did belong for nourishment. . . . These particles passing through the body of the Testicles, and being in this Athanor cohobated and reposited into a tenacious matter, at last passe through infinite Meanders through certain vessels, in which it undergoes another digestion and pelicanizing.

Highmore objects, therefore, more to Digby's theory of pangenesis than to his description of embryogeny. He goes on to give a long description of the development of the chick in the egg, mentioning in passing that the albumen corresponds to the semen and the blood of Vivipara, and the yolk to their milk.

Fabritius, who hath taken a great deal of pains in dissections . . . supposes the chick to be formed from the chalazae, that part which by our Women is called the treddle. But this likewise is false, for then every egge should produce 2 chickens, there being one treddle at each end of the egg, which serve for no other end than for ligaments to contain the yolk in an equilibrium, that it might not by every moving of the egg be shakt, broke, and confused with the white.

Highmore was the first to draw attention to the increase of brittleness which takes place in the egg-shell during incubation,[1] and he holds still to the Epicurean view that the female produces a kind of seed,[2] though he thinks that the chick embryo is nourished in the early stages by the amniotic liquid.

Perhaps the most interesting reply to Digby from the traditional angle was that of Alexander Ross. In his *Philosophicall Touchstone* he upheld the Galenic view that the liver must be first formed in generation, for the nourishment is in the blood and the blood requires a liver to make it; ergo, the liver must be the earliest organ. Such arguments could dispense with observations. Ross also mentions Digby's suggestion that the "formative virtue" was only a bundle of natural causes, but he claims that the notion was an old one in school-philosophy, being included in the phrase *causa causae, causa causati*.

It was said above that some of Digby's ideas anticipated the formulations of one of the greatest founders of modern experimental embryology, Wilhelm Roux. The most fundamental technique of modern experimental embryology is undoubtedly that of the transplantation of parts of embryos into different situations in other embryos. The problem for which it was developed by Gustav Born and Hans Spemann was that of "determination," or the onset of the fixation of the fates of parts and tissues. Will they develop, in their new environment,

---

[1] The shell loses about 7 per cent. of its lime to the interior during incubation.
[2] See p. 60.

in accordance with their original presumptive fate, or in accordance with that of the tissues of the host which immediately surround them? The first type of behaviour acquired the name *herkunftsgemäss* (or in English, "selfwise"); the second came to be called *ortsgemäss* (or in English, "neighbourwise"). As is well known, a vast branch of modern biology, which may be called experimental morphology (equivalent to the German *Entwicklungsmechanik*), has grown up since the time of W. Roux (1850–1924), and has achieved many points of contact with bio-chemistry.[1] The study of the morphogenetic hormones, or organisers, is being actively pursued to-day.

In the light of these facts it would be very desirable to have a system-atic monograph on the history of transplantation and grafting in general, but if such a treatment of the subject exists, I have not been able to find it.[2] Certainly grafting and transplantation have a long history, but because easier in plants than in animals, and in large organisms than in small embryos, they did not quickly lead to funda-mental discoveries. Moreover, in adult organisms, immunity reactions prevent the success of any but autoplastic transplantations (i.e. from place to place on the same animal). These were, however, known in the sixteenth century, as Corradi has described, and (according to Garrison and others) may be traced to ancient Indian surgery.

In the seventeenth century the concepts of "selfwise" and "neigh-bourwise" were closely approached, though in a setting of factual error, as we find from an amusing story related by Walter Charleton in 1650.

A certain inhabitant of Bruxels, in a combat, had his nose mowed off, and addressed himself to Tagliacozzus,[3] a famous Chirurgeon, living at Bononia, that he might procure a new one; and when he feared the incision of his own arme, he hired a Porter to admit it, out of whose arme, having first given the reward agreed upon, at length he digged a new nose. About thirteen moneths after his returne to his owne countrey, on a suddaine the ingrafted nose grew cold, putrified, and within a few days dropt off. To those of his friends, that were curious in the exploration of the cause of this unexpected misfortune, it was discovered, that the Porter expired near about the same punctilio of time, wherein the nose grew frigid and cadaverous. There are at Bruxels yet surviving, some of good repute, that were eye-witnesses of these occurrences. Is not this Magnetisme of manifest affinity with mumie, whereby the nose,

[1] Cf. the author's *Biochemistry and Morphogenesis* (1950).
[2] See, however, the thoughtful essay of Oppenheimer on methods and techniques in embryology.
[3] Gaspare Tagliacozzi (1546–1599). His *De Curtorum Chirurgia* was the greatest Renaissance treatise on plastic surgery. For an elaborate study of his life and times we are indebted to Gnudi & Webster.

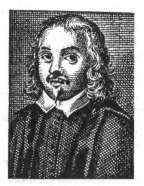

Fig. 12. Nathaniel Highmore, M.D.
(*from the title-page of his* "Corporis humani
disquisitio anatomica," *1651*).

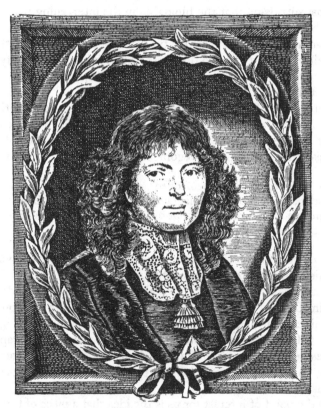

Fig. 13. René de Graaf, M.D.
(*from his* "Opera Omnia," *1677*).

enjoying, by title and right of inoculation, a community of life, sense, and vegetation, for so many moneths, on a suddaine mortified on the other side of the Alpes? I pray, what is there in this of Superstition? What of attent and exalted Imagination?

The book in which this story was related was entitled: *A Ternary of Paradoxes; The Magnetick Cure of Wounds, The Nativity of Tartar in Wine, The Image of God in Man; written originally by Joh. Bapt. van Helmont, and Translated, Illustrated, and Ampliated* by Walter Charleton. Charleton was a friend of Kenelm Digby's, and mentions him in his Prolegomena. The age was one in which men were much fascinated by magnetic phenomena such as had been described at the beginning of the century in William Gilbert's work on the lodestone (1600). The century was to end, moreover, by the triumph of the concept of attraction embodied in Newton's work on gravitation. It is therefore not in the least surprising that the biologists in the intervening period should have thought a great deal about action at a distance, and if their beliefs were sometimes rather absurd by present-day standards, this must after all to some extent be due to the great inherent difficulty of biological experimentation. Digby and Charleton, no less than van Helmont, believed in the possibility of a "magneticall" cure of wounds, the patient benefiting by the application of preparations to the sword which had caused the hurt, or the bandage which had first covered it. Hence the relevance of the transplantation story, which Charleton emphasized again in his Prolegomena, saying that he would relate

how a Tagliacotian Nose, enfeoffed with a Community of Vitality and Vegetation, by right of Transplantation, upon the face of a Gent. at Bruxels hath growne cadaverous and dropt off at the instance of that Porter's death in Bononia, out of whose arme it was first exsected.

This was an effect "magneticall," due to "the long arme of Sympathy." All this was taken quite seriously when the Royal Society began its work a decade later, and a special investigation was made of "Sir Kenelm Digby's Sympatheticall Powder for the Cure of Wounds."

Significant also is the fact that both Charleton and Digby were interested in the revival of atomism. They hoped that the rapid travel of "pestilentiall Atomes," "igneous Atomes," "mumiall Atomes," and the like, might some day explain the phenomena of attraction and action at a distance.

But the point of interest for us is the idea that a piece of transplanted tissue could long retain, though incorporated into the body of a host, properties belonging to the body from which it had been taken.

3. Thomas Browne and the Beginnings of Chemical Embryology

There are references to embryology in Sir Thomas Browne's *Pseudo-doxia Epidemica, or Inquiries into very many vulgar Tenents and commonly received Truths*, which was published at this time.[1] The twenty-eighth chapter of the third book contains a number of difficult problems in the embryology of the period, in most cases stated without any solution.

That a chicken is formed out of the yolk of the Egg was the opinion of some Ancient Philosophers. Whether it be not the nutrient of the Pullet may also be considered; since umbilical vessels are carried into it, since much of the yolk remaineth after the chicken is formed, since in a chicken newly hatched the stomack is tincted yellow and the belly full of yelk which is drawn at the navel or vessels towards the vent, as may be discerned in chickens a day or two before exclusion. Whether the chicken be made out of the white, or that be not also its aliment, is likewise very questionable, since an umbilical vessel is derived unto it, since after the formation and perfect shape of the chicken, much of the white remaineth. Whether it be not made out of the grando, gallature, germ, or tred of the egg, as Aquapendente informeth us, seemed to many of doubt; for at the blunter end it is not discovered after the chicken is formed, by this also the white and the yelk are continued whereby it may conveniently receive its nutriment from them both. . . . But these at last and how in the Cicatricula or little pale circle formation first beginneth, how the Grando or tredle, are but the poles and establishing particles of the tender membrans firmly conserving the floating parts in their proper places, with many observables, that ocular Philosopher and singular discloser of truth, Dr Harvey hath discovered, in that excellent discourse of generation, so strongly erected upon the two great pillars of truth, Experience, and Reason.

That the sex is discernable from the figure of eggs, or that cocks or hens proceed from long or round ones, experiment will easily frustrate. . . . Why the hen hatcheth not the egg in her belly? Why the egg is thinner at one extream? Why there is some cavity or emptiness at the blunter end? Why we open them at that part? Why the greater end is first excluded?[2] Why some eggs are all red, as the Kestrils, some only red at one end, as those of kites and buzzards? Why some eggs are not oval but round, as those of fishes? etc., are problems whose decisions would too much enlarge this discourse.

And elsewhere,

That [saith Aristotle] which is not watery and improlifical will not con-glaciate; which perhaps must not be taken strictly, but in the germ and spirited particles; for Eggs, I observe, will freeze, in the albuginous part thereof.

[1] See Merton.   [2] Cf. Needham (1931), p. 233.

Again,

They who hold that the egg was before the bird, prevent this doubt in many other animals, which also extendeth unto them; for birds are nourished by umbilical vessels and the navel is manifest sometimes a day or two after exclusion. . . . The same is made out in the eggs of snakes, and is not improbable in the generation of Porwiggles or Tadpoles, and may also be true in some vermiparous exclusions, although (as we have observed in the daily progress of some) the whole Magot is little enough to make a fly without any part remaining. . . . The vitreous or glassie flegm of white of egg will thus extinguish a coal.

These citations show Sir Thomas to have been more than simply the supreme artist in English prose, which is his common title to remembrance. In picking his way carefully among the doubtful points and difficult problems which previous embryologists had propounded but not answered, he usually managed to give the right answer to each. But in addition to this, he was also an experimentalist, he had made both anatomical and physical experiments on eggs, and he was prepared to put any disputed point to the test of "ocular aspection," if this could be done. His experimental contributions to embryology come out more clearly in his *Commonplace Books* which were published by Wilkin in 1836.

Runnet beat up with the whites of eggs seems to perform nothing, nor will it well incorporate, without so much heat as will harden the egg. . . . Eggs seem to contain within themselves their own coagulum, evidenced upon incubation, which makes incrassation of parts before very fluid. . . . Rotten eggs will not be made hard by incubation or decoction, as being destitute of that spirit or having the same vitiated. . . . They will be made hard in oil but not so easily in vinegar which by the attenuating quality keeps them longer from concoction, for infused in vinegar they lose the shell and grow big and much heavier then before. . . . In the ovary or second cell of the matrix the white comes upon the yolk, and in the later and lower part, the shell is made or manifested. Try if the same parts´ will give any coagulation unto milk. Whether will the ovary best ? . . . The whites of eggs drenched in saltpeter will shoot forth a long and hairy saltpeter and the egg become of a hard substance. Even in the whole egg there seems a great nitrosity, for it is very cold and especially that which is without a shell (as some are laid by fat hens) or such as are found in the egg poke or lowest part of the matrix, if an hen be killed a day or two before she layeth. . . . Difference between the sperm of frogs and eggs, spawn though long boiled, would not grow thick and coagulate. In the eggs of skates or thornbacks the yolk coagulates upon long decoction, not the greatest part of the white. . . . In spawn of frogs the little black specks will concrete though not the other. . . . In eggs we observe the white will totally freeze, the yolk, with the same degree of cold will grow thick and

PLATE VIII

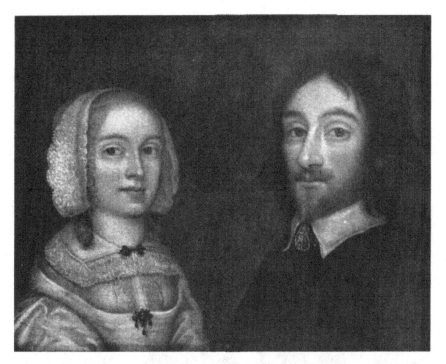

Sir Thomas Browne and his wife, Dorothy (from the portrait formerly in the possession of the Allix family at Swaffham Prior cf. Tildesley).

PLATE IX

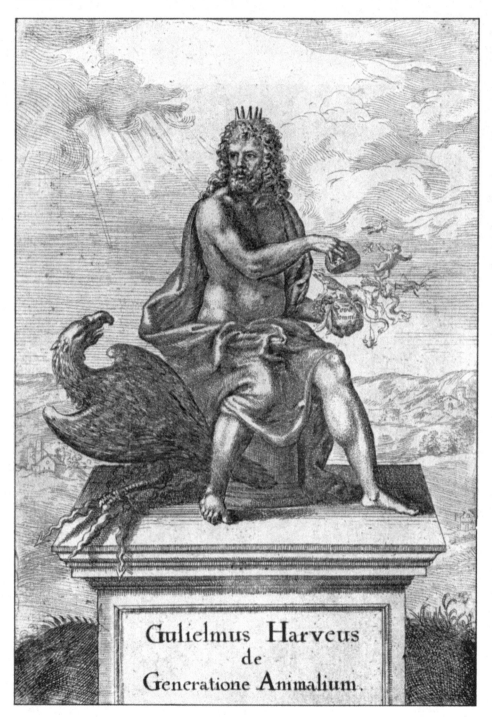

*Zeus liberating living beings from an egg (the frontispiece of William Harvey's book on the
Generation of Animals, 1651).*

clammy like the gum of trees, but the sperm or tread hold its former body, the white growing stiff that is nearest to it.

The only conclusion that can be drawn from these remarkable observations is that it was in the "elaboratory" in Sir Thomas' house at Norwich that the first experiments in chemical embryology were undertaken. His significance in this connection has so far been quite overlooked, and it is time to recognise that his originality and genius in this field shows itself to be hardly less remarkable than in so many others.[1] To study experimentally the chemical properties of those substances which afford the raw material of development was a great step for those times. It was not until some twenty-five years later that Walter Needham carried this new interest into the mammalian domain.

4. William Harvey and the Identification of the Blastoderm

The Latin edition of William Harvey's book on the generation of animals appeared in 1651, and the English in 1653. The frontispiece of the former (which is reproduced as Plate IX, opposite) is a very noteworthy picture, and derives a special interest from the fact that on the egg which Zeus holds in his hands is written *Ex ovo omnia*—a conception which Harvey is continually expounding (see especially the chapter, "That an egg is the common Original of all animals"), but which he never puts into epigrammatic form in his text, so that the saying, *omne vivum ex ovo*, often attributed to him, is only obliquely his.

The *De Generatione Animalium* was written at different times during his life, and not collected together for publication until George Ent, of the College of Physicians, persuaded Harvey to give it forth about 1650. As early as 1625 Harvey was studying the phenomena of embryology, as is shown among other evidences by a passage in his book where he says,[2]

Our late Sovereign King Charles, so soon as he was become a man, was wont for Recreation and Health sake, to hunt almost every week, especially the Buck and Doe, no Prince in Europe having greater store, whether wand-

---

[1] See Plate VIII, facing page 132. I may give two instances of Browne's awareness, isolated though he may have been at Norwich:

(1) The *Hydriotaphia* was first published in 1658. In chapter 5 occurs the famous "Life is a pure flame; we live by an invisible Sun within us." The *Tractatus Duo* of Mayow, to whom the first experimental demonstration of this is usually ascribed, was published in 1668. Patterson, however, shows that it may be found in Boyle's *Spring and Weight of the Air*, 1660. May we not conclude that Browne was in fairly close touch with the Invisible College, first mentioned in 1646?

(2) Dr Singer tells me that Browne was acquainted with the very rare work of Cesi on spores in ferns, of which no copy has been in England for many years.

[2] P. 396; this and subsequent references are to the English edition of 1653.

ring at liberty in the Woods and Forrests or inclosed and kept up in Parkes and Chaces. In the three summer moneths the Buck and the Stagge being then fat and in season were his game, and the Doe and Hind in the Autumme and Winter so long as the three seasonable moneths continued. Hereupon I had daily opportunity of dissecting them and of making inspection and observation of all their parts, which liberty I chiefly made use of in order to the genital parts.

Nor was Harvey less diligent in examining the generation of Ovipara. John Aubrey, in his *Brief Lives*, says,

I first sawe Doctor Harvey at Oxford in 1642 after Edgehill fight, but I was then too young to be acquainted with so great a Doctor. I remember that he came often to Trin. Coll. to one George Bathurst, B.D. who kept a hen in his chamber to hatch egges, which they did dayly open to discerne the progress and way of generation.

Aubrey mentions a conversation he had with a sow-gelder, a countryman of little learning but much practical experience and wisdom, who told him that he had met Dr Harvey, who had conversed with him for two or three hours, and "if he had been," the man remarked, "as stiff as some of our starched and formall doctors, he had known no more than they." Harvey seems also to have learnt all he could from the keepers of King Charles' forests, as several passages in his book show. Nor was the King's own interest lacking.

I saw long since a foetus [Harvey says] the magnitude of a peasecod cut out of the uterus of a doe, which was complete in all its members & I showed this pretty spectacle to our late King and Queen. It did swim, trim and perfect, in such a kinde of white, most transparent and crystalline moysture (as if it had been treasured up in some most clear glassie receptacle) about the bignesse of a pigeon's egge, and was invested with its proper coat.[1]

And, again—

My Royal Master, whose Physitian I was, was himself much delighted in this kinde of curiosity, being many times pleased to be an eye-witness, and to assert my new inventions.[2]

Harvey's book is composed of seventy-two exercitations, which may be divided up for convenience into five divisions. In Nos. 1 to 10 he speaks of the anatomy and physiology of the genital organs of the fowl, and the manner of production of eggs. Nos. 11 to 13 and also Nos. 23 and 36 deal with the hen's egg in detail, describing its parts and their uses, while in Nos. 14 to 22 the process of the "generation of the foetus

[1] P. 88.   [2] P. 397.

out of the hen egge" is described. The greater part of the book, comprising Nos. 25 to 62, as well as Nos. 71 and 72, is theoretical, and treats of the embryological theories held by Aristotle on the one hand, and the physicians, following Galen, on the other, instead of which it propounds new views upon the subject. Finally, Nos. 63 to 70, as well as the two appendices or "particular discourses," are concerned with embryogenesis in viviparous animals, especially in hinds and does. And just as Aristotle put much of his best embryological work into his *Historia Animalium* and not into the work with the appropriate title, so Harvey has some admirable observations on the embryonic heart scattered through his *De Motu Cordis et Sanguinis in Animalibus*.

It will be best to refer to some of the main points of interest in Harvey's discussions before trying to assess his principal contributions to the science as a whole. Harvey is the first, since Aristotle, to refer to the "white yolk" of birds.

For between the yolk which is yet in the cluster and that which is in the midst of the eg when it is perfected this is the difference in chief, that though the former be yellowish in colour and in appearance, yet its consistence representeth rather the white, and being sodden, thickeneth like it, growing compact and viscous and may be cut into slices. But the yolk of a perfect egge being boiled groweth friable and of a more earthy consistence, not thick and glutinous like the white.[1]

All of Harvey's observations on the formation of the egg in the oviduct contained in this chapter are interesting, and may with advantage be compared with the studies of Riddle and Asmundson upon the same subject, where the chemical explanation will be found for many of Harvey's simple observations.[2] Harvey's controversy with Fabricius on the question of whether the egg is produced with a hard shell or only acquires its external hardness upon standing in the air, which follows immediately on the above citation, is interesting.[3]

Fabricius seemeth to me to be in errour, for though I was never so good at slight of hand to surprise an egge in the very laying, and so make discovery whether it was soft or hard, yet this I confidently pronounce that the shell is compounded within the womb of a substance there at hand for the purpose,

[1] P. 47.
[2] A great treasury of information about the physico-chemical nature and properties of the eggs of birds and all their constituents is now available in the book of Romanov & Romanov. Nothing has yet replaced the author's systematic *Chemical Embryology* (1931) though the wealth of new knowledge won about chemical changes during embryonic development during the past twenty-six years makes this urgently necessary. Meanwhile Brachet's stimulating monograph will be found very helpful.
[3] P. 50.

and that it is framed in the same manner as the other parts of the egg are by the plastick faculty, and the rather, because I have seen an exceeding small egge which had a shell of its own and yet was contained within another egge, greater and fairer than it, which egge had a shell too.

Harvey was the first to note that the white of the hen's egg is heterogeneous, in the sense that part of it is much more liquid than the rest, and that the more viscous part seems to be contained in an exceedingly fine membrane, so that if it is sliced across with a knife, its contents will flow out. He also set right the errors of Fabricius, Parisanus and others, by showing that the chalazae were neither the seed of the cock nor the material out of which the embryo was formed, and, most important of all, by demonstrating that the cicatricula was the point of origin of the embryo. He denied, as against popular belief, that the hen contributed anything to the developing egg but heat.[1]

For certain it is that the chicken is constituted by an internal principle in the egge, and that there is no accession to a complete and perfect egge by the Hennes incubation, but bare cherishing and protection; no more than the Hen contributeth to the chickens which are now hatched, which is only a friendly heat, and care, by which she defendeth them from the cold, and forreign injuries, and helpeth them to their meat.

Whether future work will still affirm that nothing is given to the egg by the hen except heat is beginning now to be in doubt, if the results of Chattock are correct.

In the description of the development of the embryo in the hen's egg, which remains to this day one of the most accurate, Harvey says [2] with regard to the spot on the yolk, which had, of course, been seen and mentioned by many previous observers, "And yet I conceive that no man hitherto hath acknowledged that this Cicatricula was to be found in every egge nor that it was the first Principle of the Egge." Thus he unequivocally identified the blastoderm (with its primitive streak and neural folds) as the unique place of origin of the embryonic body.[3] His description[4] of the beginning of the heart, that "capering bloody point" or *punctum saliens*, is too famous to need more than a reference. He thought that the amniotic liquid was of "mighty use," "For while the embryos swim there, they are guarded and skreened from all concussion, contusion, and other outward injuries, and are also nourished by it."[5]

[1] P. 69.　　　　[2] P. 83.
[3] The term itself, *Keimhaut* (blastoderm), is of course one of those introduced by Pander in 1817.
[4] Pp. 89, 91　　　　[5] P. 88.

Thus he made no advance on the opinion which had for long been held, namely that the amniotic liquid or colliquamentum served for sustenance.

I believe [he says] that this colliquamentum or water wherein the foetus swims doth serve for his sustenance and that the thinner and purer part of it, being imbibed by the umbilicall vessels does constitute and supply the primo-genital parts, and the rest, like Milk, being by suction conveyed into the stomack and there concocted or chylified, and afterwards attracted by the orifices of the Meseraick Veins doth nourish and enlarge the tender embryo.[1]

His arguments for this are, (1) that swallowing movements take place, and (2) that the gut of the chicken is "stuft" with excrement which could hardly arise from any other source. He was thus led to divide the amniotic liquid into two quite imaginary constituents, a purer and "sincerer" part, which could be absorbed straight into the blood without chylification, and a creamless milky part, which could not be treated so simply.

About the fourth day [says Harvey] the egg beginneth to step from the life of a plant to that of an animall.[2] . . . From that to the tenth it enjoys a sensitive and moving soul as Animals do, and after that, it is compleated by degrees and being adorned with Plumes, Bill, Clawes and other furniture, it hastens to get out.[3]

These and other passages which deal with the forerunner of the theory of recapitulation are interesting, but we have already met essentially the same idea in Aristotle. Harvey contributed nothing new to it. The first point on which he went definitely wrong was the conviction he reached that the heart does not pulsate before the appearance of the blood. No doubt his lack of microscopical facilities or of the desire to use them affords the reason for this error, but it was a rather unfortunate one, for it was to a large extent upon it that he formulated his doctrine[4] "the life is in the blood." For example, he says, "I am fully satisfied that the Blood hath a being before any part of the body besides, and is the elder brother to all other parts of the foetus."[5]

The yolk, Harvey thought, supplied the place of milk, "and is that which is last consumed, for the remainder of it (after the chicken is

---

[1] P. 358. [2] P. 89. [3] P. 101.
[4] This doctrine was not peculiar to Harvey (cf. Levit. xvii. 11 and 14, Servetus, etc.). See also the elaborate study of Rüsche on the relation between blood, life and soul in ancient thought.
[5] P. 108.

hatched and walks abroad with the Henne) is yet contained in its belly."[1] He thus ranged himself with Alcmaeon and Abderhalden. All his remarks about the relationships of yolk and white in nutrition are worth consideration; in noting, for instance, that the yolk is the last to be consumed, he comes very near to anticipating the modern conception of a succession of energy-sources.

In that Physitians affirme, that the Yolke is the hotter part of the egge, and the most nourishing, I conceive that they understand it, in relation to us, as it is become our nourishment, not as it doth supply more congruous aliment to the chicken in the egge. And this appeares out of our history of the Fabrick of the chicken; which doth first prey upon and devoure the thinner part of the white, before the grosser; as it were a more proper diet, and did more easily submit to transmutation into the substance of the foetus. And therefore the yolke seems to be a remoter and more deferred entertainment than the white; for all the white is quite and clean spent, before any notable invasion is made upon the yolk.[2]

A comparison between these simple facts and our knowledge of embryonic nutrition is most interesting.

In connection with Minot's distinction of the periods of embryonic growth, it is curious that Harvey says,

And now the foetus moves and gently tumbles, and stretcheth out the neck though nothing of a brain be yet to be seen, but merely a bright water shut up in a small bladder. And now it is a perfect Magot, differing only from those kinde of wormes in this, that those when they have their freedom crawle up and down and search for their living abroad, but this worm constant to his station, and swimming in his own provision, draws it in by his Umbilicall Vessels.[3]

Sometimes Harvey confesses himself puzzled by problems which could only be solved by chemical means, yet it does not occur to him that this is the case. For instance, he enquires why heat will develop a chick out of a good egg but will only make a bad one worse.

Give me leave to add something here [he writes] which I have tried often; that I might the better discerne the scituation of the foetus and the liquors after the fourteenth day to the very exclusion; I have boiled an egge till it grew hard, and then pilling away the shell and seeing the scituation of the chicken, I found both the remaining parts of the white, and the two parts of the yolk of the same consistence, colour, tast, and other accidents, as any other stale egge, thus ordered, is. And upon this Experiment, I did much ponder whence it should come to passe that Improlifical eggs should, from the adventitious heat of a sitting Henne, putrifie and stink; and yet no such

[1] P. 105.　　　[2] P. 183.　　　[3] P. 112.

138

inconvenience befall the Prolifical. But both these liquors (though there be a Chicken in them too, and he with some pollution and excrement) should be found wholesome and incorrupt; so that if you eat them in the dark after they are boyled, you cannot distinguish them from egges that are so prepared, which have never undergone the hen's incubation.[1]

Harvey was never afraid of trying such tests on himself; in another place, for example, he says,

Eggs after 2 or 3 days incubation, are even then sweeter relished than stale ones are, as if the cherishing warmth of the hen did refresh and restore them to their primitive excellence and integrity.[2] . . . And the yolke (at 14 days) was as sweet and pleasant as that of a newlaid egge, when it is in like manner boyled to an induration.[3]

Another matter on which Harvey set Fabricius right was on the question whether at hatching the hen helps the chicken out or the chicken comes out by itself. The latter was the belief held by Harvey, who said of Fabricius' arguments on this point that they were "pleasant and elegant, but not well bottomed."[4]

On the great question of preformation *versus* epigenesis, Harvey keenly argued in favour of the latter view.

There is no part of the future foetus actually in the egg, but yet all the parts of it are in it potentially.[5] . . . I have declared that one thing is made out of another two several wayes and that as well in artificial as natural productions, but especially in the generation of animals. The first is, when one thing is made out of another thing that is pre-existent, and thus a Bedstead is made out of Timber, and a Statue out of a Rock, where the whole matter of the future fabrick was existent and in being, before it was reduced into its subsequent shape, or any tittle of the designe begun. But the other way is when the matter is both made and receiveth its form at the same time.[6] . . . So likewise in the Generation of Animals, some are formed and transfigured out of matter already concocted and grown and all the parts are made and distinguished together *per metamorphosin*, by a metamorphosis, so that a complete animal is the result of that generation; but some again, having one part made before another, are afterwards nourished, augmented, and formed out of the same matter, that is, they have parts, whereof some are before, and some after, other, and at the same time, are both formed, and grow.[7] . . . These we say are made *per epigenesin*, by a post-generation, or after-production, that is to say, by degrees, part after part, and this is more properly called a Generation, than the former.[8] . . . The perfect animals, which have blood, are made by Epigenesis, or superaddition of parts, and do grow, and attain their just future or ἀκμή after they are born.[9] . . . An animal produced by Epigenesis, attracts, prepares, concocts, and applies, the Matter at the same time, and

[1] P. 126.   [2] P. 64.   [3] P. 65.   [4] P. 129.   [5] P. 221.
[6] P. 221.   [7] P. 222.   [8] P. 222.   [9] P. 223.

is at the same time formed, and augmented.[1] . . . Wherefore Fabricius did erroniously seek after the Matter of the chicken (as it were some distinct part of the egg which went to the imbodying of the chicken) as though the generation of the chicken were effected by a Metamorphosis, or transfiguration of some collected lump or mass, and that all the parts of the body, at least the Principall parts, were wrought off at a heat or (as himselfe speaks) did arise and were corporated out of the same Matter.[2]

Nothing could be more plain than Harvey's teaching on epigenesis.

On the relation between growth and differentiation Harvey has some valuable things to say. The term "nutrition" he restricted to that which replaces existent structures, and the term "augmentation" or "increment" to that which contributes something new. That process which led to greater diversity of form and complexity of shape he called "formation" or "framing."

For though the head of the Chicken, and the rests of its Trunck or Corporature (being first of a similar constitution) do resemble a Mucus or soft glewey substance; out of which afterwards all the parts are framed in their order; yet by the same Operatour they are together made and augmented, and as the substance resembling glew doth grow, so are the parts distinguished. Namely they are generated, altered, and formed at once, they are at once similar and dissimilar, and from a small similar is a great organ made.[3]

Harvey was thus very certain that the processes of growth in size and differentiation in shape went on quite concurrently, though he had no inkling of changes in the relative rapidity of each process. On this point he goes further than Fabricius. Fabricius thought that growth was a more or less mechanical process, taking its origin from the properties of elementary substances, but that differentiation was brought about by some more spiritual or subtle activity.

Fabricius [says Harvey] affirmes amisse, that the Immutative Faculty doth operate by the qualities of the elements, namely, Heat, Cold, Moisture, and Dryness (as being its instruments) but the Formative works without them and after a more divine manner; as if (forsooth) she did finish her task with Meditation, Choice, and Providence. For had he looked deeper into the thing, he would have seen that the Formative as well as the Alterative Faculty makes use of Hot, Cold, Moist, and Dry, (as her instruments) and would have deprehended as much divinity and skill in Nutrition and Immutation as in the operations of the Formative Faculty her self. . . . I say the Concocting and Immutative, the Nutritive and Augmenting Faculties (which Fabricius would have to busie themselves only about Hot, Cold, Moist, and Dry, without all knowledge) do operate with as much artifice, and as much to a designed end, as the Formative faculty, which he affirms to possess

[1] P. 224.   [2] P. 225.   [3] P. 308.

the knowledge and fore-sight of the future action and use of every particular part and organ.[1]

Here Harvey adopts a more organic conception, being unwilling to regard growth as more mechanical than morphogenesis. "All things are full of deity (*Jovis omnia plena*)," said he,[2] "so also in the little edifice of a chicken, and all its actions and operations, *Digitus Dei*, the Finger of God, or the God of Nature, doth reveal himself."

There can be no doubt that Harvey's leanings were vitalistic. In the following passage, he argues against both those who wished to deduce generation from properties of bodies (like Digby) and the Atomists (like Highmore). Aubrey notes that Harvey was "disdainfull of the chymists and undervalued them."

It is the usual error of philosophers of these times [says he] to seek the diversity of the causes of parts out of the diversity of the matter from whence they should be framed. So Physicians affirm, that the different parts of the body are fashioned and nourished by the different materials of blood or seed; namely the softer parts, as the flesh, out of a thinner matter, and the more earthy parts as the bones, out of grosser and harder. But this error now too much received, we have confuted in another place. Nor are they lesse deceived who make all things out of Atomes, as Democritus, or out of the elements, as Empedocles. As if (forsooth) Generation were nothing in the world, but a meer separation, or Collection, or Order of things. I do not indeed deny that to the Production of one thing out of another, these forementioned things are requisite, but Generation her self is a thing quite distinct from them all. (I finde Aristotle in this opinion) and I my self intend to clear it anon, that out of the same White of the Egge (which all men confesse to be a similar body, and without diversity of parts) all and every the parts of the chicken whether they be Bones, Clawes, Feathers, Flesh, or what ever else, are procreated and fed. Besides, they that argue thus assigning only a material cause, deducing the causes of Natural things from an involuntary or casual concurrence of the Elements, or from the several disposition or contriving of Atomes; they doe not reach that which is chiefly concerned in the operations of nature, and in the Generation and Nutrition of animals, namely the Divine Agent, and God of Nature, whose operations are guided with the highest Artifice, Providence, and Wisdome, and doe all tend to some certaine end, and are all produced, for some certaine good. But these men derogate from the Honour of the Divine Architect, who hath made the Shell of the Egge with as much skill for the egge's defence as any other particle, disposing the whole out of the same matter and by one and the same formative faculty.[3]

But although these are Harvey's theories, it is significant that in his preface he says, "Every inquisition is to be derived from its causes, and chiefly from the material and efficient," thus expressly excluding formal and final considerations. Certainly, as far as his practical work went, he was unaffected by them, and in the case of the egg-shell, for example, Harvey was not the man to say, "it is present for the protection of the embryo," and then to do or say nothing more. Such an explanation, though he might gladly accept it, was no bar to further exploration both by way of experiment and observation.

Harvey not only follows Aristotle in his good discoveries and true statements about the egg, but also, unfortunately, in his less useful parts, as, for example, when he devotes several pages to the discussion of how far the egg is alive, and whether there is any soul in subventaneous or unfruitful eggs. He decides that there is only a vegetative soul. On the other hand, he admirably refutes the opinion of those physicians—who were not few in number—who declared that the foetal organs were all functionless during foetal life.

But while they contende that the mother's Blood is the nutriment of the foetus in the womb, especially of the *Partes Sanguineae*, the bloody parts (as they call them) and that the Foetus is at first, as if it were a part of the mother, sustained by her blood and quickened by her spirits, in so much that the heart beats not and the liver sanguifies not, nor any part of the Foetus doth execute any publick function, but all of them make Holy-Day and lie idle; in this Experience itself confutes them. For the chicken in the egge enjoyes his own Blood, which is bred of the liquors contained within the egge, and his Heart hath its motion from the very beginning, and he borrow-eth nothing, either blood or spirits from the Hen, towards the constitution either of the sanguineous parts or plumes, as those that strictly observe it may plainly perceive.[1]

We have already seen how the Stoics in antiquity believed that the embryo was a part of the mother until it was born; from this idea the transition would be easy to the belief that all the organs in the embryo were functionless and dependent on the activity of the corresponding ones in the maternal organism.[2]

One of Harvey's most important services to thought lay in his abolishing for good the controversy which had gone on ever since the sixth century B.C. about which part of the egg was for nutrition and which for formation. He had the sense to see that the distinction was a useless and baseless one—

There is no distinct part (as we have often said) or disposed matter out of which the Foetus may be formed and fashioned. . . . An egge is that thing, whose liquors do serve both for the Matter and the Nourishment of the foetus. . . . Both liquors are the nourishment of the foetus.[3]

[1] P. 173.
[2] Other physicians had also refuted this Stoic vestige, so Daniel Winckler in 1630.
[3] P. 220.

As regards spontaneous generation, Harvey considered that even the most imperfect and lowest animals came out of eggs.

We shall show that many Animals themselves, especially insects, do germinate and spring from seeds and principles not to be discerned even by the eye, by reason of their contract invisible dimensions (like those Atomes, that fly in the aire) which are scattered and dispersed up and down by the winds; all which are esteemed to be Spontaneous issues, or born of Putrefaction, because their seed is not anywhere seen.[1]

Unfortunately, he never did return to this subject, for, as he himself informs us in another place, all the papers and notes in his house in London were destroyed at the time of the Civil War, so that what he had written on the generation of insects irretrievably perished.[2]

Another point on which Fabricius had been in error was the appearance of bone and cartilage in the embryo. According to him, "Nature first stretcheth out the Chine Bone, with the ribbes drawn round it, as the Keel, and congruous principle, whereon she foundeth and finisheth the whole pile."[3] This armchair conceit Harvey was easily able to destroy by a mere appeal to experience, but by experience also he came upon a fact less easy to be explained, namely that the motion of the foetus began when as yet there was hardly any nervous system. "Nor is it less new and unheard of, that there should be sense and motion in the foetus, before his brain is made; for the Foetus moves, contracts, and extends himself, when there is nothing yet appears for a braine, but clear water."[4] On the basis of this paradox Harvey may be said to be the discoverer of myogenic contraction, but he could already claim that distinction, for the first heart-beats are accomplished long before there are any nerves to the heart, as he himself points out. "We may conclude from this fact," he remarks,[5] "that the heart and not the brain is the first principle of embryonic life," and he gives instances of physiological actions not under the conscious control of the individual, such as the reflexes, as we should call them, of the intestinal tract, and the emetic action of infusion of antimony which cannot be tasted much and "yet there passeth a censure upon it by the Stomack"[6] and a vomit ensues. Thus, twenty-five years before Francis Glisson, Harvey had formulated, from embryological studies, the view that irritability was an intrinsic property of living tissues.

[1] P. 205.
[2] There is some obscurity in Harvey's attitude on spontaneous generation, as Redi pointed out in 1668, for if the "seeds" from which insects originate are not always necessarily derived from previous insects of the same species, they do not differ so greatly from the Stoic-Kabbalistic "seeds" (see pp. 66 and 80 passim), and hence shade into Epicurean atoms.
[3] P. 313.   [4] P. 345.   [5] P. 348.   [6] P. 349.

Both Harvey and Fabricius were very puzzled about the first origin of the blood. "What artificer," says Harvey,[1] "can transform the two liquors into blood, when there is yet no liver in being ?" It was to be a long time before this question was answered by Wolff's discovery of the blood islands in the blastoderm, and, even now, the chemistry of the appearance of haemoglobin is one of the most obscure problems of chemical embryology. The older observers explained it by considering the yolk to be akin to blood and ready to turn into it at the slightest inducement.

Another problem which neither Fabricius nor Harvey did anything to solve was the nature of the air-space at the blunt end of the egg.

Fabricius recounts several conveniences arising from it, according to its several magnitudes, which I shall declare in short, saying, It contains aire in it, and is therefore commodious to the Ventilation of the egge, to the Respiration, Transpiration, and Refrigeration, and lastly to the Vociferation of the Chicken. Whereupon, that cavity is at the first very little, afterwards greater, and at last greatest of all, according as the several recited uses do require.[2]

As regards the placenta, Harvey took the side of Arantius and denied any connection between the maternal and foetal circulations.

The extremities of the umbilicall vessels are no way conjoined to the extremities of the Uterine vessels by an Anastomosis, nor do extract blood from them, but are terminated in that white mucilaginous matter, and are quite obliterated in it, attracting nourishment from it.[3] . . . Wherefore these caruncles may be justly stiled the Uterine Cakes or Dugs, that is to say, convenient and proportionate organs or instruments designed for the concocting of that Albuginous Aliment and for preparing it for the attraction of the veins.[4]

He criticises van Spieghel for not going far enough in this.

There came forth a book of late, wrote by one Adrianus Spigelius, wherein he treateth concerning the use of the umbilicall arteries and doth demonstrate by powerfull arguments that the Foetus doth not receive its Vital Spirits by the arteries from the Mother, and hath fully answered those arguments which are alledged to the contrary. But he might also as well have proved by the same arguments that the blood neither is transported into the Foetus from the mother's veines by the propagations of the umbilicall veins, which is made chiefly manifest by the examples drawn from the Hen-Egge and the Caesarean Birth.[5]

From all this it would appear that Harvey regarded the uterine milk as the special secretion of the placenta, conveyed to the foetus through the umbilical cord. The nature and constitution of the uterine milk is still

[1] P. 376.   [2] P. 382.   [3] P. 439.   [4] P. 439.   [5] P. 537.

very imperfectly understood. Its discovery is usually attributed to Walter Needham, but various remarks in this chapter (Ex. No. 70) seem to show that Harvey was well acquainted with it. In later times it was regarded by some (Bohnius and Charleton in 1686, Zacchias in 1688 and Franc in 1722) as the sole source of foetal nourishment. Mercklin spoke of it in 1679 as *materia albuginea, ovique albo non absimili.*

The least satisfactory parts of Harvey's book are Exercitations Nos. 71 and 72 on the innate heat and the primigenial moisture. Here he becomes very wordy and speculative, giving us little but confused and puzzled argument. He devotes many pages to proving that the innate heat is the blood and to drawing distinctions between blood and gore, the one in the body, the other shed.[1] In one place he speaks of the processes of generation as so divine and admirable as to be "beyond the comprehension and grasp of our thoughts or understanding." Two centuries previously Frascatorius had said precisely the same thing about the motion of the heart, and it was ironical that the very man who shed a flood of light on cardiac physiology should in his turn have despaired of the future of our knowledge of embryonic development.

Harvey did not say much about foetal respiration, and his few remarks are contained in one of the "additional discourses." He was puzzled exceedingly by the question. But he came very near indeed to the truth when he said,

Whosoever doth carefully consider these things and look narrowly into the nature of aire, will (I suppose) easily grant, that the Aire is allowed to animals, neither for refrigeration, nor nutrition sake. For it is a tryed thing, that the Foetus is sooner suffocated after he hath enjoyed the Aire, than when he was quite excluded from it, as if the heat within him, were rather inflamed than quenched by the aire.[2]

Had Harvey pursued this line of thought, and looked still more narrowly into the nature of air, he might have anticipated Mayow. He does say that he proposes to treat of the subject again, but he never did.

5. The Riddle of Fertilisation

The mainspring of Harvey's researches on the does and hinds can be understood by a reference to Rueff's figures in Fig. 10. According to the Aristotelian theory, the uterus after fertile copulation would be full of menstrual blood and semen; according to the Epicurean theory (held

[1] Here Harvey was standing at the boundary beyond which no one could go without chemical thought and experiment. "Innate heat" and "primigenial moisture," crude terms though they were, recognised phenomena which we now know to be those of that concert of enzyme actions constituting metabolism, and the complex of factors which prevent the denaturation of protein molecules in the living body.
[2] P. 483.

145

by the "physitians") it would be full of the mixed semina. If this coagulated mass exists, said Harvey, it ought to be possible to find it by
dissection, and this was what he tried to do.[1] It soon became plain, as
may be read in Ex. No. 68, not only to Harvey but to the King and the
King's gamekeepers, that no such coagulum existed, and the result was
made still more certain by means of segregation experiments which the
King carried out at Hampton Court.[2] Accordingly there was nothing to
be done but to abandon all the older theories completely, and have
recourse to some sort of hypothesis in which an *aura seminalis*, an
"incorporeal agent" or a "kinde of contagious property" should bring
about fertilisation. This was a perfectly sound deduction from Harvey's
experiments, and did not then appear anything like so unsatisfactory as
it does now, for Gilbert of Colchester was not long dead, the "lodestone" was beginning to be investigated by the virtuosi,[3] and even such
extravagances as Sir Gilbert Talbot's Powder "for the sympatheticall
cure of wounds" were only with difficulty distinguishable from the real
effects of magnetic force.[4]

But to Harvey himself the subject of the action of the seed was hid
in deep night, and he confessed that, when he came to it, he was "at a
stand." Some very interesting light is thrown upon his mind in this
connection by a copy of the *De Generatione Animalium* annotated by
himself, and now in the possession of Dr Pybus, by whose courtesy and
by that of Dr Singer, who has transcribed the notes, I have been enabled

[1] See pp. 199, 228, 251, 416.
[2] The account given by Harvey himself (1653, p. 416) cannot be omitted: "When
I had often discovered to His Majesties sight this alteration in the Womb, and having
likewise plainly shewed that all this while no portion of seed or conception either was
to be found in the Womb, and when the King himself had communicated the same as
a very wonderful thing to diverse of his followers, a great debate at length arose: The
Keepers and Huntsmen concluded, first, that this did imply, that their conception
would be late that year, and thereupon accused the drought; but afterwards when they
understood that the rutting time was past and gone; and that I stood stiffly upon that,
they peremptorily did affirm, that I was first mistaken my selfe, and so had drawn the
King into my error; and that it could not possibly be, but that something at lest of the
Conception must needs appear in the Uterus: untill at last, being confuted by their
own eyes, they sate down in a gaze and gave it over for granted. But all the Kings
Physitians persisted stiffly, that it could no waies be, that a conception should go forward unless the males seed did remain in the womb, and that there should be nothing
at all residing in the Uterus after a fruitfull and effectuall Coition; this they ranked
amongst their 'ἀδύνατα.
"Now that this experiment which is of so great concern might appear the more
evident to posterity; His Majestie for tryal-sake (because they have all the same time
and manner of conception) did at the beginning of October separate about a dozen
Does from the society of the Buck and lock them up in the Course neer Hampton
Court. Now lest any one might affirm that doubtlessly there did continue the seed
bestowed upon them in Coition (their time of Rutting being then not past) I dissected
diverse of them, and discovered no seed at all residing in their Uterus; and yet those
whom I dissected not, did conceive by the virtue of their former Coition (as by Con-
tagion) and did Fawn at their appointed time."
[3] See p. 81.   [4] Cf. p. 130.

146

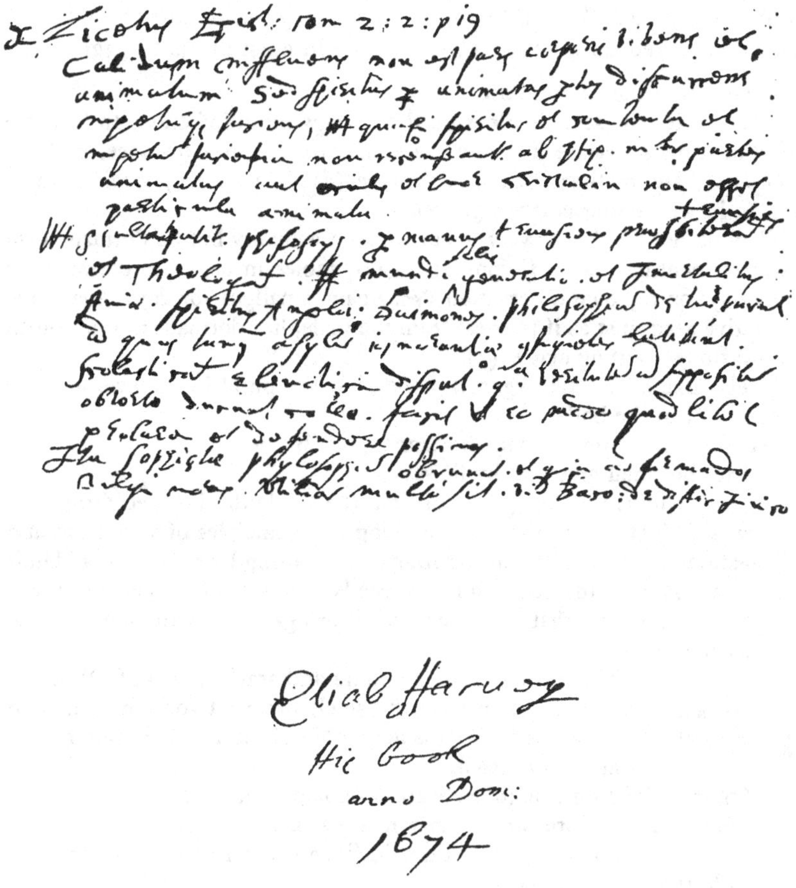
Eliab Harvey
His book
anno Dom:
1674

Fig. 14. Manuscript notes of Dr. William Harvey.

to study it. It was given by Harvey to his brother Eliab, whose name it still bears. The notes, which are on the fly-leaves, are written in much the same way as those famous ones which Harvey used for his lectures at the College of Physicians in London, and which have been reproduced in facsimile. There is the same mixture of Latin and English, and the same signs, such as WH, to denote thoughts claimed as original. A page is reproduced in Fig. 14.

For the most part, the notes are uninteresting and nothing but a confusion of Aristotelian terms, yet one page is concerned with the mode of action of the seed, and here we can, as it were, see Harvey's mind wrestling with this most difficult of problems. He thinks that odour and the sense of smell may give a clue.[1] That his thoughts on this point were doomed to oblivion as soon as egg-cells and spermatozoa were discovered does not detract from the interest of his struggle.

Quod facit semen fecundum

What makes the seed fertile is on the analogy of an infection. In fact, the infection causes disease in many cases, and that from a distance, both by another ... and by the same ... △ Venereal (?) disease corrupts coitus with a woman in whose uterus is the poison.

They do not [or do not yet?] come forth in actuality but lie dormant as in warm fermenting matter [? fomite]. Again, rabies in dogs lies dormant for many days on my own observation W⊣. Again, smallpox for days. Again, the generative seed, just as it (passes) from the male, lies dormant in the woman as in warm fermenting matter (?).

Or else like a . . ., like light in stone . . ., the pupil in the eye, in sense motion, . . . in the body.

Like ferment, vapour, odour, rottenness . . . by rule.

Or like the smell given off by flowers.

Like heat, inflammation (?) △ in lime (heat?) both the wet form. . . . Like what is first . . . in the art of cooking . . . principles of vegetation and propagation. △ Dormice by hibernating . . . cleansing by water and all kinds of lotions, again for insects, as for their seeds as well (?) Or when a soul is a god present in nature, that is divine which it brings about without an organic body by means of law.

See Aristotle on sense and the objects of sense. Marvels concerning odours and smells given off. Whether everything that can be smelt gives off something and so disperses (?) what is not without heat, or by destroying ... attracts to itself.

△ Amongst inflammable (objects are) fire, naphtha, paper. . . .

△ W⊣ manus et odore car . . . anatomia manair. . . .

△ Anat . . . post 4ᵒʳ poras. otium inclinente die rursus quod prius et olefrere vid. . . . Galen. . . .

△ Mr. Boys spainel in Paris lay all ye third night and morning in getting dogg. Whelping dogg's sent (scent) are a stronger sent, vesting in vestigio alios   ord . . . gr . . . lepris odore lepris esse libidine esse. Hors, the mare, *hors*, the cow, a bull per mutta millsa.

△ . . . si lepra fracedo in farioli fader cupidinitus. Dogg ye otter in aquas fracedo vasorum ex sulpore?

Such were the thoughts on action at a distance, on particles, odorous or contagious, flying from place to place, on fermentation and latency,

---

[1] And that there may be some analogy between fertilisation and the transmission of an infectious disease. On this point John Nardi of Florence, one of Harvey's correspondents, held the same opinion, as the letters between them, printed by Willis at the end of his edition of Harvey, show (1847, pp. 603, 610, 615). Nardi's *Noctes Geniales* (Bologna, 1655) contains a reference to the point. A parallel between the penetration of egg-cells by spermatozoa and other cells by invasive bacteria was really not so far off the mark.

which thronged to Harvey's mind as he wrestled with the problem of fertilisation unaided by that triumphant tool the microscope.

6. Harvey's Achievements and Influence

Summarising now Harvey's influence on embryology, we must admit that it was in certain respects reactionary.

1. He did not break with Aristotelianism, as a few of his predecessors had already done, but on the contrary lent his authority to a moribund outlook which involved the laborious treatment of unprofitable questions.

2. His dislike of atomism and "chymistry" precluded any close co-operation between his followers and those of the Descartes-Gassendi tradition.

But these failings are far outweighed by his positive services.[1] It must again be remembered that he used no compound microscope, and was content to rely, like Riolan, on "perspectives," or simple lenses of very low power.

1. There can be no doubt that the doctrine *omne vivum ex ovo* was an advance on all preceding thought. Harvey's scepticism about spontaneous generation antedated by nearly twenty years the experiments of Redi.[2] It is important to note that he was led to his idea of the mammalian ovum by observations on small embryos surrounded by their chorion no bigger than hen's eggs, for the follicle was not discovered until the time of Stensen and de Graaf, and the true ovum not till the time of von Baer.[3]

2. Extending this doctrine downwards as well as upwards, he denied the possibility of generation from excrement and from mud, saying that even vermiparous animals had eggs.

3. He identified definitely and finally the cicatricula on the yolk membrane as the spot from which the embryo originated.

[1] Attention is drawn by Bilikiewicz (p. 25) to the peculiarly empirical tradition of English philosophy described e.g. by Wentscher, and Harvey is placed in a line of descent incorporating Roger Bacon, Duns Scotus, William of Occam and Francis Bacon. On Harvey's knowledge of his predecessors, see Fraser-Harris.

[2] The crucial words in Redi's *Generation of Insects* ought not to be omitted: "I began to believe that all worms found in meat were derived directly from the droppings of flies, and not from putrefaction, and I was still more confirmed in this belief by having observed that before the meat grew wormy flies had hovered over it, of the same kind that later bred in it. But belief would be vain without the confirmation of experiment, hence in the middle of July I placed a snake, some fish, some eels of the Arno, and a slice of milk-fed veal in four large, wide-mouthed flasks; having well closed and sealed them, I then filled the same number of other flasks in the same way, only leaving these open. It was not long before the meat and the fish, in these second vessels, became wormy, and flies were seen entering and leaving at will; but in the closed flasks I did not see a worm, though many days had passed since the dead flesh had been put in them."

[3] See Sarton and Corner.

4. Discussing the question of metamorphosis (preformation) and epigenesis, he decided plainly for the latter, at any rate for the sanguineous animals.

In addition to these achievements, there are others, perhaps less noticed hitherto, but equally important.

5. He destroyed once and for all the Aristotelian (semen-blood) and Epicurean (semen-semen) theories of early embryogeny. This was perhaps the greatest blow he gave to the Peripatetic teaching on development. In spite of it, Sennertus, van Linde and Sylvius adhered to the ancient views, and Cyprianus in 1700 had the distinction of being the last to support them in a scientific discussion, though Sterne in *Tristram Shandy*,[1] as late as 1759, referred to them in a way that shows they still lived on in popular thought.[2]

6. He handled the question of growth and differentiation better than any before, anticipating the ideas of the present century.

7. He settled for good the controversy which had lasted for 2200 years as to which part of the egg was nutritive and which was formative, by demonstrating the unreality of the distinction.

8. He set his predecessors right on a large number of detailed points, such as the nature of the placenta.

9. He made a great step forward in his theory of foetal respiration, though here he did not consolidate the gain.

10. He affirmed that embryonic organs were active, and that the embryo did not depend on external aid for its principal physiological functions.

But all these titles to remembrance, great as they are, do not account for the peculiar fascination of Harvey. A little of it is perhaps due to his imaginative style, which comes out clearly in Martin Llewellyn's English version.[3] A word of censure is due to Willis for transmuting it in his translation into the dull and pedestrian style of 1847. No one who reads the 1653 edition of Harvey can ever forget such metaphors as this, "For the trunck of the body hitherto resembles a skiff without a deck, being in no way covered up by the anteriour parts,"[4] or the vigour of diction which promotes such remarks as, "In a hen-egge after the tenth day, the heart admits no spectators without dissection,"[5] or again,

---

[1] Book I, ch. 20.
[2] Verbally, it was still quite possible to support the Hellenistic view that the embryo was formed from menstrual blood, in the post-Harveian period, if it were admitted that this blood flowed little by little through the umbilical vessels. This was the position of John Freind in his treatise on menstruation, *Emmenologia* (1700–1730). See p. 179.
[3] As Keynes points out, there is no proof that Llewellyn was the translator. Whoever it was deserves the applause of posterity.
[4] P. 333.   [5] P. 333.

"For while the foetus is yet feeble, Nature hath provided it milder diet and solider meats for its stronger capacity, and when it is now hearty enough, and can away with courser cates, it is served with commons answerable to it. And hereupon I conceive that perfect eggs are not onely party-coloured, but also furnished with a double white,"[1] or, lastly, "An egge is, as it were, an exposed womb; wherein there is a substance concluded, as the Representative and Substitute or Vicar of the breasts."[2]

In this connection, it would be a pity not to quote from the verses which Llewellyn prefixed to his translation of Harvey's book.[3] After describing the controversies that followed the *De Motu Cordis*, he wrote

> A Calmer Welcome this choice Peice befall,
> Which from fresh Extract hath deduced all,
> And for Belief, bids it no longer begg
> That Castor once and Pollux were an Egge;
> That both the Hen and Housewife are so matcht,
> That her Son born, is only her Son hatcht;
> That when her Teeming hopes have prosp'rous bin,
> Yet to conceive, is but to lay, within.
> Experiment, and Truth both take thy part:
> If thou canst 'scape the Women! there's the Art.
>
> Live Modern Wonder, and be read alone,
> Thye Brain hath Issue, though thy Loins have none.
> Let fraile Succession be the Vulgar Care;
> Great Generation's Selfe is now thy Heire.

Curiously enough, the "calmer welcome" which Martin Llewellyn hoped for actually happened. Harvey's book was so well reasoned and

---

[1] P. 301.   [2] P. 369.

[3] One of Harvey's epitaphs is of interest to the embryologist. It was an inscription, in a strange Latin style, attached to his statue in the Royal College of Physicians, and it perished with the building in the fire of 1666.

Gulielmo Harveo
viro
monumentis suis immortali
hoc insuper
R.
Collegium Medicorum Londiniensium
Qui enim Sanguini motum
Ut et animalibus ortum dedit
meruit esse
Stator perpetuus

—presumably "he who gave motion to the blood, even as he allotted to animals their origin, has deserved to stand here for ever as their tutelary deity." An interesting recent account of Harvey's life and times is that of Heringham. Since the above account of Harvey's work on embryology was written, A. W. Meyer's valuable *Analysis of the De Generatione Animalium of Harvey* has appeared.

based on such good observations that it produced only three answers, and they were of little importance. Janus Orcham took exception to Harvey's finding no seed in the uterus and suggested that it had vaporised like a steam, but his Aristotelian leanings were promptly detected and castigated by Rallius. Matthew Slade, taking the pseudonym of Theodore Aldes, published in 1667 his *Dissertatio epistolica contra D. G. Harveium*, which was, in his own words, "a detection of one or two errors in that golden book on the generation of animals of William Harvey, greatest of physicians and anatomists." The errors were purely anatomical, and ab Angelis defended Harvey against Slade's attack, claiming that the "errors" were not errors at all. A manuscript work of Slade's appears to be extant.

During the first printing of this book there came to my notice the attack of Alexander Ross on Harvey's *De Generatione*. As described on p. 127 Ross also wrote a polemic against Digby (the *Philosophicall Touchstone*, see p. 281), and the following title shows the breadth of his objections to any advanced thought: *Arcana Microcosmi; or, the hid secrets of man's body discovered; in an anatomical duel between Aristotle and Galen concerning the parts thereof; . . . with a refutation of Dr Brown's Vulgar Errors, the Lord Bacon's Natural History, and Dr Harvy's book De Generatione, Comenius, and others; whereto is annexed a letter from Dr. Pr. to the Author and his answer thereto, touching Dr Harvy's book De Generatione; by A. R.* (Newcomb, London, 1652). This book upholds the Aristotelian theory of embryogenesis from menstrual blood (p. 28) and the doctrine of spontaneous generation (p. 155); it also attacks Harvey's speculations on fertilisation (p. 232). On p. 230 there is a passage which may bear a preformationist interpretation: "The egge is not altogether a body inorganicall actually, seeing it hath different parts." The letter from Dr. Pr. is thus introduced: "Good reader, I met yesternight with this learned letter, which I have briefly answer'd, and have annexed to this Appendix, that thou mayst know how offensive Dr Harvey's opinion is to others as well as to myself." It appears that Harvey's magnetic analogies were more than Ross and his friend could bear. Ross' polemic against Browne bore the title *Medicus Medicatus; or, the Physician's Religion cured by a lenitive or gentle Potion; with some animadversions upon Sir Kenelm Digbie's Observations on Religio Medici, by A. R.* (Young, London, 1645).

Harvey's influence was evidently speedily felt by his contemporaries. Strauss soon wrote a rather poor book on the bird's egg in imitation of him. But the best instance is that in 1655, very soon after the publication of Harvey's book, William Langly, "an eminent senator and physician of Dordrecht," made a great many experiments on the development of the hen's egg. Buffon says that he worked in 1635, i.e. before Harvey, but this is not the case, for in his observations which were published by Julius Schrader in 1674 the later date is given several times. Langly mentions Harvey more than once, and evidently followed his example in careful observation, for his text is concise and accurate and his drawings very noteworthy (see Fig. 15).

Julius Schrader included Langly's work in a composite volume containing a well-arranged epitome of Harvey's book on generation and some observations of his own on the hen's egg. The book was dedicated to Matthew Slade and J. Swammerdam. On the practical side Schrader added nothing memorable to Harvey and Langly, but it is noteworthy that the mammalian embryo was throughout these centuries more popular material than that of the chick. Out of fifty embryologists between Harvey and Haller, the names of Langly, Schrader, Malpighi, Maître-Jan and Snape practically exhaust the list of those who studied the egg of the hen. This orientation of mind doubtless sprang from the strong influence of medicine, and especially obstetrics, on seventeenth- and eighteenth-century embryology.

One of the most interesting English followers of Harvey was Andrew Snape, farrier to Charles II, who in 1683 published as an appendix to his treatise on the anatomy of the horse an excellent account of the development of the chick and the rabbit. Often naming Harvey in the text, he accepts the doctrine of *ex ovo omnia*, and of course identifies the whole blastocyst with the mammalian egg, as Harvey had done. Following Highmore, he first describes the germination of plant seeds. His plate of the generation of the rabbit is copied without acknowledgment from de Graaf.

Snape is perhaps of interest as illustrating the influence of animal breeding on embryology. Just as the needs of practical obstetrics called forth the compilations of Bauhin and Spach in the sixteenth century, so after the destruction of the feudal economy in the English civil war, the needs of stockraisers stimulate Snape.[1]

7. Atomist Theories of Embryonic Development; Gassendi and Descartes

Harvey's death took place in 1657. The following year saw the publication of Pierre Gassendi's *Opera Omnia*, and thus brought in an entirely new phase in embryology.[2] Together with René Descartes'

---

[1] For Snape's rather dubious position in the history of comparative anatomy, see F. Smith, vol. 1, p. 334.
[2] The important treatise of Marcus Marci, whose significance was first realised by W. Pagel, might have been discussed here, but since that somewhat solitary thinker stands in close relation to the Kabbalah, he has been treated of on pp. 80–1. He was much more modern in his views than either Gassendi or Descartes.

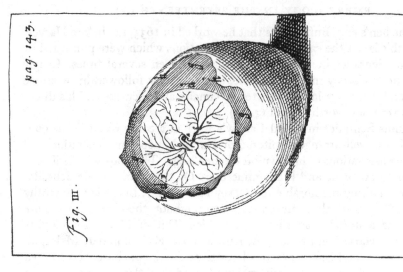

pag. 143.

Fig. III.

B. Fig. III.

The observations of William Langly, made in 1655, were published by J. Schrader in 1674, perhaps stimulated by the work of Malpighi, who is referred to in the preface. The frontispiece shows birds and an infant arising from eggs, and also a form of magnifying glass or perspicilium, but there is no mention of its use in Langly's text. Langly's figures, one of which is here reproduced, are therefore of interest in that they closely resemble the pictures which would have been needed for Harvey's book had it been illustrated.

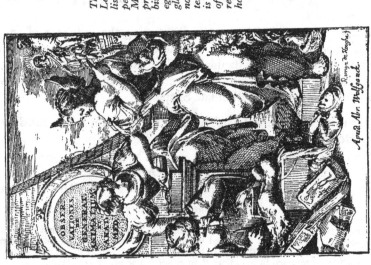

A. Frontispiece.

Apud Abr. Wolfgand.

R.vrijn Pelkogher.f

Fig. 15. From J. Schrader's "Observationes et Historiae, etc.," Amsterdam, 1674.

154

treatise on the formation of the foetus, Gassendi's *De generatione animalium et de animatione foetus* marks a quite different attitude to the subject.[1] Harvey had adopted a rather contemptuous position about the "corpuscularian or mechanical philosophy," which was then coming in, and had expected even less help from it in the solution of his problems than from his equally despised "chymists." Gassendi now set out to show that the formation of the foetus could be explained on an atomist basis: and, using the Galenic physiology and the new anatomy as a framework, he set forth his theory in full. As we read it through at the present day, however, we cannot avoid the conclusion that it was not a success. In spite of his frequent quotations from Lucretius and his persuasive style, it does not carry conviction. The truth of the matter was that the time was not ripe for so great a simplification. The facts were insufficiently known, and that Gassendi is not quite as interested in them as he is in his theory is shown by the circumstance that he only mentions Harvey once.

Gassendi examines in turn the Aristotelian and the Epicurean doctrines of embryogeny and rejects them both, the former on the ground that the change from egg to hen is too great and difficult for anything so shadowy and ghostlike as a "form" to accomplish, and the latter because it leaves no room for teleology. He therefore adopts as the basis of his system atomism and panspermic preformationism, alleging that the germs of all living things were made at the Creation, but that they come to their perfection as atomic congregations in an atomistic universe. Thomas' monograph is a valuable help to the study of this very interesting thinker.

At exactly the same time, Descartes was speculating on the same subject. Added to his posthumous *De Homine Liber* (1662) is a treatise on the formation of the foetus. He may also have written a work *On the generation of animals*, for a manuscript with that title was found among his papers after his death, and was believed to be in his handwriting. There is evidence, however, that it is not his, and though it was published in Cousin's edition of his works, we may safely neglect it, agreeing, in the words of that editor, that it is "a fragment in which very mediocre and often quite false ideas struggle to light through the medium of a style devoid alike of clarity and grandeur." It must be admitted, however, that even his main treatise is very confused. It suffers from the fact that its earlier part contains much which really belongs to the physiological text-book immediately preceding it. Thus it begins abruptly in the middle of a disquisition on the error of attributing bodily functions to the soul. Before long, however, it warms to its theme, and a conception of growth is outlined.

[1] *Opera*, vol. 2, Sect. III, Bk. IV, pp. 260 ff.

When one is young, the movement of the little threads which compose the body is less slow than it is in old age, because the threads are not so tightly joined one to the other, and the streams in which the solid particles run are large, so that the threads become attached to more matter at their roots than detaches itself from their extremities, so that they grow longer and thicker, in this way producing growth.[1]

The fourth part of the book is called, strangely enough, a Digression, in which the formation of the animal is outlined. The mixture of seeds is then described, and a theory of the formation of the heart attempted by means of an analogy with fermentation. The explanation is unconvincing, but has a certain interest as showing chemical notions beginning to permeate biological thought. Indeed, Descartes' way of looking at development was thoroughly novel, as is illustrated by the following citation.

How the heart begins to move. . . . Then, because the little parts thus dilated tend to continue their movement in a straight line, and because the heart now formed resists them, they move away from it and take their course towards the place where afterwards the base of the brain will be formed. They enter into the place of those that were there before, which for their part move in a circular manner to the heart, and there, after waiting for a moment to assemble themselves, they dilate and follow the same road as the aforementioned ones, etc.

Descartes, in fact, with premature simplification, was trying to erect an embryology *more geometrico demonstrata*.[2] That he failed in the attempt was as obvious to his contemporaries as it is to us—"We see," said Garden, "how wretchedly Descartes came off when he began to apply the laws of motion to the forming of an animal." In doing so, he was many years before his time.

But in the history of embryology these men and their writings have a very great significance.[3] Impressed by the unity of the world of phenomena, they wished to derive embryology as well as physics from fundamental laws. This attempt, which resulted in a Galen-Epicurus synthesis on the one hand and a Galen-Descartes synthesis on the other, must be regarded as a noble failure. Its authors did not realise

[1] Time's mutations have a trick of justifying speculations of a materialist character in ways unexpected not only to their original authors, but to men of generations just preceding our own. Here, for example, Descartes' imaginative language sounds more interesting in 1957 than it did in 1927, for the intervening years have brought so much new knowledge of the fibrillar character of many protein particles and molecules, not least those of embryonic cells.

[2] He would have been fascinated indeed by the great treatise of d'Arcy Thompson (1917) submitting embryonic, as all other, life, to rigorous mathematical treatment— so Cartesian, yet at the same time free from all preconceived theory.

[3] See Heussler, de St Germain and Berthier.

what a vast array of facts would have to be discovered before a mechanical theory could with any justice be applied to explain them. Gassendi and Descartes were like the Ionian nature-philosophers, propounding general laws before particular instances were accurately known. Their ineffectiveness arises from the fact that they did not themselves appreciate this, and consequently worked out their ideas in prolix detail, the whole of which was inevitably doomed to the scrap-heap from the very beginning. But the spark was not to die; and if anywhere in this history we are to find the roots of physico-chemical embryology, we must pause to recognise them here.

Much less well known, but not without interest, was the *Dissertatio de vita Foetus in Utero* of Gregorius Nymmanus, which was reprinted in the same year as the second edition of Descartes' book, 1664. Nymmanus writes with a very beautiful Latin style, and expresses himself with great clearness. His proposition is, he says, "That the foetus in the uterus lives with a life of its own evincing its own vital actions, and if the mother dies, it not uncommonly survives for a certain period, so that it can sometimes be taken alive from the dead body of its mother." In supporting this thesis, Nymmanus answers the arguments of those who had held that the lungs and heart of the foetus were inactive *in utero*. Fabricius, Riolanus and Spigelius all proved, says Nymmanus, that the mother and the foetus by no means necessarily die at the same time. "The essential life," he says, "is the soul itself informing and activating the body; the accidental life is the acts of the soul which it performs in and with the body." Though the foetus cannot be said to have life in the latter sense, it can in the former. The foetus, says Nymmanus, prepares its own vital spirits and the instruments of its own soul; there is no nerve between it and its mother. If, he says, the foetal arteries got their sphygmic power from the maternal heart, they would stop pulsating when the umbilical cord was tied, but this is not the case. The pulse of the embryo is therefore due to the foetal heart itself. Galen, says Nymmanus, was aware of this, but did not understand the meaning of it. Again, the foetus *in utero* moves during the mother's sleep, and *vice versa*. Nymmanus' dissertation is an interesting study in the transition from theological to scientific embryology which took place all through the seventeenth century, and may be followed in the writings of Varandaeus, de Castro, Dolaeus, Hildanus, Scultetus, Ammanus, Augerius and Garmannus. The problem of animation-time, a more metaphysical aspect of the same question, was still being handled, but less attention was being paid to it than formerly.

Honoratus Faber's *De Generatione Animalium* of 1666 does not belong to its period. Its author, a Jesuit, proceeds in scholastic fashion to lay down four definitions, three axioms, one hypothesis and seventy-seven propositions, in the last of which he summarises his conclusions. He is interesting in that he displays a disbelief in spontaneous generation, thereby anticipating Redi, and he is careful to mention the work of Harvey, but nevertheless his treatise is of little value. His chief importance is that he is an epigenesist, and therefore demonstrates to us how that opinion was becoming accepted, when Malpighi's brilliant observations and bad theory sent it out of favour, and prepared the way for the numerous controversies of the following century.

8. Fixatives and Uterine Milk; Robert Boyle and Walter Needham

It was in 1666 also that the following appeared in the *Philosophical Transactions of the Royal Society*:

A way of preserving birds taken out of the egge, and other small faetus's: communicated by Mr. Boyle.

When I was sollicitous to observe the Processe of Nature in the Formation of the Chick, I did open Hens Eggs, some at such a day, and some at other daies after the beginning of the Incubation, and carefully taking out the Embryo's, embalmed each of them in a distinct Glass (which is to be carefully stopt) in Spirit of Wine; Which I did, that so I might have them in readinesse to make on them, at any time, the Observations, I thought them capable of affording; and to let my Friends at other seasons of the year, see, both the differing appearances of the chick at the third, fourth, seventh, fourteenth, or other daies, after the eggs had been sate on, and (especially) some particulars not obvious in chickens, that go about, as the hanging of the Gutts out of the Abdomen, etc. How long the tender Embryo of the Chick soon after the Punctum saliens is discoverable, and whilst the bodie seems but a little organized Gelly, and some while after that, will be this way preserv'd, without being too much shrivel'd up, I was hindred by some mischances to satisfie myself; but when the Faetus's, I took out, were so perfectly formed as they were wont to be about the seventh day, and after, they so well retained their shape and bulk, as to make me not repent of my curiosity; And some of those, which I did very early this Spring, I can yet shew you..

Boyle said in conclusion that he sometimes also "added Sal Armoniack, abounding in a salt not sowre but urinous."

In the following year (1667) there appeared the *De Formato Foetu* of Walter Needham. Needham was a Cambridge physician who went to Oxford to study in the active school of physiological research which such men as Christopher Wren, Richard Lower, John Ward and Thomas Willis were making famous. His book on the formation of the embryo, written later (and dedicated to Robert Boyle), after he had been in practice in Shropshire for some time, is important because it is the

PLATE X

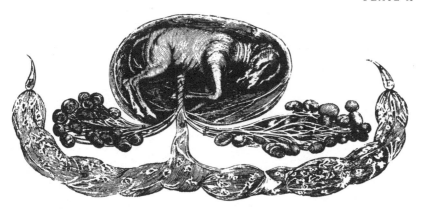

(A) Exhibet foetum bubulum cum membranis suis, artificiose separatis.

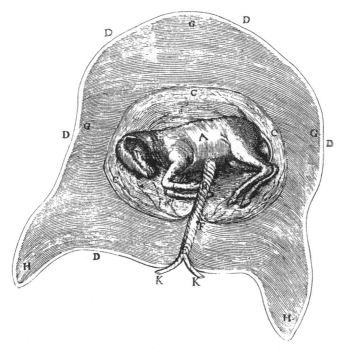

(B) Exhibet foetum equinum quem, quia ad manus non erat chalcographo ostendendus,
ego ex memoria descripsi.

Illustrations from Walter Needham's De Formato Foetu *of 1667. The upper one is very
similar to, but not, as Lewis suggests, identical with, Fig. 29 of Plate XIV in*
De Formato Foetu *of Fabricius (Venice, 1600).*

first book in which chemical experiments on the developing mammalian embryo are reported, and also because it contains the first practical instructions for dissections of embryos (see Plate X, facing page 158).[1]

Sir Thomas Browne had, as we have already seen, made experiments of a chemical nature on the constituents of birds' eggs and of the eggs of Amphibia, but he did not analyse them after any development had been allowed to take place. He may therefore be regarded as the father of the static aspect of physico-chemical embryology, while Walter Needham may be regarded as the founder of the dynamic aspect. The practical difficulties of these pioneers of animal chemistry may be seen in such a book of practical instructions as Salmon's *General Practise of Chymistry* of 1678. They had no satisfactory glassware, no pure reagents, the methods of heating were incredibly clumsy, and there were no means of measuring either heat or atmospheric pressure.

In the review of Needham's book which is to be found in the *Philosophical Transactions of the Royal Society* for September 1667 there occurs the sentence, "These humours (the amniotic, allantoic, etc.) he saith, he hath examined, by concreting, distilling, and coagulating them; where he furnishes the Reader with no vulgar observations." What were these observations? They are to be found in the chapter entitled "The nature of the humours":

I now proceed to speak of this other nutritive liquor round about the urine itself which latter is plainly separated by the kidneys and the bladder. These liquors also proceed from the blood and seem similar to its serum but yet they are different from it. For when fire is applied to them in an evaporating basin (*cochlea*) they do not coagulate, as the blood-serum always does. Indeed, not even the colliquamentous liquid of the egg itself coagulates in this manner, although it is formed from juices which are evidently liable to coagulation—in the same way humours differ among themselves before and after digestion, filtration, and the other operations (*mangonia*) of nature. All, when distilled, give over a soft and mild water (*mollem et lenem*) very like distilled milk. This property is common to the liquor of the allantoic space, along with the rest. Because when the salts are not yet made wild and exalted the serum of the blood remains still quite soft and does not give proof of a tartaric or saline nature. Indeed, the first urine of an infant is observed by nurses to be not at all salt, but in older animals, when I distilled it in an alembic, I seemed to observe a little volatile salt at the small end (*in capitello*). Coagulations attempted by acids happened differently in respect of the different humours. For when I poured a decoction of alumina into the liquor of the cow's amnios it exhibited a few rather fine coagulations but they were clearly white. The allantoic juice, however, was precipitated like urine. Spirits of vitriol and

---

[1] Some information concerning Walter Needham and his friends, especially John Ray, the botanist, is contained in Raven's book on the latter.

vinegar brought about less results than alumina in each case. Spontaneous concretions I found also in the later months; these I discovered in both places. They are more frequent and larger, however, within the allantoic membrane.

From the above excerpt, which contains the account of all that Needham did on the chemical composition of the embryonic liquids, it can be seen that he treated the whole matter more dynamically than Browne. He was the first to describe the solid bodies in the amniotic fluid (*hippomanes*, see Jenkinson) and his chemical experimentation was all pioneer work.

His book has other merits, however. In the first chapter he refutes the theory which Everard had propounded, that the uterine milk was identical with the contents of the thoracic duct, conveyed by lymphatic vessels from the lacteals of Aselli to the uterus, instead of elsewhere; and he shows that arteries must be the vessels bringing the material to the womb. The second chapter deals with the placenta,

where he giveth a particular account of the double Placenta or Cake, to be found in Rabbets, Hares, Mice, Moles, etc., and examines the learned Dr Wharton's doctrine, assigning a double placenta to at least all the viviparous animals, so as one half of it belongs to the Uterus, the other to the Chorion, shewing how far this is true, and declaring the variety of these Phaenomena. Where do occur many uncommon observations concerning the difference of [uterine] Milk in ruminating and other animals, the various degrees of thickness of the uterin liquor in oviparous and viviparous creatures.[1]

He describes the human placenta correctly enough.

The use of the placenta is known to be to serve for conveighing the aliment to the foetus. The difficulty is only about the manner. Here are examined three opinions, of Curvey, Everhard, and Harvey. The two former do hold that the foetus is nourished only from the Amnion by the mouth; yet with this difference, that Curvey will have it fed by the mouth when it is perfect, but whilst it is yet imperfect, by filtration through all the pores of the body, and by a kind of juxtaposition: but Everhard, supposing a simultaneous formation of all the instruments of nutrition together and at first, and esteeming the mass of bloud by reason of its asperity and eagerness unfit for nutrition, and rather apt to prey upon than feed the parts, maintains, that the liquor is sucked out of the amnion by the mouth, concocted in the stomack, and thence passed into the Milky Vessels even from the beginning. Meantime they both agree in this, that the embryo doth breath but not feed through the umbilical vessels. This our Author undertakes to disprove; and having

[1] Needham was thus an important precursor of that comparative study of placental structure and function which reached definitive rationality in the classification of Grosser (1927).

asserted the mildness of, at least, many parts of the bloud, and consequently their fitness for nutrition, he defends the Harveyan doctrine of the colliqua-tion of the nourishing juyce by the Arteries and its conveyance to the foetus by the veins.

In the third chapter Needham gives the first really comparative account of the secondary apparatus of generation, enunciating the rather obvious rule that in any given case the number of membranes exceeds the number of separate humours by one.[1] He affirms that all the humours are nutritive save the allantoic. It had previously been held that all fish eggs were of one humour only, but he points out that a selachian egg has its white and yolk separate. He gives the results of his chemical experiments at this point, and suggests that the noises heard from embryos *in utero* and *in ovo* may be due to the presence of air or gas in the amniotic cavity, thus forming a link between Leonardo and Mazin. In his fourth chapter he deals with the umbilical vessels and the urachus, and here he claims priority over Stensen for the discovery of the *ductus intestinalis*[2] in the chick, referring to Robert Boyle, Robert Willis, Richard Lower and Thomas Millington, to whom, he says, he showed the duct before Stensen published his observations on it. The fifth chapter is concerned with the *foramen ovale*, and the arterial and venous canals, and with the foetal circulation in general. The sixth is about respiration or "biolychnium," and in it Needham writes against the conception of a vital flame, alleging cold-blooded animals, etc. in his favour, but here he takes a retrograde step, for he argues that the use of the lungs is not for respiration but to "comminute the bloud and so render it fit for a due circulation."

The seventh and last chapter contains a direction for the young Anatom-ists, of what is to be observed in the dissection of divers animals with young; and first, of what is common to the viviparous, then, what is peculiar to severall of them, as, a sow, mare, cow, ewe, she-goat, doe, rabbet, bitch, and a woman, lastly, what is observable in an Egg, skate, salmon, frog, etc. All is illustrated with divers accurate schemes.

[1] For the seventeenth-century and later folklore of the embryonic membranes (cf. the "Silly How," etc.) see Brand, esp. p. 406.
[2] The *ductus intestinalis*, which connects the avian yolk with the gut of the embryo, has a peculiar importance in the history of embryology, since it provided one of the main arguments on the preformationist side at the climax of that debate (see p. 199; and Fig. 22).
As Adelmann rightly remarks, it was known to Aristotle (*Historia*, 562ᵃ 5, *Generat.* 753ᵇ 20), and to Coiter, who speaks of an outgrowth from intestine to yolk. No mention of it is made by Aldrovandus, Fabricius or Harvey. In 1664 appeared Stensen's *De vitelli in intestina pulli transitu Epistola* (bound up with his *De Musculis et Gland. Observationum Specimen*) in which the rediscovery was made, but W. Needham had a priority of ten years, as described in the text. See May.

The subsequent course of chemical embryology in the seventeenth century may be put in a very few words. Marguerite du Tertre incorporated in her obstetrical text-book of 1677 the results of some similar experiments to those of Needham. "If you heat the (amniotic) liquor," she says, "it does not coagulate, and if you boil it it flies away leaving a crass salt like urine, but if you heat the serosity of blood, it solidifies as if it were glue." The same observation was recorded by Mauriceau in 1687, who concluded, with some common sense, that, as there was so little solid matter present, the liquid could not be very nutritive; and by Case in 1696, who said,

In this juice the plastic and vivifying force resides, for although to our eyes it looks in colour and consistency like the serum of the blood, yet it is absolutely (*toto coelo*) different; for if a little of the former is slowly evaporated (*si in cochleari super ignem detines*) no coagulation will ever appear.

Lister said this once more in 1711, but with Boerhaave's work of 1732 the subject entered a new phase.[1]

9. The Discovery of the Follicles of the Mammalian Ovary

In 1664 Nicholas Stensen, that great anatomist, later a bishop, who was also in many ways the founder of modern geology, produced his *De musculis et glandulis specimen*, in which Coiter's observations on the vitelline duct and the general relations between embryo and yolk in the hen's egg were made again and confirmed. About this time also Deusingius described his case of abdominal pregnancy, and was thus the first anatomist to draw attention to this phenomenon.

In 1667 Stensen published his *Elementorum myologiae specimen*, in which he described the female genital organs of dogfishes. He demonstrated the follicles in the ovaries and affirmed that the "testis" of women ought to be regarded as exactly the same organ as the "ovary" or "roe" of Ovipara. At the time he carried the suggestion no further, and it is surprising that it did not arouse more interest, for it was exactly what Harvey had been looking for. Nothing obvious having been found in the uteri of King Charles' does, and the conviction yet being very strong that viviparous conceptions really came from eggs, Stensen's minute ova supplied the fitting answer to the question. Thus Harvey and Stensen between them substituted the modern concept of mammalian ova for the ancient theory of the coagulum all in the space of fourteen years.

In 1670 Theodore Kerckring published a curious work on foetal

[1] Ebstein has written the history of the boiling test for protein in urine.

osteology (see Fig. 16), and, two years later, de Graaf and Swammerdam described in detail the follicles of mammalia (see Fig. 17), thus demonstrating the truth of Stensen's suggestion of some years before.[1] It is important to note that these workers mistook the "Graafian follicles" for eggs—a mistake which was not rectified till the time of von Baer. Stensen himself not long after also published an account of these "eggs," but he was by then too late to gain the priority of demonstration. Portal's claim that Ferrari da Grado, who lived in the fifteenth century, was the true discoverer of mammalian ova has been disproved by Ferrari,[2] and, although it is true that Volcher Coiter mentioned what we now call the Graafian follicles, he did not recognise in any way their true nature.

De Graaf's discovery was confirmed in 1678 by Caspar Bartholinus, and, in 1674, by Langly, whose original observations had been made, so it was said, in 1657, the year of Harvey's death. If this is true, Langly has the priority of observation, Stensen of theory and de Graaf of demonstration.[3]

The concept of biological homology originates from Harvey, Stensen and de Graaf, according to Tur. The mammalian ovary was recognised as homologous with the ovary of the oviparous animals. In this connection, the work of Nuck in 1691 is very important, as one of the earliest instances of experimental procedure. He ligatured the uterine horns after copulation in a dog, and observed pregnancy afterwards, implantation having taken place above the ligature. His conclusion was that the embryo was derived from the ovary and not from the sperm— *animal ex ovo generari experimento probatur*. His work was repeated almost exactly 100 years later by Haighton, who drew almost exactly the same conclusion from it.[4]

10. The Micro-iconographers and Preformationism; Marcello Malpighi and Jan Swammerdam

In the year 1672, Marcello Malpighi, who had for many years previously been working on various embryological problems with the aid of the simple microscope,[5] published his tractates *De Ovo Incubato*

---

[1] See Maar. The words *mulierum testes ovaris analogi sunt* appear in *Hist. Dissect. Piscis*, Maar's edition, vol. 2, p. 153.
[2] *Une Chaire de Médecine . . .*, pp. 115 ff.
[3] See Tur. Cole (p. 48) believes that the first use of the term "ovum" for the ovarian follicles of mammals in print is in van Horne's *Prodromus* of 1668. The idea was evidently widely current in these two decades.
[4] See pp. 209–10 and 230.
[5] Bibliography of the history of the microscope by O. W. Richards. Of the large literature on this subject we may mention only the introductions of Rooseboom and Hintzsche; and the paper of Hughes on achromatism.

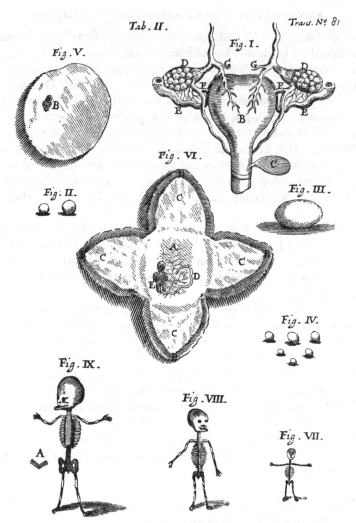

Fig. 16. *Theodore Kerckring's imaginative drawings of human foetal development (1670) taken from* Phil. Trans. Roy. Soc., 1672, no. 81, pp. 4018 ff.

Fig. I. *"a* Matrix *with its chief dependances."*

Fig. II. *"Eggs of different bigness, as Dr Kerkringius affirms to have found them in the testicles of a Woman."*

Fig. III. *"A bigger Egg."*

Fig. IV. *"Smaller Eggs from the testicles of a cow"—(Graafian follicles).*

Fig. V *"represents an Egg, which Dr Kerkringius affirms to have opened 3 or 4 days"* [sic] *"after it was fallen into the* Matrix *of a woman, and in which he saw that little embryon marked B, whereof he found the head begun to be distinguished from the body, yet without a distinct preception of the organs."*

Fig. VI *"a bigger egg, opened a fortnight* [sic] *after conception."*

Figs. VII, VIII & IX. *" The sceletons of Infants 3 weeks, 4 weeks and 6 weeks after conception* [sic]."

Kerckring simply drew reduced copies of the skeleton of the newborn infant. (Bilikiewicz, p. 96.)

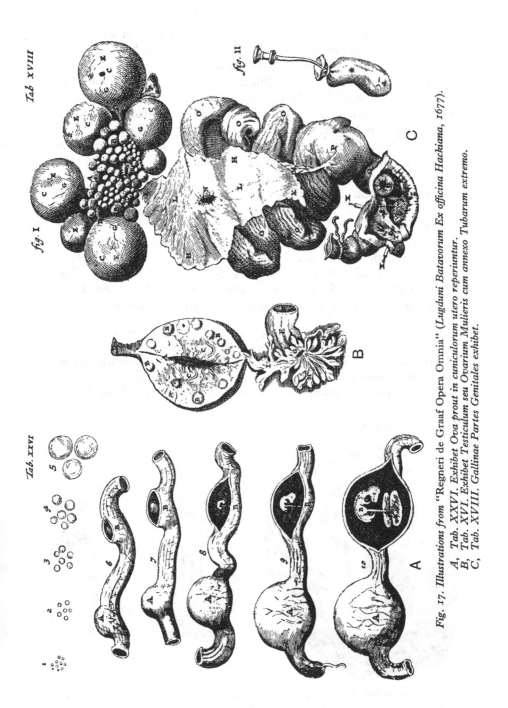

Fig. 17. Illustrations from "Regneri de Graaf Opera Omnia" (Lugduni Bataorum Ex officina Hackiana, 1677).

A, Tab. XXVI. Exhibet Ova prout in cuniculorum utero reperiuntur.
B, Tab. XVI. Exhibet Testiculum seu Ovarium Mulieris cum annexo Tubarum extremo.
C, Tab. XVIII. Gallinae Partes Genitales exhibet.

and *De Formatione Pulli in Ovo*. In spite of its great importance, it was anything but a voluminous work. The plates in which Malpighi represented the appearances he had seen in his examination of the embryo at different stages are beautiful, and I reproduce some of them here (Fig. 18, below and Plate XI, opposite). Description of the embryo was now pushed back into the very first hours of incubation, and it is interesting to note that Malpighi could not have done his work without Harvey, whose name he mentions on his first page, and who pointed out the cicatricula as the place where development began, and therefore, as Malpighi must have reasoned, the place where microscopic study would be most profitable. Now for the first time the blastoderm was described, the neural groove, the optic vesicles, the somites and the earliest blood-vessels.

Malpighi appears to have been anticipated, as regards the first description of the chick's heart pulsating in colourless blood, by Henry Power, M.D., of Halifax (a friend of Sir Thomas Browne's), whose charmingly written *Experimental Philosophy* appeared in 1664. Power confirmed microscopically the opinion of Parisanus (see p. 116).

For view but an Egge [he says on p. 60] after the second days Incubation, and you shall see the cicatricula in the Yolk, dilated to the breadth of a groat or six-pence into transparent concentrical circles; in the Centre whereof is a white Spot, with small white threads (which in futurity proves the Heart with its Veins and arteries) but at present both its motion and circulation is

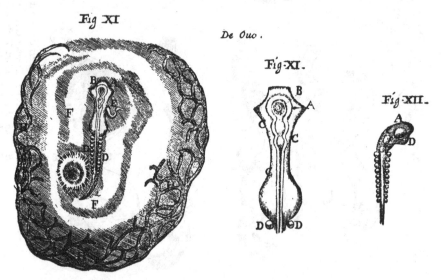

Fig. 18. Malpighi's drawings of the early stages of development in the chick embryo.

PLATE XI

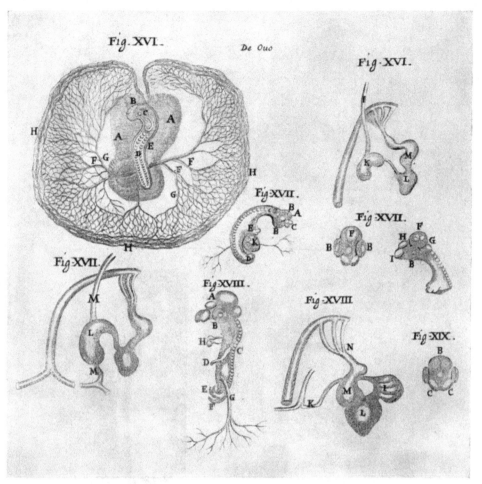

Illustrations from Malpighi's De Ovo Incubato *of 1672 showing the early stages of the development of the chick (compare with Lillie's monograph).*

Fig. XVI (left) shows the *area vasculosa* and the embryo at about 85 hours' incubation; at F and G the vitelline vessels, at H the marginal vein, at B the anterior vitelline veins, at D the somites of which 20 have been drawn. Figs. XVI (right), XVII and XVIII illustrate the formation of the heart, as Malpighi saw it. They are of great interest as they show the aortic arches. In Fig. XVII the lower M represents the confluence of the two omphalomesenteric veins coming from the yolk-sac, and leading into the ductus venosus, L. It is joined above by the Duct of Cuvier (upper M) from the cardinal vein of the embryonic body (cf. Lillie, Fig. 115). In Fig. XVIII the vessel K will ultimately become the vena cava, I is the auricle, L the ventricle and M the bulbus (cf. Lillie, Fig. 199). At N are shown three aortic arches, connecting the heart with the aorta. Their signifi-cance was not appreciated till the time of Rathke, who in 1825 demonstrated the fish-like gill-slits and gill-arches in the embryos of birds and mammals.

PLATE XII

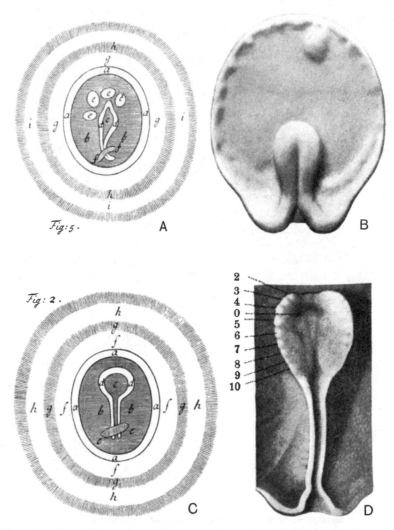

Fig: 5. A

B

Fig: 2. C

2
3
4
0
5
6
7
8
9
10

D

Illustrations from "The curious and accurate observations of Mr Stephen Lorenzini of Florence on the Dissections of the Cramp-Fish : *containing the comparative anatomy of that and some other Fish, with Experiments. Dedicated to his Most Serene Highness the Prince of Tuscany, and now done into English from the Italian, with Figures after the Life, by J. Davis, M.D. Jeffery Wale, London*", *1705.*

A. Table III, Fig. 5 (the earlier stage), the egg of the cramp-fish. *aaaaa*, the white Circle or Cicatrix; *bb*, a certain Colliquamentum of a leaden colour; *c*, the first rude Draught of the Animal; *dd*, a white stripe or Selvadge; *eeee*, little Bladders of various Figures and different Bigness; *ff* a certain little Bag; *gggg*, a large Swathe or Bordering, in some places of a Sulphureos colour; *hh*, another circle of the Colliquamentum; *ii*, a white Belt or Girdle.

C. Table IV, Fig. 2 (later).

B and D are taken from photographs of Ziegler's, see text.

undiscernable to the bare eye, by reason of the feebleness thereof, and also because both the Liquor and its Vessels were concolour to the white of the Eggs they swum in; but the Heart does circulate this serous diaphanous Liquor, before (by a higher heat) it be turned into bloud. And one thing here I am tempted to annex, which is a pretty and beneficial Observation of the Microscope, and that is, That as soon as ever you can see this red pulsing Particle appear (which Doctor Harvey conceited, not to be the Heart, but one of its Auricles) you shall most distinctly see it, to be the whole Heart with both Auricles and both Ventricles, the one manifestly preceding the pulse of the other (which two motions the bare eye judges to be Synchronical) and without any interloping perisystole at all; So admirable is every Organ of this Machine of ours framed, that every part within us is entirely made, when the whole Organ seems too little to have any parts at all.

The cloven hoof of preformationism may be observed in the last few lines, and their chronological position should be noted.

Recently Cole has brought to light another anticipation of Malpighi, even more interesting, if not so reputable, as the preceding. On March 14th, 1671, William Croone deposited with the Royal Society a manuscript paper on the development of the chick; in the following year a brief abstract of it was published in the *Philosophical Transactions*, but it did not appear in full till 1757. Croone examined by dissection the cicatricula of the hen's egg, and gave an illustration purporting to represent the preformed embryo, but obviously recognisable to modern eyes as a fragment of vitelline membrane accidentally caricaturing the features of a bird. "Croone's paper," says Cole, "is important, not on account of its merits, which are negligible, but because it is the first reasoned attempt, based on observation and illustration, to establish the corporeal existence of a preformed foetus in the unincubated egg." Croone rather naïvely admits his preconceived bias in favour of preformation, or rather of "instantaneous generation," followed by "metamorphosis," but does not indicate whence he derived it. Joseph de Aromatari, Swammerdam, Highmore, were all possible sources.

Among the immediate followers of Malpighi was Lorenzini (see also p. 207), a Tuscan investigator whose merit has apparently been overlooked. A pupil of Nicholas Stensen and Francesco Redi, he published in 1678 (six years only after Malpighi's *De Ovo Incubato*) a description of the anatomy of the elasmobranch fish *Torpedo*, plentiful then no doubt as now at Naples. An English translation appeared in 1705.

Lorenzini recognised the ovary of this fish as homologous with that of the hen, and studied the early development of the eggs, giving two semi-diagrammatic pictures of the blastodisc. These are reproduced in Plate XII, facing page 167. In the earlier one, shown side by side with a modern representation of Ziegler's, the medullary groove is seen growing forward over the surface of the blastodisc, and Lorenzini has tried to indicate the presence of the little distinct swellings which are formed by the segmentation cavity. In the second picture he has correctly shown the outspread cephalic end of the medullary plate, which closes later than the rest of the neural tube, though he does not figure the neuromeres. No explanation is available for what he describes as a "little bag" (*f, f*, in the first figure, *e, e*, in the second), unless it was a turned-up fragment of the blastodisc.[1]

It is always considered that the modern phase of the controversy over preformation *versus* epigenesis began with Malpighi, though the firmness of his convictions on this question have been much exaggerated. Embryogeny, preformationists held, is not comparable to the building of an artificial machine, in which one part is made after another part, and all the parts gradually "assembled," but takes place rather by an unfolding of what was already there, like a Japanese paper flower in water. Malpighi was led towards this belief by the fact that development goes on after fertilisation as the egg passes down the oviduct, and in the most recently laid eggs gastrulation is already over, so that in his researches he could never find an absolutely undeveloped germinal spot. It is curious to note that he says his experiments were done *mense Augusti, magno vigente calore*, so that a more than usual degree of development would have taken place overnight. Had he examined the cicatriculae in hen's eggs before laying, he would very probably not have formed this theory, and the epigenesis controversy might have been settled with Harvey. Another influence which was unfavourable to the epigenetic position was that it was Aristotelian, and therefore unfashionable. Yet Malpighi's view was much more sensible than many which succeeded it, for he did not maintain a perfectly equal swelling up of all parts existing at the start, but rather an unequal unfolding, a distribution of rate of growth at different times and in different regions of the body. Thus he says,

Now, as Tully says, Death truly belongs neither to the living nor to the dead, and I think that something similar holds of the first beginnings of animals, for when we enquire carefully into the production of animals out of their eggs, we always find the animal there, so that our labour is repaid and we see an emerging manifestation of parts successively, but never the first origin of any of them.

[1] We owe to Oppenheimer a special study of the history of the embryology of fishes. Lorenzini was not the only seventeenth-century anatomist who contributed to it; Duverney (1648–1730), for example, studied the heart of the carp and its development.

What had been unfounded speculation for Seneca in antiquity and for Joseph de Aromatari and Everard in late times was now set upon an apparently firm experimental basis by Malpighi.[1]

It is most instructive to note the difference in the attitudes of Langly and Schrader respectively towards the preformation question. Langly has no doubts about it, nor has Faber; they both follow Harvey and epigenesis unquestioningly, but Schrader, though he believes in epigenesis on the whole, is not at all certain about it. His friend, Matthew Slade, he says, brought the epistle of Joseph de Aromatari to his attention, and what with that, and the unexplained observations of Malpighi on the pre-existence of the embryo, he is not willing to deny all value to preformationist doctrine. Others were bolder. It was immediately seized upon by Malebranche, the Streeter of his age, who, in his *Recherche de la Vérité* of 1672, realised its philosophical possibilities, and gave it a kind of metaphysical sanction. That mystical microscopist, Swammerdam, made use of it as an explanation of the doctrine of original sin. In a remarkably short space of time it was a thoroughly established piece of biological theory.

Malebranche refers to it in his *Recherche de la Vérité* in the chapter where he treats of optical illusions and emphasises the deceitfulness and inadequacy of our senses.

We see in the germ of a fresh egg which has not been incubated an entirely formed chicken. We see frogs in frogs' eggs and we shall see other animals in their germs also when we have sufficient skill and experience to discover them. We must suppose that all the bodies of men and animals which will be born until the consummation of time will have been direct products of the original creation, in other words, that the first females were created with all the subsequent individuals of their own species within them. We might push this thought further and belike with much reason and truth, but we not unreasonably fear a too premature penetration into the works of God. Our thoughts are, indeed, too gross and feeble to understand even the smallest of his creatures.

Malebranche, who was a priest of the Oratory of the Cardinal de Bérulle, took an ardent interest in the scientific life of his time[2]—for example, in a letter to Poisson, the Abbé Daniel wrote, "Reverend Father, M. Malebranche has written to me saying that he has installed an oven in which

[1] For the earlier part of this train of thought, see pp. 66 and 121; for the later, see pp. 213 ff.

[2] Just as Christian theology led some seventeenth-century thinkers to take an active interest in embryological phenomena, so in earlier centuries Buddhism in China had stimulated speculation and some observation on metamorphosis in plants and animals (see *Science and Civilisation in China*, vol. 2). Plate XIII, facing page 170, shows this element in Buddhist iconography, the "putting off of the 'old man' " in deliverance from illusion.

he has hatched eggs. He has already opened some and has been able to see the heart formed in them and beating, together with some of the arteries."[1]

Swammerdam's support for preformation came from a different angle. He had been investigating insect metamorphosis, and, having hardened the chrysalis with alcohol, had seen the butterfly folded up and perfectly formed within the cocoon. He concluded that the butterfly had been hidden or masked (*larvatus*) in the caterpillar, and thence it was no great step to regard the egg in a similar light. Each butterfly in each cocoon must contain eggs within it which in their turn must contain butterflies which in their turn must contain eggs, and so on. Before long, Swammerdam extended this theory to man. "In nature," he said, "there is no generation but only propagation, the growth of parts. Thus original sin is explained, for all men were contained in the organs of Adam and Eve. When their stock of eggs is finished, the human race will cease to be."

In 1684 Zypaeus reported that he had seen minute embryos in unfertilised eggs, and there were other similar claims. *Hinc recentiores physiologi*, said Schurigius in 1732, *hominem in ovulis delineatum quoad omnes partes in exiguis staminibus ante conceptionem existere statuunt*.

Swammerdam cannot be regarded simply as one of the principal pillars of the preformation theory. His own embryological researches, which were made chiefly on the frog, were remarkable in many ways. He was the first to see and describe the cleavage of the egg-cell and later segmentation. He said that there was a time during the development of the tadpole when its body consisted of granules (*greynkens* or *klootkens*), but as these grew smaller and much more numerous they escaped his penetration (see Fig. 19). Leeuwenhoek also saw these cells,[2] and his account was published long before Swammerdam's, but his observations on the rotating embryos of *Anodon* and the eggs of fleas were equally interesting.

11. Foetal Respiration and Composition; John Mayow and Robert Boyle

In 1674 John Mayow, a young Oxford physician, published his tractate, *De Respiratione Foetus in Utero et Ovo*, which was included as one of the parts of his *Tractatus Quinque medico-physici* in that year. Mayow was the first worker to realise that gaseous oxygen, or, as he

---

[1] Blampignon, p. 9; Schrecker.
[2] See Plate XIV, facing page 171. Dobell's book on Leeuwenhoek, though marked by certain lapses of taste, is probably the most considerable and ingenious study of any seventeenth-century biologist extant. Unfortunately, he confined himself to the transcription and evaluation only of the protozoological and bacteriological observations.

PLATE XIII

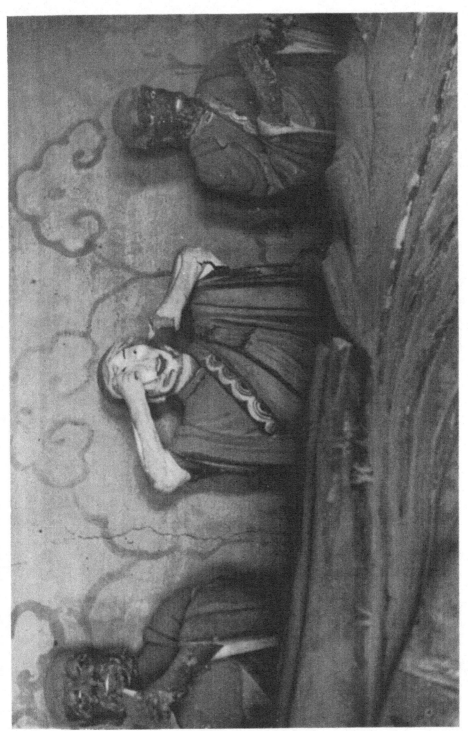

Metamorphosis in Buddhist iconography; statues in the Sleeping Buddha temple at Suchow (Chiu-ch'üan), Kansu province, China. (Original photograph, 1943.)

PLATE XIV

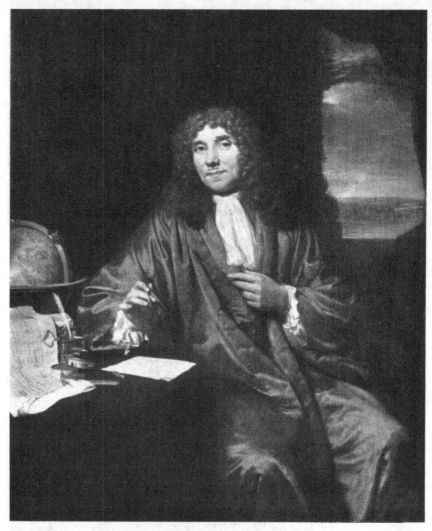

Portrait of Anton van Leeuwenhoek (1632–1723) by Jon. Verkolje (1650–93) in 1686, now in the Rijksmuseum, Amsterdam.

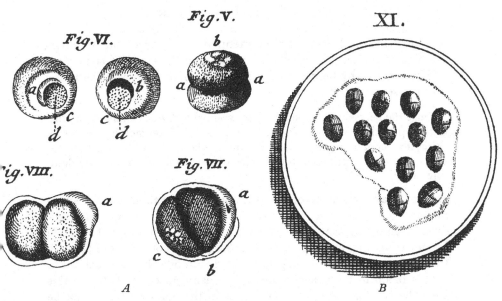

Fig. 19. Observations on the cleavage of the amphibian egg.

A. *The first pictures of the 2-cell stage, from* "Johannis Swammerdammii Biblia Naturae" (*Leyden, apud Isaacum Severinum, Balduinum Vander Aa, Petrum Vander Aa, 1738*).

Blastomeres of the frog's egg at the 2-cell stage are shown in Tab. XLVIII, figs. V, VI, VII, VIII.

(p. 813) "*in re fig. V aa, Porro observabam, Ranunculum universum, notabili admodum sulco sive plicatura, in duas veluti partes dividi a, a*..........*Haecce autem observatio sulci vel plicaturae corporis Ranunculi; quam quidem, casu saltem fortuito primitus a me animadversam, in vivis postmodum Ranunculis quoque detexi; plurimum mihi dein adferebat lucis ad certius existimandum de subita illa corpusculi Ranunculorum expansione et elongatione, quae die quarto, cum Embryo sese explicat, evenire cernitur. Crediderim hinc, quod altera illa explicati Ranunculi pars in Caput et Thoracem accrescat; altera vero in Abdomen atque Caudam, quae pedetentim magis augetur.*"

(p. 814) "*in re fig. VII. . . . In medio hujus Ovi manifeste rursus descriptum ante sulcum b conspiciebam.*"

These observations were made between 1665 and 1675. In 1676 Oligerus Jacobaeus published his "De Ranis Observationes" (*Billaine, Paris*). *His illustrations show the tail-bud stages but no blastomeres. On preformation he appears to agree with Swammerdam rather than with Harvey.*

B. *The first pictures of the 4-cell stage, from* "Expériences pour servir à l'histoire de la génération des animaux et des plantes"; *par M. l'Abbé Spallanzani (ed. Senebier), Barthelemi Chirol, Geneva, 1786.*

(p. 36). "*Ils ressemblent à de petits globes noirs qui paroissent ronds à l'œil nud et avec une lentille foible; mais si on les observe avec une forte lentille, on les voit sillonnés de quatres sillons que ce coupent à angles droits comme la peau à demi-ouverte des châtaignes ou des marons, Fig XI. Quoique ces petits sillons ne soient pas nuds, mais couverts d'une membrane très-subtile qui enveloppe étroitement le reste de l'œuf; si l'on ôte cette membrane, on voit à découvert la peau apparente de l'œuf qui est noire et qui se déchire par le plus léger attouchement, avec l'intérieur de l'œuf dont la substance est presque fluide, d'une couleur presque blanche, homogène, ou similaire en apparence, composée de petites particules globuleuses quand on l'observe avec un microscope.*" (*Is this the earliest mention of yolk-platelets?*)

termed it, the "nitro-aerial" vapour, was the essential factor in the burning of a candle and the respiration of a living animal. His work was forgotten until Beddoes drew attention to it in 1790, but since then many have praised it and Schultze makes him the equal of Harvey.[1]

The reason why he became interested in embryology is given in the opening sentences of his work.

Since the necessity of breathing is so essential to the sustaining of life that to be deprived of air is the same as to be deprived of common light and vital spirit, it will not be out of place to enquire here how it happens that the foetus can live though imprisoned in the straits of the womb and completely desti-ture of air.

He first of all gives an account of the opinions held about foetal respira-tion and the umbilical cord. He says that he disagrees (1) with the view that the embryo breathes *per os* while it is in the womb, for there is no air in the amnion and the *suctio infantuli* proves nothing; and (2) with the view propounded by Spigelius that the umbilical vessels existed to supply blood to the placenta for the nourishment of the latter. If this were the case, he says, the membranes in the hen's egg could not be formed before the vitelline vein, as they are, and in cases of foetal atrophy the placenta would always die and be corrupted too, which does not happen. Nor does he support the view of Harvey (3) that the um-bilical vessels supply blood for the concoction and colliquation of the food of the foetus, for why should not the embryonic body prepare its own nutritious juice before birth just as it does afterwards. He further thinks the theory (4) that the umbilical vessels are for carrying off surplus foetal nourishment quite untenable and as little likely as the theory (5) that they exist for the object of allowing a foetal circulation—for this could just as well be accomplished through the vessels which exist in the embryonic body.

Mayow decides therefore for the opinion of *divinus senex Hippocrates* and Everard that the umbilicus is a respiratory mechanism, carefully dissociating himself, however, from the hypothesis of Riolanus that the umbilical cord with all its windings is so arranged to cool the blood passing through it. He then says,

We observe, in the first place, that it is probable that the albuminous juice exuding from the impregnated uterus is stored with no small abundance of aerial substance, as may be observed from its white colour and frothy charac-ter [Needham's uterine milk]. And in further indication of this, the primi-genial juices of the egg, which have a great resemblance to the seminal juice of the uterus, appear to abound in air particles. For if the white or the yolk of

[1] For an extreme view in the opposite direction see Patterson.

an egg be put into a glass from which the air is exhausted by the Boylian pump, these liquids will immediately become very frothy and swell up into an almost infinite number of little bubbles and into a much greater bulk than before—a sufficiently clear proof that certain aerial particles are most intimately mixed with these liquids. To which I add that the humours of an egg when thrown into the fire give out a succession of explosive cracks which seem to be caused by the air particles rarefying and violently bursting through the barriers which confined them. Hence it is that the fluids of the egg are possessed of so fermentative a nature. For it is indeed probable that the spermatic portions of the uterus and its carunculae are naturally adapted for separating aerial particles from arterial blood. These observations premised, we maintain that the blood of the embryo, conveyed by the umbilical arteries to the placenta or uterine carunculae, brings not only nutritious juice, but along with this a portion of nitro-aerial particles to the foetus for its support, so that it seems that the blood of the infant is impregnated with nitro-aerial particles by its circulation through the umbilical vessels quite in the same way as in the pulmonary vessels. And therefore I think that the placenta should no longer be called a uterine liver but rather a uterine lung.

These splendid words, informed by so much insight and scientific acumen, show that, by the time of Mayow, chemical embryology had certainly come into being. He died at the early age of thirty-six, and we may well ponder how different the subsequent course of this kind of study would have been if he had lived a little longer.

The second part of Mayow's treatise is concerned with respiration in the hen's egg during its development, and it may be noted that his observations on the air contained in the liquids before development probably account for the facts which have been reported at one time and another concerning an alleged anaerobic life of embryos in early stages. Mayow was wrong in supposing that the gas which he pumped out from white and yolk was purely "nitro-aerial," but he shows the greatest good sense in his reminder that the amount of nitro-aerial particles required by embryos must be comparatively small owing to their small requirement for "muscular contraction and visceral concoction." His remarks on the effect of heat on the developing egg are not so clear as the remainder of the treatise, but he seems to mean that the heat will disengage the nitro-aerial particles from the liquids, and so aid in respiration, an idea which was later used by Mazin. His fundamental mistake here was that he failed to realise that the egg-shell was permeable to air; and this vitiates all his reasoning about the respiration of the egg. "It will not be irrelevant," he says, "to enquire here whether the air which is contained in the cavity in the blunter end of every egg contributes to the respiration of the chick." He first notes that the cavity in question lies between two membranes and not between the shell-membrane and the shell as Harvey himself had supposed; and then he goes on to say that he disagrees with the opinion of Fabricius, who had asserted that the air in the air-space serves for the respiration of the chick. His reasons are (1) that there would not be enough there for the needs of the embryo, which would use it, as it were, at one gulp, and (2) that the air in it cannot pass through the inner membrane, an error into which he was led by observing that if an egg-shell with its contents removed and its air-space intact was put into a vacuum, the air-space would swell up until it was as big as the egg itself. Mayow sees now what had escaped the attention of all previous observers, namely that the egg-contents are not "rarefied or expanded, but are on the contrary condensed and forced into a narrower space than before." Such a condensation could, he thinks, take place in four ways: (a) by an increase in propinquity of discrete particles, (b) by a subsidence of motion on the part of a congregation of particles into rest, (c) by the extraction of some subtle spirit from amongst the particles, and (d) by a decrease in elasticity on the part of some elastic substance previously present. We should at the present time choose the third alternative as being the truest, in view of the loss of water and carbon dioxide which the egg suffers as it develops,[1] but Mayow chose the fourth, thinking it probable that the "air distributed among the juices of the egg loses its elastic force on account of the fermentation produced among these juices by incubation." Now since the egg-contents are compacted into smaller bulk by the process of incubation, a vacuum would be created somewhere if Nature had not, with her customary prudence, inserted a small amount of air into the air-space which might in due course expand and avoid this. His proof for this was an inaccurate observation; he thought he saw, in eggs at a late stage, when the contents were removed, the air-space collapse to the normal size which it occupies in unincubated eggs. He expressly says that his theory does not depend upon the conception of *horror vacui*, but that, by the compressive action of the imprisoned air, the fluids of the egg are forced into the umbilical vessels, and the particles composing the embryonic body packed more tightly together. "The internal air appears to perform the same work as the steel plate bent round into numerous coils by which automata are set in motion."

With this ingenious but erroneous supposition Mayow concludes what is undoubtedly the first great contribution to physiological or biophysical embryology.[2] His views on foetal respiration were soon

[1] See Fig. 20, p. 176.
[2] For modern knowledge on metabolism and growth during ontogenesis, see the treatise of Brody.

generally accepted, as the writings of Zacchias, Viardel, Pechlin and John Ray[1] show, but Sponius as late as 1684 was asserting that the lungs of the foetus were functional *in utero*, absorbing from the amniotic liquid the nitro-aerial particles which P. Stalpartius supposed the placenta to be secreting into it. It is interesting to note that by Mayow's own air-pump method Bohn found nitro-aerial particles in the uterine milk in 1686, and Lang found them in the amniotic liquid in 1704. The problem had by then arrived at a stage beyond which it could not progress in the absence of quantitative methods.

The year 1669 saw the publication of Nicholas Hoboken's useful treatise on the anatomy of the placenta, and of the English edition of P. Thibaut's *Art of Chymistry*.[2] I mention the latter here because of a reference to the special conditions of embryonic life which is found in it,[3] but as yet no real help was being given to embryology by contemporary chemistry.

About this time also Francis Willoughby published his famous book on birds, an attempt to bring Aldrovandus up to date, in which a good picture is given of the embryological knowledge of the time, although no new observations or theories appear. Another contemporary review is that of Barbatus.

In 1677 spermatozoa were discovered, as announced by Ham and Leeuwenhoek[4] in the *Philosophical Transactions of the Royal Society*, though Hartsoeker afterwards claimed that he had seen them as early as 1674, but had not had sufficient confidence to publish his results.[5] There is a reference to this in the letters of Sir Thomas Browne, who, writing to his son, Dr Edward Browne, on December 9th, 1679, said,

I sawe the last transactions, or philosophicall collections, of the Royal Society. Here are some things remarkable, as Lewenhoecks finding such a vast number of little animals in the melt of a cod, or the liquor which runnes from it; as also in a pike; and computeth that they much exceed the number of men upon the whole earth at one time, though hee computes that there may bee thirteen thousand millions of men upon the whole earth, which is very many.[6] It may bee worth your reading.

At the same time as these events were taking place, Robert Boyle,[7] at Oxford and London, was engaged in continuing those experiments in chemistry which had led him not long before to write his *Sceptical Chymist*. It is not generally known that in this work, which appeared

---

[1] *Wisdom of God in Creation*, p. 73.   [2] See Ferguson.   [3] *Art*, p. 207.
[4] On this subject see Cole; and Meyer (1938); von Buddenbrock; and Hughes for further details.
[5] On this see Dobell, pp. 69 ff.
[6] Too many, to convince the ovists; see p. 223.
[7] See Plate XV, facing page 176.

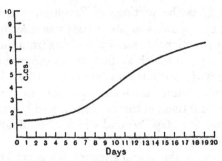

Fig. 20. *The increase in the size of the air-space of the hen's egg during development, due to the loss of water and CO_2 from the egg.*

in 1661, and which set the key for the whole spirit of subsequent physico-chemical research, Boyle has a reference to embryology, and curiously enough in connection with a point which, though it is easily seen to be of the highest importance, has been quite overlooked by the commentators upon him. One of the main views he was trying to urge was that until some system could be proposed which would give a means of quantitative estimation of the constituents of a mixture, no further progress would be made. He was asking, in fact, that chemistry should become an exact science, and his demand is only veiled by the unfamiliarity of his language. His preference for the "mechanical or corpuscularian" philosophy was mainly due to his realisation that, unless chemistry was going to start measuring something, it might as well languish in the obscurity to which Harvey would willingly have relegated it. Thus he says,

But I should perchance forgive the Hypothesis I have been all this time examining [that of the alchemists], if, though it reaches but to a very little part of the world, it did at least give us a satisfactory account of those things which 'tis said to teach. But I find not that it gives us any other than a very imperfect information even about mixt bodies themselves; for how will the knowledge of the *Tria Prima*[1] discover to us the reason why the Loadstone drawes a Needle, and disposes it to respect the Poles, and yet seldom *precisely* points at them? how will this hypothesis teach us how a Chick is formed in the Egge, or how the seminal principles of mint, pompions, and other vegetables, can fashion Water into various plants, each of them endow'd with its peculiar and determinate shape and with divers specifick and discriminating Qualities? How does this hypothesis shew us, *how much* Salt, *how much* Sulphur, *how much* Mercury must be taken to make a Chick or a Pompion? and if we know that, what principle is it, that manages these ingredients and con-

[1] The salt, sulphur and mercury of the alchemists.

176

PLATE XV

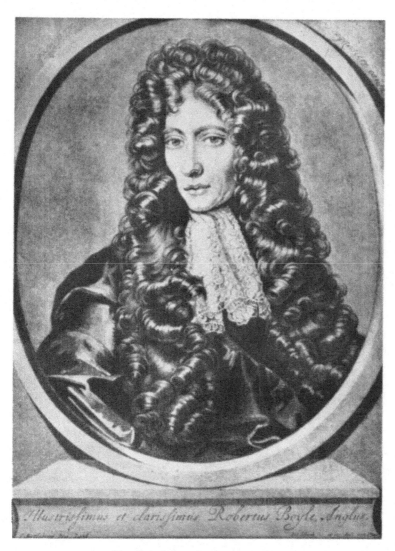

The Hon. Robert Boyle (1627–1691).

trives, for instance, such liquors as the White and Yolke of an Egge into such a variety of textures as is requisite to fashion the Bones, Arteries, Veines, Nerves, Tendons, Feathers, Blood and other parts of a Chick; and not only to fashion each Limbe, but to connect them altogether, after that manner which is most congruous to the perfection of the Animal which is to consist of them? For to say that some more fine and subtile part of either or all the Hypostatical Principles is the Director in all the business and the Architect of all this elaborate structure, is to give one occasion to demand again, *what proportion and way of mixture* of the *Tria Prima* afforded this Architectonick Spirit, and what Agent made so skilful and happy a mixture?[1]

Boyle's instance of the magnetic needle pointing nearly, not exactly, at the north, and his use of the expressions "how much", "how many", "proportion", "way of mixture," indicate that he was moving towards a quantitative chemistry, and by obvious implication a quantitative embryology. Elsewhere he says that he thinks the *Tria Prima* will hardly explain a tenth part of the phenomena which the "Leucippian" or atomistic hypothesis is competent to deal with. Thus, although Boyle made few experiments or observations on embryos, he occupies a very important position in the history of embryology.

During the last two decades of this century, the Oxford Philosophical Society was occupied on a good many occasions with problems relating to embryology. It is extremely interesting to note, in connection with what we have just seen in Boyle, that John Standard of Merton College reported on February 10th, 1685,

the following obbs. concerning y[e] weight of y[e] severall parts of Henn's eggs; done with a pair of scales which turned with $\frac{1}{2}$ a grain.[2]

	ozs.	dr.	scr.	grns.
A henn's egg weighed	2	–	1	15
The skin weighed	–	–	–	16
The shell	–	2	2	4
The yolk	–	5	1	–
The white	1	1	–	6
Loss in weighing				9

Another early quantitative observation was that of Claude Perrault, who found about 1670 that incubated ostrich eggs lost one-ninth of their weight in five weeks.[3] The Oxford Philosophical Society, however,

[1] Italics mine.
[2] The full appreciation of the balance as a tool of investigation did not, of course, come until the second half of the eighteenth century, though Sudhoff has found in Paracelsus a hint of it.
[3] *Mém, Hist. Nat.* (1671), vol. 2, p. 138; (1676), vol. 2, p. 177.

preferred as a rule to consider more unusual things, such as "the egges of a parrot hatched in a woeman's bosome, a hen egg figur'd like a bottle, a hen egg that at the big ende had a fleshie excrescence, another hen-eg, monstrous, a suppos'd cocks egg, and the egs of a puffin, an elligug, and a razor-bill." Mention of these different kinds of eggs reminds us that the systematic collection and classification of eggs had been begun some years before by Sir Thomas Browne (as may be seen in John Evelyn[1]) and by John Tradescant. About this time R. Waller made some noteworthy observations on the "spawn of frogs and the production of Todpoles therefrom," extending the work begun by Swammerdam not long before. Mauriceau now gave a description of the phenomenon of sterile foetal atrophy. The century fittingly closes with the treatises of Ettmüller and Gibson, in which the embryological work of the seventeenth century is summarised with considerable accuracy. Ettmüller supported the moribund menstruation theory of embryogeny with the argument that animals do not menstruate because they are more prolific than men, and therefore all their blood is required for generation.[2] Garmann's *Oologia curiosa*, which appeared in 1691, is worth mention also, as a review of the knowledge of the time. But that his work was what the booksellers' catalogues describe as "curious" is shown by the following chapter-headings "De ovo mystico, mythico, magico, mechanico, medico, spagyrico, magyrico, pharmaceutico." Finally this was the time when embryonic monsters began to receive a really scientific description. We take an illustration (Plate XVI, facing page 178) from an unusual source, Robert Plot's *Natural History of Staffordshire* (1686); it shows a teratoma with the well-formed teeth and hair so characteristic of such cystic growths. Dr Plot surmised that "dame Nature in this birth at first intended Twinns" but did not know "how she came thus to miscarry in her plastics."

[1] *Diary*, vol. 2, p. 69.   [2] *Opera*, p. 170.

PLATE XVI

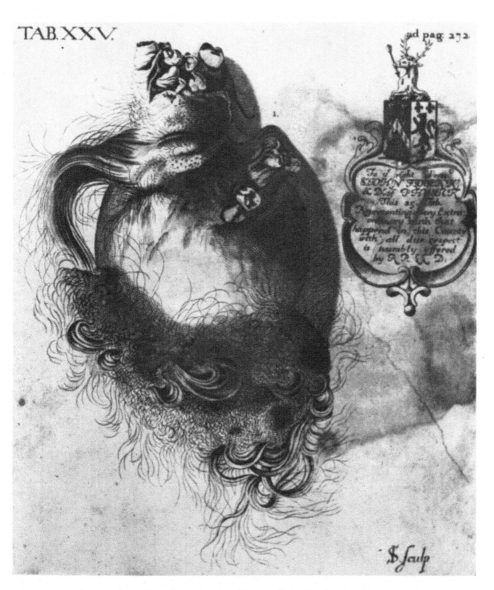

A teratoma with well-formed teeth and hair
(*from Robert Plot's* Natural History of Staffordshire, *1686*).

CHAPTER IV

EMBRYOLOGY IN THE EIGHTEENTH CENTURY[1]

1. Theories of Foetal Nutrition

DURING the course of the seventeenth, and the first quarter of the eighteenth, century, many theories were propounded concerning foetal nutrition. It is convenient to classify them (Table I).

At this point the *Emmenologia* of John Freind[2] deserves special reference. This was a book which dealt with all aspects of menstruation.[3] As has already been mentioned (p. 150 n. 2) he supposed that the blood passing through the placenta to the embryo was distinctively menstrual blood. This view he supported by an arithmetical argument. Calculating the amount of menstrual blood evacuated in nine months, he said,

> The quantity of Blood which the Mother may bestow upon the nourishment of her Offspring will be *lib.* 13 *ozs.* 2⅓, which will outweigh the new-born Foetus with all its Integuments, if they should be put into a balance; and leave no room to doubt, its being able to bestow very proper nourishment on the Embrio. For the mean weight of a new-born Foetus is about 12 *lib.*, sometimes it is found greater, and very often less.

This quantitative outlook forms a parallel to Harvey's approach in his famous calculation about the circulation of the blood.

Freind's view that the maternal and foetal circulations were continuous was derived from the experiments of Rayger and Gayant, who had injected a blue dye into the foetal circulation and found it again in the maternal. Work of this kind had begun as far back as about 1555, when apparently Amatus Lusitanus had made similar observations on a woman, and in the *Crocologia* of J. F. Hertodt, published in 1671, where under the heading "An crocus foetum tingat in utero ?" we find a description of the public dissection of a pregnant dog to which this dye had been given in the diet. The embryos were markedly yellow.

---

[1] Cf. the interesting recent résumé of W. Schopfer.
[2] Biographical details of Freind in an essay by Greenwood.
[3] Müller-Hess has written a monograph on the development of knowledge on menstruation from the sixteenth century onwards.

TABLE I

I. That the embryo was nourished directly by menstrual blood.

Beckher, 1633.

Plempius, 1644. Plempius did not deny that the umbilical cord was functional, but insisted that the blood passing through it was menstrual. In 1651 Harvey's work was published.

Sennertus, 1654. F. Sylvius, 1680.

Seger, 1660. Cyprianus, 1700.

van Linde, 1672.

II. That the embryo was nourished through its mouth.

(a) By the amniotic liquid.

(i) In addition to the umbilical blood.

Harvey, 1651.	Linsing, 1701.
W. Needham, 1667.	Pauli, 1707.
de Graaf, 1677.	Barthold, 1717.
C. Bartholinus, 1679.	S. Middlebeek, 1719.
van Diemerbroeck, 1685.	Teichmeyer, 1719.
Ortlob, 1697.	Gibson, 1726.
D. Tauvry, 1700.	

(ii) Alone; the umbilical blood being regarded as unnecessary or of minor importance.

Moellenbrock, 1672.	P. Stalpartius, 1687.
Everardus, 1686.	Bierling, 1690.

Case, 1696. Case thought the embryo arose entirely out of the amniotic liquid like a precipitate from a clear solution; see p. 184.

Berger, 1702.

These writers assumed as their principal experimental basis reports of embryos born without umbilical cords, e.g. those of:

Rommelius, 1675 (in Velsch).

Valentinius, 1711.

(b) By the uterine milk or *succum lacteo-chylosum*.

Mercklin, 1679.	J. Waldschmidt, 1691.
Drelincurtius, 1685.	Tauvry, 1694.
Bohnius, 1686.	Franc, 1722.
Zacchias, 1688.	Dionis, 1724.

TABLE I (*continued*)

III. That the embryo was nourished through the umbilical cord only.
  (*a*) By foetal blood (the circulations distinct).

Arantius, 1595.	Snelle, 1705.
Harvey, 1651.	Falconnet, 1711.
W. Needham, 1667.	F. Hoffman, 1718.
Ruysch, 1701.	Monro, 1734.

      It is to be noted that Bierling, P. Stalpartius, Berger, Barthold and Charleton, who supported the discontinuity theory of the circulations, were all upholders of the theory of foetal nourishment *per os*, so that their reasons for doing so were not those on account of which we agree with Hoffmann and Needham at the present time.

  (*b*) By maternal blood (the circulations continuous).

Laurentius, 1600.	Hamel, 1700.
de Marchette, 1656.	de Craan, 1703.
Rallius, 1669.	Lang, 1704.
Muraltus, 1672.	van Horne, 1707.
Blasius, 1677.	Freind, 1711.
Veslingius, 1677.	

      de Méry, 1711. De Méry combated Falconnet's view of the separate circulations. He said that he had not himself tried Falconnet's experiments, but that some students had, and could not repeat them.

      Aubert, 1711. Narrative of a case in which the umbilical cord had not been tied at the maternal end and the mother had nearly bled to death through it.

Nenterus, 1714.	Wedel, 1717.

      Bellinger, 1717. Bellinger believed that the maternal blood was transformed by the embryonic thymus gland into proper nourishment for itself, after which it was secreted into the mouth by the salivary ducts and so went to form meconium without the necessity for deglutination. Heister's comments on this extraordinary theory are worth reading. Perhaps Bellinger was indebted to Tauvry for his idea of the importance of the thymus gland. Tauvry had drawn attention in 1700 to its diminution after birth.

de Smidt, 1718.	Dionis, 1724.

(*continued overleaf*)

TABLE I (*continued*)

(*c*) By menstrual blood.
      Plempius, 1644.

(*d*) By uterine milk.
      Ent, 1687.
      Camerarius, 1714. (*Opinio conciliatrix!*)
      F. Hoffmann, 1718.

(*e*) By the amniotic fluid.
      Vicarius, 1700.   Goelicke, 1723.

IV. That the embryo was nourished through pores in its skin.
      Deusingius, 1660.   Stockhamer, 1682.
      Nitzsch, 1671.

> This was suggested on the ground that in the earlier stages of development there is no umbilical cord. In 1684 de St Romain argued against it on the ground that, if it were true, the embryo would dissolve in the amniotic liquid.

During this period also there were continued disputes about the origin of the amniotic liquid. Van Diemerbroeck and Verheyen considered that it could not be the sweat of the embryo, for the embryo was always much too small to account for it, and, moreover, du Tertre had described cases where the secundines had been formed with the membranes but in the absence of the embryo. Dionis affirmed that whatever it was it could not be urine, for urine will not keep good for nine days, *a fortiori* not for nine months. Drelincurtius put forward a theory that the embryo secreted it from its eyes and mouth by crying and salivating, while Bohn and Blancard derived it from the foetal breasts. Lang, Berger and de Gouey criticised this notion without bringing forward anything constructive, and de Gouey was in his turn annihilated by D. Hoffmann, who with Nenter and König supported the modern view, namely, that it was a transudation from the maternal blood-vessels in the decidua. The question was complicated further by the alleged discovery by Bidloo in 1685 of glands in the umbilical cord, and by Vieussens in 1705 of glands on the amniotic membrane. J. M. Hoffmann and Nicholas Hoboken supported the view that these were the important structures. There the problem was left during the eighteenth century, various writers supporting different opinions from time to time, and it is still not fully solved.

2. Growth and Differentiation; Stahl and Maître-Jan

Very early in the eighteenth century (1708) there appeared a work by G. E. Stahl, van Helmont's most famous follower, which struck the keynote of the whole period. Stahl's *Theoria Medica Vera*, divided as it was into physiological and pathological sections, belonged in essence to the *a priori* school of Descartes and Gassendi. It differed from them profoundly, however; for instead of trying to explain all biological phenomena, including embryonic development, from mechanical first principles, it started out from first principles of a vitalistic order, and, having combined all the *archaei* into one informing soul, it sought to show that the facts could be convincingly explained on this basis. The spiritual kinship of Stahl with Descartes and Gassendi is due to an atmosphere which can only be called doctrinaire, and which was common to them all. Like the methodist school of Hellenistic medicine, they subordinated the data to a preconceived theory.

Stahl is also interesting in that he represents a trend of thought which favoured what has been called "instantaneous generation followed by metamorphosis." Cole calls this the "precipitation" theory[1] but I cannot altogether accept his account of it.

"Metamorphosis" was defined by Harvey (1653, pp. 222 ff.) as the bringing into being of a formed object from a mass of material previously possessing no form; as opposed to "epigenesis," where assumption of form and increase of mass proceed simultaneously.

Artificial productions are perfected two several waies; one, when the artificer cuts and divides the matter which is provided to his hands, and so by paring away the superfluous parts doth leave an Image remaining behinde, as the Statuary doth; the other, when the Potter formes the like Image of Clay, by adding more stuff, or augmenting, and so fashioning it, so that at one and the same time, he provides, prepares, fits, and applies his materials.

Harvey's "metamorphosis" we should now call "differentiation without growth" and his "epigenesis" we should call "differentiation plus growth." It should be carefully noted that to epigenesis Harvey does not oppose "preformation," for he was writing some thirty years before Malpighi's unfortunate summer-time experiments, and Joseph de Aromatari's seed had not yet sprouted. "Preformation" in modern terms would correspond to "growth without differentiation," all the complexity of the finished form being supposed to be present initially. "Metamorphosis" in Harvey's mind was nothing more nor less than the Aristotelian blood-and-seed theory, and his description of a sculptor making a statue out of a pre-existent mass can best be understood in the light of Rueff's drawings (Fig. 10). Harvey opposed Fabricius pre-

[1] P. 205.

cisely because the latter ventured to point to the chalazae in the hen's egg as the homologue of the mammalian blood-and-seed.

But the relations between growth and differentiation were still open to different opinions in the eighteenth century and many believed that the former was by far the more important of the two. If the differentiation process was pushed far enough back in the life of the embryo, the distinction between epigenesis and preformation tended to disappear. We have already had (p. 167) in Croone an example of a preformationist who believed illogically that "instantaneous generation" was followed by "metamorphosis," and Stahl is an example of an epigenesist who thought that the governing *archaeus* provided by the semen organised whatever it found in the uterus into the form of the body, after which there was pure growth and no further differentiation. The distinction thus became almost academic.

After the mysterious organising process

the entire remaining business of generation [said Stahl[1]] is taken up with the formation of the body, which from the first rudiment, so to speak, is nothing afterwards but nutrition; namely, such as is carried on from this time up to old age; while in the body what is once completely shaped is not merely preserved by a perpetual supply, nor, if it perchance fails, is it merely rebuilt, but in fact it continually grows until it is completely formed in all its parts. A perpetual assimilation everywhere accompanies apposition, or rather the apposition itself is set up immediately in such order and situation that assimilation is brought about and exists because of that very position. . . . That Principle which unfolds its activity primarily in the brain and the nerves presides over the formation of the body, and those parts which constitute the only immediate instrument of its actions being formed first of all, make it probable for that reason that something ought to, or at least can, be provided by themselves alone. . . . As for how the blood is generated, if we are to believe the theories commonly held to-day, it is thought to be born from a spontaneous gliding-together and chance meeting of particles uniting themselves mutually.

Thus:

(A) EPIGENESIS ≡ Differentiation + Growth   Harvey
(B) PREFORMATION ≡ Growth alone   Malpighi, Swammerdam, etc.
(C) METAMORPHOSIS ≡ Differentiation alone   Aristotle, Fabricius
(D) PRECIPITATION ≡ (A) in the very early   Stahl, Case
     stages, followed by (B)
(E)   (B) in the very early stages, followed   Croone
     by (C)
(F)   (C) in the very early stages, followed   Buffon
     by (B)

Theoria, pp. 425 ff.

In 1722 Antoine Maître-Jan published his book on the embryology of the chick, the only one on this subject between Malpighi and Haller. It was an admirable treatise, illustrated with many drawings which, though not very beautiful, were as accurate as could be expected at the time. Perhaps its most remarkable characteristic is its almost complete freedom from all theory—Maître-Jan says hardly a word about generation in general, and is far from putting forward a "system" in the usual eighteenth-century manner. He contents himself with the recital of the known facts including those added by his own observations. He gives no references, and writes in an extremely modern and unaffected style.

The only traces of theoretical presupposition which can be found in him are Cartesian, for he speaks of the activity of ferments in blood-formation. He is an epigenesist, and long before Brooks, he gives the right explanation of Malpighi's error, affirming that the hot Italian summer was responsible for some development in Malpighi's eggs before Malpighi examined them. Although Maître-Jan's book must have been accessible both to Buffon and Haller, they perpetuated Malpighi's mistake till nearly the end of the century.

In technique, Maître-Jan was pre-eminent. He was the first embryologist to make practical use of Boyle's suggestion regarding "distilled spirits of vinegar" for hardening the embryo so that it could be better dissected.[1] He also used "weak spirits of vitriol"; after treating blastoderms with it, he said, "I saw with pleasure an infinity of little capillary vessels which had not appeared to be there before" (see Plate XVII, facing page 186). He made a few chemical experiments also, noting that vinegar would coagulate egg-white, and estimating quantitatively the difference in oil-content of different yolks—though for this he gives no figures.

His theory he relegated to an appendix entitled *Objections sur la génération des animaux par de petits vers*. There were sixteen of them, but the most cogent one was that, as little worms had been found under the microscope in pond-water, vinegar and all kinds of liquids, there was no reason to suppose that those in the semen were in any essential way connected with generation. For his time, this argument was an

---

[1] His actual words are as follows:

p. 101. "Si l'on verse dans cet œuf (70 hours) ou dans un autre de pareil tems de couvée, du vinaigre distillé, on verra en peu de tems le fœtus blanchir et devenir plus solide et si opaque, qu'on ne sçauroit plus distinguer au travers les vésicules du cœur, ni même les vaisseaux qui y aboutissent, hors celui qui règne le long du corps."

p. 148. "Je dirai enfin que quoiqu'on ne découvre qu'assez obscurément la plûpart des principales parties intérieures, hors le cœur et quelques vaisseaux (144 hours), à cause de leur trop de molesse et de la viscosité de tout le fœtus, elles ne laissent pas que d'avoir déjà quelque forme, comme on le connoîtra en faisant infuser le fœtus dans le vinaigre distilé."

excellent one, and was open to no demur save on the ground of filtration experiments which had not yet been made (see pp. 211–12).

About this time there was some controversy over the circulation of blood, the *foramen ovale*, etc., in the embryo. From 1700 to 1710, Tauvry and de Méry were engaged in a polemic on this subject, and the latter also corresponded with Duverney, Silvestre and Buissière in a controversy which recalls that of Laurentius and Petreus a hundred years before. Nicholls wrote later on the same subject. Daniel Tauvry was interesting, however, for other reasons. He was an epigenesist, and wrote vigorously against the view that the soul constructed during embryogeny a suitable home for itself.

Nine years later two books appeared which form very notable landmarks in the history of embryology. One was Martin Schurig's *Embryologia*, and the other the *Elementa Chemiae* of Hermann Boerhaave.

The former, however, gave to the world no new experiments or observations; it was the first of what we should now call the typical "review" kind of publication. Schurig saw that he was living at the end of a great scientific movement following the Renaissance, and set himself accordingly for many years to compile large treatises on specific physiological subjects, taking care to give all references with meticulous accuracy, and to omit no work, significant or insignificant. His *Spermatologia* was the first to appear (in 1720), and it was followed in 1723 by *Sialologia* (on the saliva), *Chylologia* (1725), *Muliebria* (1729), *Parthenologia* (1729), *Gynaecologia* (1731) and *Haematologia* (1744). His *Embryologia* was the last but one of the series. In it he treated compendiously of all the theories which had been advanced about embryology during the immediately preceding two centuries, and his chapters on foetal nutrition and foetal respiration throw a flood of light on the "intellectual climate" in which Harvey and Mayow worked. Schurig's bibliography is a very striking part of his book, extending to sixteen pages, and including five hundred and sixty references, it was the first attempt of its kind.

3. Chemical and Quantitative Approaches to the Origin of Organisation; Boerhaave, Hamberger and Mazin

Hermann Boerhaave was a more prominent figure, a professor at Leiden for many years, and renowned for his encyclopaedic learning on all subjects remotely connected with medicine. His *Elementa Chemiae*, which became the standard chemical book of the whole period, demonstrates throughout the exceedingly wide outlook of its author, and contains in the second volume what must be regarded as the first detailed account of chemical embryology. I reproduce here the

PLATE XVII

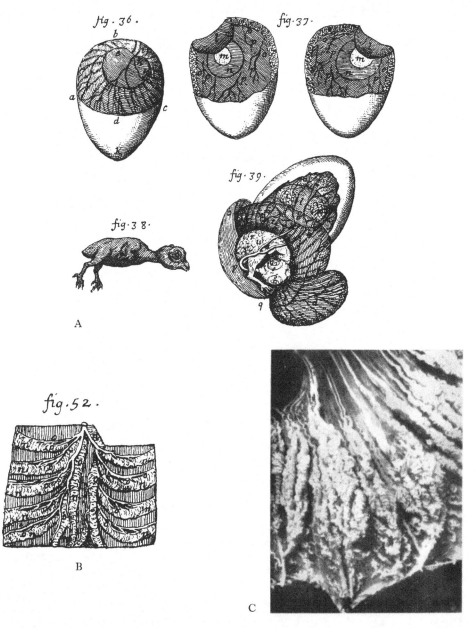

Illustrations from Antoine Maître-Jan's Observations sur la formation du poulet, où les divers changemens qui arrivent à l'œuf à mesure qu'il est couvé, sont exactement expliqués et représentés en Figures. *D'Houry, Paris, 1722.*

A. Drawings of embryos of from 200–250 hours' incubation.
B. The first drawing of the villosities on the interior of the yolk-sac.
(p. 232) "une pièce de la seconde membrane de jaune sur la superficie intérieure de laquelle on voit plusieurs rangées de ces petites vaisseaux entortillées de diverses grandeurs et différemment disposées" [379 hrs.].
C. Photograph of the villosities, from Remotti. They play an important part in the absorption of the yolk.

relevant passages in full because of their great interest. It will be noted that they are cast in the form of lecture addresses, as if they had been taken down direct from the lectures of the professor, a fact which gives them a peculiar charm when it is remembered how many great men must have listened to them, among them Albrecht von Haller and Julien de la Mettrie. In considering what follows, it should be noted that Boerhaave's interest is biological all the time, and that he does not treat the liquids of the egg, as nearly all the chemists before him had done, as substances of curious properties indeed, but quite remote from any question relating to the development of the embryo. Another interesting point is that he deals only with the white, and hardly mentions the yolk; this is perhaps to be explained by the Aristotelian theory[1] that the embryo was formed out of the white, and only nourished by the yolk (*ex albo fieri, ex luteo nutriri*), a theory which was still alive, in spite of Harvey, in the first half of the eighteenth century. If this was what was at the bottom of Boerhaave's mind, then it is obvious that the egg-white would be to him the liquid inhabited more particularly by the plastic force. This, then, is what he has to say about the biochemistry of the egg.

Op. Chem. in Animalia. (Processus 109.) *The albumen of a fresh egg is not acid, nor alkaline, nor does it contain a fermented spirit.* The white of a fresh egg, separated from the shell, the membranes and the yolk, I enclose in clean glass vessels, and into each of these I pour different acids, and shake them up, mixing them, and no sign of ebullition appears however I treat them. Therefore I lay these vessels aside. Now in these other two vessels I have two fresh portions of albumen, and I mix with them in one case alkaline salt and in the other volatile alkali. You see they are quiet without any sign of effervescence. Now behold a remarkable thing, in this tall cylindrical vessel is half an ounce of the albumen of an egg and two drams of spirits of nitre, in this other vessel is half an ounce of egg-white, together with four and a half ounces of oil of tartar *per deliquium* both heated up to 92 degrees. Pray observe and behold, with one movement I pour the alkaline albumen into the acid albumen, with what fury they boil up, into what space they rarefy the mass, so that they stream out of the vessel although it is ten pints in size (*decupli capace*). They have scarcely changed their colour. But when the effervescence has abated how suddenly they return to the limits of space occupied before. But now if more egg-white is heated to 100 degrees in a retort (*cucurbita*) an insipid water containing no spirit is given off. If egg-white is applied to the naked eye or naked nerve it does not give the smallest sense of pain, and scarcely affects the smell; nothing more inert and more insipid can be put on the tongue. It appears mucous and viscid to the touch, not at all penetrable. Hence in the fresh white of an egg there is no alkali or acid, or both together. It is indeed

[1] *Historia*, 561ᵃ 25.

a thick, sticky, inert, and insipid liquor, yet from this truly vital liquid at a heat of 93 degrees within the space of 21 days the chick grows in the incubated egg from a tiny mass hardly weighing a hundredth of a grain into the perfect body of an animal, weighing an ounce or more. We have learnt therefore of a liquid distinct from all others, from which by inscrutable causes fibres, membranes, vessels, entrails, muscles, bones, cartilages, and all the other parts, tendons, ligaments, the beak, the claws, the feathers, and all the humours can be produced—and yet in this liquid we find softness, inertia, absence of acid, alkali, and spirit, and no tendency to effervesce. Indeed, if there were the slightest effervescence in it, it would certainly break the eggshell; therefore we see from how slow and inactive a mass all the solid and fluid parts of the chick are constructed. And yet this itself is rendered absolutely useless for forming the chick by greater heat. It scarcely bears 100 degrees with good effect but at a less temperature never brings forth a chick, for under 80 degrees will not suffice. But by a heat kept between these limits, there is brought about so marvellous an attenuation of the mucous inactivity that it can exhale a great part through the shell of the egg and the two membranes, the yolk and chalazae alone remaining along with the amniotic sac. For the yolk, the uterine placenta of the chick, takes little part in the nourishment. Meanwhile Malpighius has shown that this albumen is not a liquid of a homogeneous kind, as the blood-serum flowing through the vital vessels is, but that it is a structure composed of numerous membrane-like and distinct small saccules, filled with a liquid of their own, in the same way as in the vitreous humour of the eye.

(Processus 111.) *Exploration of the egg-white with alcohol.* In this transparent vessel is the albumen of an egg, and into it, as you perceive, I gently pour the purest alcohol, so that it descends down the sides of the vessel and reaches the albumen. I do this deliberately and with such solicitude that you may see the surface of the albumen which, touching the alcohol, holds it up, being immediately coagulated, while the lower part remains liquid and transparent. As I now gently shake them together, it appears evident that wherever the alcohol touches the albumen a concretion is formed. Behold now, while I shake them up thoroughly together, all the egg-white is coagulated. If alcohol previously warmed is employed in this experiment, the same result is brought about but more rapidly. It appears therefore that the purest vegetable spirits immediately coagulate the plastic and nutrient material.

(Processus 112.) *The fresh albumen of an egg is broken up by distillation.*These fresh eggs have been cooked in pure water till they become hard. I now take the shining white separating off all the other things and break it up into small pieces. I put these, as you see, into a clean glass retort (*cucurbita*) and I duly cover it by fitting on an alembic and add a receiver. By the rules of the [chemical] art I place the whole retort in a bath of water and I apply to it successive degrees of fire until the whole bath is boiling. No vaporous streaks (*striae*) of spirits are given off but simple water in dewy drops and this in incredible quantity, more than nine-tenths. I continue so with patience until by the heat of boiling water no more drops of this humour are given off.

Then this water shows no trace of oil, salt, or spirit; it is perfectly transparent and tasteless, except that it eventually grows rather sour. It is odourless, save that towards the end it gives off a slight smell of burning. It shows absolutely no sign of the presence of any alkali, when I test it in every way, as you can see for yourselves; nor does it reveal any trace of acid, when tried how you will. Here you see pounds of this water, but in the bottom of the now open retort see, I beg of you, how little substance remains. Behold, there are fragments contracted into a very small space in comparison with the former quantity. They are endowed with a golden colour especially where they have touched the glass, but yet they are transparent after the manner of coloured glass. When I take them out I find them very light, very hard, quite fragile, and breaking apart with a crack, smelling slightly of empyreuma, with a taste rather bitter from the fire, and without any flavour of alkali or acid. This is the first part of the analysis. Now I take these remaining fragments in a glass retort (*retortam*) in such a way that two-thirds remain over. I put the retort into a stove of sand, first arranging a large receiver. Then thoroughly luting all the joints I distil by successive grades of fire and finally by the highest which I call *suppressionis*. There ascends a spirit, running in streaks [*striatim*] fat and oily, and at the same time, volatile salts of solid form everywhere on the walls of the vessel, rather plentiful in proportion to the dried fragments but small in proportion to the whole albumen before the water had been removed from it. Finally an oil appears besides the light golden material mixed with the first, black, thick, and pitchy. When by the extreme force of the fire this oil is finally driven forth, then the earth in the bottom, closely united with its most tenacious oil, swells up and is rarefied and rises right up to the neck of the retort so that had the retort been overfull it would have entered into the neck and clogged it up even causing it to burst with danger to the bystanders. The operation is to be continued till no more comes out. That first spirit, oily and fatty, is clearly alkaline by every test, as you may tell from the way it effervesces when acid is poured on it. If we rectify it we resolve it into an alkaline volatile salt, an oil, and inert foetid water. The salt fixed to the walls is completely alkaline, sharp, fiery, oily, and volatile; and the final oil is specially sharp, caustic, and foetid. The black earth which remains in the retort is shiny, light, thin, and fragile, foetid from the final empyreumatic oil, and soft because of it. If then it is burnt on an open fire, it leaves a little fixed earth which is white, insipid, tasteless, and odourless, from which scarcely any salt can be extracted, but only a very heavy dusty powder (*pollinem*).[1]

(Processus 113.) *The fresh albumen of an Egg will putrefy.* Sound eggs kept at 70° for some days will become foetid and stink. . . . We have learnt then that this is the nature of the material which will shortly be changed into the structure, form, and all the parts of the animal body. Repose and a certain degree of heat produce that effect in that material. We observe therefore the spontaneous corruption and change of the material, and what is extremely remarkable, if an impregnated egg is warmed in an oven (*in hypocaustis*) to a

[1] Cf. the dry distillation of egg-white by Pictet & Cramer in 1919.

heat of 92 degrees it employs these attenuated parts changed by such a heat to nourish, increase, and complete the chick for 21 days. But in this chick nothing alkaline, foetid, or putrid is found, hence observe, O doctors (*medici*) the remarkable manifestations of Nature—by repose and a certain degree of heat a thick substance becomes thin, a viscous substance becomes liquid, an odourless substance becomes foetid, an insipid substance becomes sour and extremely acrid and bitter to the taste, a soothing substance becomes caustic, a non-alkali becomes alkaline, a latent oil becomes sweet and putrid. Let these results be compared with the observations of Marcellus Malpighius on the incubated egg, and we shall observe things which shall surprise us. I took care to investigate only the albumen of the egg first of all, separating the other parts off where possible, for the albumen alone forms the whole of the material which proceeds to feed (*in pabulum*) the embryo. The other constituents of the egg only assist in changing the albumen, so that when it is changed, it may be applied to forming the structure of the chick.

Boerhaave's treatment of these subjects has only to be compared with that of Joachim Beccher, who wrote in 1703, to show how thoroughly modern in outlook it is. Beccher's *Physica Subterranea* contains a whole section devoted to the growth of the embryo, but it is extremely confused and very alchemical in its details.[1] The advance made in the thirty years between Beccher and Boerhaave was immense, but, if the biochemistry of development advanced so fast, its biophysics was not far behind, as is shown by the work of G. E. Hamberger and J. B. Mazin.

Hamberger's most important contributions, contained in his *Physiologia Medica* of 1751, were his quantitative observations on the water-content of the embryo and its growth-rate, in which he had no forerunners. Hamberger showed

that there are much less solid parts in the foetus than in the adult. The cortical substance of the brain of an embryo loses 8694 parts in 10,000 on drying but in the adult it only loses 8096 and that of the cerebellum from 81 parts is reduced to 12. The maxillary glands of the embryo lose out of 10,000 parts 8469, the liver 8047, the pancreas 7863, the arteries 8278 and even the cartilages lose four-fifths of their weight decreasing from 10,000 to 8149½.

The corresponding figures for the adult were: liver 7192, and heart 7836. These figures do not widely differ from those obtained in recent times.

J. B. Mazin published his *Conjecturae physico-medico-hydrostaticae de Respiratione Foetus* in 1737 and his *Tractatus Medico-mechanica* in 1742. In the first of these works Mazin supports what is essentially Mayow's theory of embryonic respiration, without, however, mentioning Mayow more than once. It had not been popular since 1700, though Pitcairn

[1] Bk. 1, sect. iv, ch. 4, p. 207, "De mixtione animali."

had defended it. Mazin put the liquids of eggs under an air-pump, and observing that air could be extracted from them affirmed that the air was hidden in them and that the embryo could therefore respire. He spoke of "aerial particles" in the amniotic liquid, and discussed the respiration of fishes in connection with this. The specific gravity of the embryo also interested him, and he did a great deal of calculation and experiment on it. His most interesting passage, perhaps, is that in which he mentions the "eolipile" of the Alexandrians, the primitive form of the steam-engine, and says that just as the heat of the fire makes the water boil, so the heat of the viscera makes the amniotic liquid boil, giving off respirable vapours. The time-relations of this analogy are interesting, for by 1712 Thomas Newcomen had succeeded in making a steam-engine which worked with considerable precision, and the question of steam-power was widely discussed. Possibly Mazin was acquainted with the Marquis of Worcester's *Century of the Names and Scantlings of Inventions*, which had been published in 1663, and which had contained an aeolipile or "water-commanding machine." England was the centre of this movement and other countries employed Englishmen as engineers; Humphrey Potter, for instance, erected a steam-engine for pumping at a Hungarian mine in 1720.

As for the discovery of oxygen, it was near at hand, and Scheele in 1773 and Priestley in 1774 were soon to supply the knowledge without which Mazin could not proceed further.

In his second book, Mazin reported many quantitative observations on the specific gravity of the embryo. He found that it diminished as development proceeded, being to the amniotic liquid as 282 to 274 in the fourth month and as 504 to 494 in the fifth month. His work on this subject was continued by Joseph Onymos, whose *De Natura Foetus* appeared in 1745.

R. J. Raisin also contributed to this wave of precise measurement in embryology. His dissertation of 1753 took account of the difference between the pulse rates of infants and adults, and contained an arithmetical argument about the prenatal secretion of the foetal kidneys. But it also gave a list of the relative weights of organs, showing that some decreased and others increased relatively to the weight of the body as a whole. Thus the brain was one-tenth part of the body in the foetus and one-twenty-fifth part in the adult (see Table II, overleaf). It was the first mention of heterauxetic growth,[1] save for the isolated observations of Leonardo (see p. 98).

About this time, we get occasional references to the obscure mechanisms controlling animal growth. Although the brilliant speculations of Marci (see p. 81) had long been forgotten, some writers, such as

TABLE II

	Fetus	Adultus
Cerebrum .	1/10	1/25
Pulmo .	1/66	1/17
Thymus .	1/324	1/4560
Cor .	1/189	1/114
Hepar .	1/23	1/21
Lien .	1/324	1/175
Pancreas .	1/907	1/445
Ventriculus vacuus .	1/767	1/212
Renes .	1/154	1/136
Surrenales glandulae .	1/324	1/3040

James Parsons, were groping about for the morphogenetic controls. In his *Philosophical Observations* of 1752 Parsons had a good deal to say about "primary" and "subordinate organisations," notions which have a certain resemblance to the field theories of modern embryology, for a short account of which the article of Waddington may be consulted. Parsons said of his organisations:

There can be no more natural Way of answering a Question proposed by a Gentleman of Penetration in Philosophical Knowledge, which is Why do not Animals and Vegetables grow on without End? Why do not Seeds, when they are perfectly form'd, grow on in their Pods, Husks, or other Receptacles? Because, says he, when a Body has once begun to grow, the same Propensity for growing on ought still to continue, and, the Particles of Matter increasing too, it ought not to cease.

The answer of Parsons was that the organisation comes to "its full Power of Distention, so far as is consistent with its natural Form," after which further nourishment becomes useless and the structures all rigidify.[2] Parsons was on the verge of a field theory, for he gave much consideration to the regeneration experiments carried out by Trembley and others on fresh-water coelenterates (cf. Baker). But he did not develop his idea far enough to escape the objection that the "organisations" were mere abstract simulacra of the visible forms of the animals and plants themselves. For the rest, he was a convinced ovist, accepting Nuck's experiment (see p. 163) in the wrong sense (contrast with Massuet, see comment on p. 209), and desirous of explaining all generation as budding or "propagation." Like Galen long before him, he conducted a lively polemic against all formulations of the *vis plastica*, but in favour, unfortunately, of the direct action of God. In the successive action of his primary and secondary organisations, however, we

---

[1] The classical modern treatment of the relative growth-rates of parts of organisms is of course that of Huxley.
[2] Pp. 94 ff.

approach rather closely the modern conception of a succession of organisers or inductors in development (see Aristotle's ideas on this, p. 48 passim, and the references to modern embryology there given).

These writers, together with Haller himself and J. C. Heffter, who handled the problem of embryonic growth rate, contribute to one of the best, because most quantitative, aspects of eighteenth-century embryology.

4. Albrecht von Haller and the Rise of Techniques

Boerhaave's greatest pupil was Albrecht von Haller.[1] Like Oliver Wendell Holmes at Harvard, Haller occupied a "settee" rather than a "chair" at Göttingen, and taught not only physiology but also medicine and surgery, botany, anatomy and pharmacology as well. Nor did he merely deal with so many subjects superficially; in each case he published what amounted to the best and most complete text-book up to then written. Haller was made professor in 1736, and for many years worked at Göttingen, devoting much of his time to embryological researches, which, with those of his opponent Wolff, stand out as the greatest between Malpighi and von Baer. In 1750 he published a series of dissertations and short papers on all kinds of physiological subjects, which would have been the direct ancestors of the modern compilations by groups of experts, had they been more systematically arranged. The volume on generation repays some study. The contributions relevant to the present discussion had been written at various times during the previous seventy years, and may be summarised selectively as follows:

IV. Christopher Sturmius, *De plantarum animaliumque Generatione* (first published 1687). In this paper Sturmius argues on behalf of the preformation theory, "which in our times does not lack supporters," quoting Perrault, Harvey and Descartes. He contents himself with countering arguments which had been urged against it, as, (*a*) spontaneous generation, (*b*) annual recurrence of plants, (*c*) insect metamorphosis, (*d*) generation without copulation.

V. Rudolf Jacob Camerarius,[2] *Specimen Experimentorum physiologico-therapeuticorum circa Generationem hominis et animalium.* The most interesting thing about this is that Camerarius mentions the observations of D. Seiller, a sculptor, who had ascertained that the body is five times the size of the head in the embryo but seven and a half times the size of it in the adult. This is in the direct line between Leonardo and Scammon.

XV. Philip Gravel, *De Superfœtatione* (first published 1738).

[1] See d'Irsay.
[2] Afterwards famous as the discoverer of sexuality in plants.

XVIII. Adam Brendel, *De Embryone in ovulo ante conceptum prae-existante* (first published 1703). Brendel "stands for the Graafian hypothesis." Unfortunately, he was also a preformationist and believed that every limb, organ and function existed not potentially but actually in the unfertilised egg before its passage down the Fallopian tube.

XXII. Camillus Falconnet, *Non est fetui Sanguis Maternus alimento* (first published 1711). This is the first of the French contributions to the book; they are all very markedly shorter than the German ones and much less heavily ornamented with irrelevant quotations. Falconnet is concerned to prove that the maternal and foetal circulations are separate, and he describes in an admirably concise manner an experiment in which he bled a female dog to death, after which, opening the uterus, he discovered that the embryonic blood-vessels were full of blood although those of the mother had none in at all. Arantius was therefore justified. Falconnet was soon confirmed by Nunn.

XXIII. Jean de Diest's *Sui Sanguinis solus opifex Fetus est* (first published 1735) was written to prove a similar point. He refers to the experiment of Falconnet and the injections of F. Hoffmann, and criticises Cowper's experiment in which mercury had been injected into the umbilical vessels and found in the maternal circulation, on the grounds that mercury is so "tenuous and voluble" that it might pass where blood could not pass normally. He also objects to the view that the foetus is nourished by the amniotic liquid.

XXIV. Francis David Herissant, *Secundinae fetui Pulmonis praestant officia, et sanguine materno Fetus non alitur* (first published in 1741). An excellent paper in which the respiratory function of the placenta is proved by the observation that the foetal blood-vessel leading to the placenta is always full of dark venous blood, while that leading away from the placenta is light and arterial (*floridiori coccineoque colore, ut ipsemet observavi*). Herissant adduces also the cases of acephalic monsters, such as that of Brady, which could not possibly have drunk up any amniotic fluid, and yet were fully formed in all other respects. He concludes that the umbilical cord serves for respiration and nutrition.

XXV. After these three French workers, there is a great drop to Johannes Zeller, whose *Infanticidas non absolvit nec a tortura liberat Pulmonum Infantis in aqua subsidentia* (first published 1691) is a long-winded discussion of the floating lung test in forensic medicine. His memory deserves a word of obloquy for his vigorous insistence upon death and torture for infanticide even during puerperal insanity. Perhaps it was Zeller who called forth the noble answer of de la Mettrie to this inhumanity in his *Man a Machine*.[1]

XXVI. Zeller's *De Vita humana ex Fune pendente* (first published 1692) is no

[1] For a detailed historical account of this test and its unreliability, see Krammer.

better, though at the time, perhaps because of its striking title, it was famous. It deals with the ligation of the umbilical cord at birth.

Such were some of the typical papers printed by Haller in his 1750 collection. He retired from the Göttingen chair three years later, and in 1757 the first volume of his *Elementa Physiologiae* was published, probably the greatest text-book of physiology ever written. It appeared only by slow degrees, so that it was not until 1766 that the embryological section was available. This volume contains a discussion of a mass of literature, most of which had arisen during the preceding twenty-five years, for although many of the names mentioned by Haller occur also in Schurig, many are quite new.

Haller himself published in 1767 a volume of his collected papers on embryology, most of which were concerned with the developing heart of the chick, which he worked out very thoroughly, in collaboration with Kuhlemann. Kuhlemann had already shown in the sheep what Harvey had proved for the doe. But Haller was a convinced preformationist, a fact which was largely due to his researches on the hen's egg, where he observed that the yolk had a much more intimate connection with the embryo than had previously been supposed. Since the whole yolk was part of the embryo, as it were, the preformation theory seemed to him to fit the facts better than epigenesis.[1]

Haller went further than Schurig in that he usually gave an opinion of his own after summarising those of other people, but his views were by no means always enlightened, and the atmosphere of Buffon is, on the whole, more congenial to us than that of Haller. Haller, for example, believed that the amniotic liquid had nutritious properties, and that the nutrition of the embryo in mammalia was accomplished first of all *per os* and afterwards *per umbilicum*. He denied that the placenta had any respiratory function, and indeed his whole teaching on respiration was retrograde. He mentions, however, an experiment of Nicolas Lemery's, in which it had been found that indigo would penetrate the shell of a developing hen's egg from the outside. Consequently, air might do so too, and Vallisneri had shown that, if an egg was placed in boiled water under an air-pump, the air inside would rush out through the shell and appear in the form of bubbles.

Haller was much more progressive in holding the origin of the amniotic liquid (according to him a subject of extraordinary difficulty—*solutionem non promittam*) to be a transudation from the maternal blood-vessels. He followed Noortwyck in asserting the separateness of the maternal and foetal circulations in mammalia. He opposed the

---

[1] See pp. 198-9.

DIES.	TIBIA.	FEMUR.	PARS OSSEA TIBIÆ.	PARS OSSEA FEMORIS.	CUBUS TIBIÆ.	CUBUS FEMORIS.
Sextus.		8				512
Septimus	$10\frac{7}{10}$	$8\frac{1}{2}$	0	0	$1224\frac{445}{1000}$	$614\frac{1}{8}$
Octavus	20	14	0	0	8000	2744
Nonus	24.prox.	18.prox.	10		13824	5832
Decimus	30	$22\frac{2}{7}$			27000	10161
Undecimus	$41\frac{2}{3}$	$31\frac{5}{3}$	11	7	72301	29791
Duodecimus	$43\frac{1}{3}$	$32\frac{5}{3}$	$17\frac{1}{2}$	$12\frac{1}{2}$	80624.prox.	30568
Decimus Tertius	48	37	30	24	110592	50653
Decimus Quartus	55.prox	44. prox.	43. prox.	30. prox.	166375	85284
Decimus Quintus	79	50			500149	125000
Decimus Sextus	82*	$63\frac{2}{7}$	39**	29	551368	257505
Decimus Septimus	$91\frac{1}{2}$	$67\frac{1}{2}$	73	48	766061	320047
Decimus Octavus	$100\frac{5}{2}$	$72\frac{1}{2}$	74	53	1017575	378040
Decimus Nonus	103	$75\frac{1}{2}$	70	52	1098712	446675
Vigesimus	$110\frac{1}{2}$	$78\frac{1}{2}$	75	60	1324260	483736
Vigesimus Primus	113	83			1422897	571787
Vigesimus Secundus	$117\frac{2}{3}$	$83\frac{1}{3}$	100	72	1628406	576381

Fig. 21. Facsimile of a table in A. von Haller's "Elementa Physiologiae" of 1766, containing some of his observations on the growth in length and weight of embryonic bones in the chick.

existence of eggs in Vivipara—"We may conclude from all this," he said, "that the ovarian vesicles are not eggs and that they do not contain the rudiments of the animal." But he accepted it in the restricted sense that the embryonic membranes resembled an egg, thus:

If we call an egg a hollow membranous pocket full of a humour in which the embryo swims, we may admit the opinion of the older authors who derive all animals from eggs with the exception of the tiny simple animals of which we have already spoken. It was in this sense that Aristotle and Empedocles before him, said that even trees were oviparous. This has also been confirmed by the experiments of Harvey on insects, fishes, birds, and quadrupeds.

Haller's most original work was in connection with the growth-rate of the embryo; here he struck out, for once, into entirely new country. He made a beginning with the quantitative description of embryonic growth, and one of his tables showing the changing lengths of the bones is reproduced herewith (Fig. 21). He wrote:

The growth of the embryo in the uterus of the mother is almost unbelievably rapid. We do not know what its size is at the moment of its formation, but it is certainly so small that it cannot be seen even with the aid of the best microscopes, and it reaches in nine months the weight of ten or twelve pounds. In order to clear up this speculation, let us examine the growth of the chick in the egg. In this case again we are unable to measure its size at the moment when the egg is put to incubate but it cannot be more than $\frac{4}{100}$ in. long, for if it were, it would be visible, and yet 25 days later it is 4 ins. long. Its relation is therefore as 64 to 64 millions or 1 to 1 million. This growth takes place in a singular manner; it is very rapid in the beginning and continually diminishes in speed. The growth on the first day is from 1 to $91\frac{1}{8}$, and what Swammerdam calls a worm grows in one day from one twentieth or one thirtieth of a grain to seven grains, i.e. it increases its weight by 140 to 240 times. On the second day the growth of the chick is from 1 to 5, on the third day, from 1 to not quite 4, on the fifth day from 1 to something less than 3. Then from the sixth to the twelfth day, the growth each day is hardly from 4 to 5, and on the twentyfirst day it is about from 5 to 6. After the chick has hatched, it grows each day for the first 40 days at an approximately constant rate, from 20 to 21 on each day. The increase of the first twentyfour hours is therefore in relation to that of the last as $546\frac{3}{4}$ to 5 or 145 to 1. Now as the total increase in weight in the egg is to that of the whole growth period (up to the adult) as 2 to 24 ozs. all the post-embryonic growth is as 1 to 12, i.e. it is to the growth of one day alone early in incubation as 1 to $7\frac{1}{2}$.... The growth of man, like that of the chick, decreases in rapidity as it advances. Let us suppose that a man, at the instant of conception, weighs a hundred-thousandth of a grain and that a one-month-old embryo weighs 30 grains; then the man will have acquired in that time more than 300,000 times the weight that he had to begin with. But if a foetus of the second month weighs 3 ozs. as it approximately does, he will only now have acquired 48 times the weight he had at the beginning of the period. This is a prodigious decrease in speed, and at the end of the ninth month he will not weigh more than about 105 ozs. which is not more than an average increase of 15 per month. A child three years old is about half the size of an adult. If then the adult weighs 2250 ozs. the three-year old child only weighs 281 ozs. which is an eighth of the adult weight. Now from birth to 3 years he will grow from 105 to 281 or as 5 to 14, but in the following 22 years he will only accumulate 2250 ozs. or eight times what he had at 3 years. The growth of a man will therefore be in the first month of intra-uterine life as 1 to 300,000, in the second as 1 to 48, in each of the others as 1 to 15. In the first 3 years of extra-uterine life his growth will be from 164 to 281 and in the succeeding 22 years from 281 to 384, and the growth of the first month to the last will be as 300,000 to $\frac{28}{456}$ or 136,800,000 to 28, or 4,885,717 to 1. The whole growth of man will consequently be as 108,000,000 to 1.

In spite of the rather unfamiliar language in which these facts are described, and the theory of the growth of the heart which Haller subsequently put forth to explain them, they remain fundamental to embryology. Their quantitative tone is indeed remarkably modern. In my opinion, when all the voluminous writings of Haller are carefully searched through, nothing more progressive and valuable than these figures can be found. Haller and Hamberger stand thus between Leonardo on the one hand and Minot and Brody on the other. That they stood so much alone is only another indication of the extraordinary reluctance with which the men of past generations assented to the truth contained in Robert Mayer's immortal words, "Eine einzige Zahl hat mehr wahren und bleibenden Wert als eine kostbare Bibliothek von Hypothesen."[1]

Of development as a whole, Haller spoke thus,

In the body of the animal therefore, no part is made before any other part, but all are formed at the same time. If certain authors have said that the animal begins to be formed by the backbone, by the brain, or by the heart, if Galen taught that it was the liver which was first formed, if others have said that it was the belly and the head, or the spinal marrow with the brain, adding that these parts make others in turn; I think that all these authors only meant that the heart and the brain or whatever organ it was, were visible when none of the other parts yet were, and that certain parts of the embryonic body are well enough developed in the first few days to be seen while others are not so until the latter part of development; and others again not till after birth, such as the beard in man, the antlers in the stag, the breasts and the second set of teeth. If Harvey thought he descried an epigenetic development, it was because he saw first a little cloud, then the rudiments of the head, with

[1] *Kleinere Schriften und Briefe*, p. 226.

the eyes bigger than the whole body, and little by little viscera being formed. If one compares his description with mine, one will see that his description of the development of the deer corresponds exactly with mine of the development of the chick. If more than twenty years ago, before I had made many observations upon eggs and the females of quadrupeds, I employed this reasoning to prove that there is a great difference between the foetus and the perfect animal, and if I said that in the animal at the moment of conception one does not find the same parts as in the perfect animal, I have realised abundantly since then that all I said against preformation really went to support it.

The reasons for this change of opinion are not clearly given in Haller's writings, and Dareste concluded that it would always remain a mystery.

This mystery has, however, been almost completely elucidated by F. J. Cole. In 1744 Haller was certainly an epigenesist,[1] in 1758 undoubtedly a preformationist; in the intervening period he had made his own embryological researches. How was it that they had the unfortunate effect of carrying him further from the truth rather than towards it?

In Cole's words:[2]

The yolk, Haller asserts, is the continuation of the intestine of the embryo chick. The inner membrane of the yolk is continuous with the inner membrane of the intestine, and is thus identical with the inner membrane of the gut generally and the skin and the ectoderm. The external membrane of the yolk is an extension of the external membrane of the intestine, and is hence continuous with the mesentery and peritoneum. The envelope which covers the yolk during the last ten days of development is the skin of the foetus. Therefore it is no absurdity to say that from the beginning, and before fertilisation, the intestine of the foetus is no more than a small hernia of the membrane of the yolk. Now if the yolk is continuous with the skin and intestine of the foetus it must be contemporaneous with it, and is truly a part of the foetus. But the yolk was present in the abdomen of the hen, and was a part of the hen, independently of any congress with the cock. Hence the foetus, enclosed in the amnion, must have existed at the same time, though invisible on account of its smallness and transparency.

It is not difficult, with the aid of Fig. 22, to follow Haller's argument. The "inner membrane of the yolk" is the endoderm, which it is true does become continuous with the skin and epidermis *after* the gut cavity has been completed. The "external membrane of the yolk" is the splanchnic mesoderm, and the "envelope which covers the yolk during the last days of incubation" is the allanto-chorion, which, however, is *not* the skin of the foetus. Haller's procedure is typical of the time, in which observation and inference had only the remotest relations with one another. For example, the statements "Now if the yolk is continuous with the skin and the intestine of the foetus, it must

[1] See his notes on Boerhaave's *Praelectiones*, vol. 5, pt. II, pp. 497 ff. (1744 ed.).
[2] *Early Theories . . .*, p. 88.

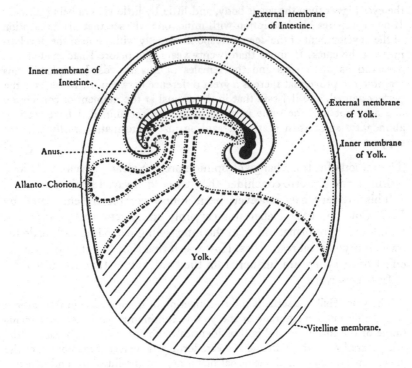

Fig. 22. Diagram of the membranes of the chick embryo, to illustrate Haller's arguments (from F. J. Cole).

be contemporaneous with it" and "the yolk must have arteries and veins as without them it could not have been brought into existence" are pure assumptions, and beg the very question he has set out to prove. If these assumptions can be shown to be baseless, as they are, the whole argument collapses.

In a word then, Haller confused the vitelline membrane with the yolk-sac, and assumed *a priori* that foldings, outgrowths, etc., of cell-layers could not take place, i.e. that epigenetic processes did not exist. Substantially the same argument as Haller's had been used some twenty years before (in 1722) by Maître-Jan, according to Cole.

The *emboîtement* aspect of preformation presented no difficulties to Haller. Speaking of the generation of *Volvox*, he said,

It follows that the ovary of an ancestress will contain not only her daughter but also her granddaughter, her greatgranddaughter and her greatgreat-granddaughter, and if it is once proved that an ovary can contain many generations, there is no absurdity in saying that it contains them all.

The following passage is interesting.

We must proceed to say what is the efficient cause of the beautiful machine which we call an animal. First of all let us not attribute it to chance, as Ofrai[1] would have us do, for although he pretends that all animals come from earth, he is not attached to the ancient opinion, and nobody now believes what Aelian says, namely that frogs are born from mud. . . . Vallisneri has found the fathers and mothers of the little worms in galls, a quest of which Redi despaired, and Redi[2] in his turn has made with exactitude and precision those experiments which Bonannus, Triumphet, and Honoratus Faber had only sketched out imperfectly. Moreover, no seed, no clover. . . . This was the received opinion but in our century a proscribed notion has been revivified and some great men have pretended that there are little animals which are engendered by an equivocal generation, without father and mother, and that all the viscera and all the parts of these animals do not exist together, but that the nobler parts are formed first by epigenesis and that then the others are formed little by little afterwards.

This is an admirable illustration of how the ideas of spontaneous generation and of epigenesis were bound up together. Haller goes on to say:

M. Needham does not admit an equivocal generation but he does admit epigenesis, and a corporeal non-intelligent force, which constructs a body from a tiny little germ furnishing the necessary matter for it. He says that there are only the primitive germs which were made at the original creation and that germs organised like animals do by no means pre-exist, for if they did, *molae uterinae*, encysted tumours, and the like, could not come into being.

Haller then goes on to describe Needham's experiments with meat broths, etc., and objects to his "system," largely on the ground that "blind forces without any intelligence, could hardly be able to form animals for ends foreseen and ready to take their places in the scheme of beings." He considers that Needham's theories are completely disproved by experiments such as those of Spallanzani, though, curiously enough, he does not quote the latter author in this connection. I shall return to this later (p. 211). He continues,

Nobody has upheld epigenesis more than M. Wolff, who has undertaken an examination to demonstrate that plants and animals are formed without a mould out of matter by a certain constant force which he calls "essential" (in his *Theoria Generationis*). . . . I have indeed seen many of the phenomena which he describes, and it is certain that the heart seems to be formed out of

[1] Is this not Julien Offray de la Mettrie? Haller had a habit of using Christian names, e.g. Turberville for J. T. Needham.
[2] See R. Cole.

a congealed humour and that the whole animal appears to have the same consistency. But it does not follow that because this primitive glue which is to take on the shape of the animal does not appear to possess its structure and all its parts, that it has not effectively got them. I have often given greater solidity to this jelly by the use merely of spirits of wine and by this means I saw that what had appeared to me to be a homogeneous jelly was composed of fibres, vessels, and viscera. Now surely nobody will say that the *vis essentialis* of the spirit of wine gave an organic structure to an unformed matter, on the contrary it is rather in the removal of transparency and the accession of greater firmness to the extremities, as well as the making of a more obvious boundary to the contour of a viscus that one could see the structure of a cellular tissue, which was ready to be formed but which the transparency had previously hidden and the wetness not allowed to be circumscribed by lines. . . . Finally, to cut a long story short, why does this *vis essentialis*, which is one only, form always and in the same places the parts of an animal which are so different, and always upon the same model, if inorganic matter is susceptible of changes and is capable of taking all sorts of forms? Why should the material coming from a hen always give rise to a chicken, and that from a peacock give rise to a peacock? To these questions no answer is given.

This was the case because Wolff was not a theorist, but rather an experimentalist; his writings are marked by their abstention from the discussion of speculative points. The above passage is very interesting. It reminds us of the great difficulties with which the embryologists of this epoch had to contend. Serial section cutting was unknown, the staining of thin layers and reconstruction were unheard of; even the hardening of the soft embryonic tissues was only just discovered, as is indicated by Haller above. Hertwig has excellently discussed[1] the advances in embryological technique which took place during this and the following century. It is true that dyes were beginning to be used, as some instances already given demonstrate, and as is seen from the use of madder in the staining of bones, which began about this time, and was later much used by the Hunters. Hertodt's *Crocologia* is important in this connection. Hertodt, by injecting saffron into the maternal circulation, found it afterwards in the amniotic fluid,[2] and his experiment was cited by Haller in support of that theory of the origin of the liquid. But the most important advance in technique was the progress in artificial incubation. The art, though lost throughout the Middle Ages and the seventeenth century, was now to be revived.

During this period much work was done on it. As far back as 1600, de Serres had mentioned some experiments of this nature, but they were not successful.[3] "The chicks," he said, "were usually born deformed,

[1] And more recently Oppenheimer.   [2] Quaestio IV, p. 278.   [3] Bk. v, ch. 2.

202

defective or having too many legs, wings, or heads, nature being inimitable by art." Birch, in his *History of the Royal Society*, speaks similarly.[1] "Sir Christopher Heydon [a relative of Digby's Sir John?] together with Drebell, long since in the Minories hatched several hundred eggs but it had this effect, that most of the chickens produced that way were lame and defective in some part or other." Antonelli states that similar trials were made at the court of the Grand-Duke Ferdinand II at Florence about 1644, while Poggendorff and Antinori relate that the Accademia d. Cimento, inspired by Paolo del Buono, made trial of artificial incubation between 1651 and 1667.

But the most famous of all the attempts to make artificial as successful as natural incubation were those of de Réaumur, whose book *De l'art de faire éclore les Poulets* of 1749 achieved a wide renown. He devotes many chapters to a detailed description of incubators of very various kinds (see Plate XVIII, facing page 204): but he nowhere gives any indication of his percentage hatch. It was probably low. He speaks also of the "funestes effets" of the vapours of the dung on the developing embryos, without, however, furnishing any foundation for an exact teratology. In the second volume he describes those experiments on the preservation of eggs by varnish which caught the imagination of Maupertuis and were held up to an immortal but by no means deserved ridicule by Voltaire in his *Akakia*. For the details of this amusing but irrelevant issue, see Miall and Lytton Strachey.

After de Réaumur, there were numerous continuations of the work which he had started, in particular by Thévenot, La Boulaye, Nelli, Porta and Cedernhielm. Much the most interesting of these was the work of Beguelin, who attempted to incubate eggs with part of the shell removed so as to form a round window. He was not, however, successful in the carrying out of this very modern idea. Probably the most peculiar investigation made on developing eggs at this time was that of Achard, who is mentioned in a passage of Bonnet's.

M. de Réaumur did not suspect in 1749 that some day one would try to substitute the action of the electric fluid for his borrowed heat. This beautiful invention was reserved for M. Achard of the Prussian Academy who excels as an experimentalist. He has not so far succeeded in actually hatching a chick by means of so new a process, but he has had one develop up to the eighth day, when an unfortunate accident deranged his electrical apparatus.

Bonnet goes on to say that this substitution of electricity for heat gives him hope that by electrical means an artificial fertilisation will one day become possible.

[1] Vol. 3, p. 455.

References to these experiments and to those of many minor investigators will be found in Haller. By the beginning of the nineteenth century a great mass of literature had developed on the subject, and it had become possible to hatch out eggs more or less successfully from furnaces, though the losses were still great. Early in the nineteenth century Bonnemain and Jouard referred to the large number of monsters produced, and in 1809 Paris wrote,

During the period that I was at College, the late Sir Busick Harwood, the ingenious Professor of Anatomy in the University of Cambridge, frequently attempted to develope eggs by the heat of his hotbed, but he only raised monsters, a result which he attributed to the unsteady application of the heat.[1]

5. Embryos and Theologians

This is the most convenient place to mention theological embryology again. See pp. 22, 65–6, 75. Its place in the eighteenth century was small, and in the nineteenth, with the general recognition that whatever the soul might be it was not a phenomenon, it altogether disappeared from serious general discussion. F. E. Cangiamila's *Embryologia Sacra*, however, ran through several editions between 1700 and 1775. Cagniamila or Cangiamila[2] (*Panorm. Eccl. Can. Theol. et in toto Sicil. Regno contra haereticam pravitatem Inquisitore Provinciali*) deals very fully with the time of animation, quoting a host of writers such as St Gelasius, St Anselm, Hugh of St Victor and Pico della Mirandola. His mind retains a quite mediaeval conformation, as the following curious passage illustrates: *Quot non foetus abortivos ex ignorantia obstetricum et matrum excipit latrina, quorum anima, si Baptismate non fraudaretur, Deum in aeternam videret, esset decentius tumulandum!* His instructions for the baptism of

[1] *Observations*, p. 366.
[2] Cangiamila, whose strange personality has recently been sympathetically reviewed by Hutchinson and by Boldrini, deserves a little biographical notice. Born at Palermo in 1702, he became Archpriest at Girgenti in 1731 and had the distinction of baptising the first infant delivered by Caesarean section in Sicily. He was lecturer at Palermo in 1742 and Vicar-General and provincial Inquisitor in 1755. His *Embryologia Sacra* was a best-seller (see Bibliography) and was even translated into modern Greek for the benefit of those Orthodox who desired to study the lengths to which Reason and the Latin mind could go. Cangiamila's main formula was conditional; *Si tu es capax, ego te baptizo* (even to the amnion). His anxiety to baptise the embryo led him to the advocacy of frequent Caesarean section both on the living and the dead. Two centuries earlier theology had been more modest, and the Roman *Rituale* of 1584 contented itself with an edifying *De Benedictione foetus in utero matris*. Nevertheless the condemnation of the unbaptised infant to eternal torment goes back to a very early stage of Latin theology and is deeply embedded in the teaching of Councils, saints and popes, as has been learnedly shown by Coulton in his study of Infant Perdition. The doctrine does humanity no credit.
Jewish thought on this subject has an echo in Cohen's book on the Talmud (p. 392), Byzantine in the paper of Stur.
Current speculation regarding the ethics of foeticide may be found in Arendt; Glenn; and Hughes.

PLATE XVIII

De Réaumur's illustration of his Incubators (from De l'art de faire éclore les poulets, 1749).

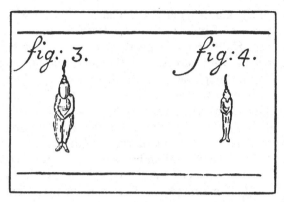

Fig. 23. Dalenpatius' drawings of human spermatozoa (from Leeuwenhoek).

monsters are also very odd. But theological embryology probably reached its climax in the report of the doctors of divinity at the Sorbonne on March 30, 1733, in which intra-uterine baptism by means of a syringe was solemnly recommended. This is included in Deventer's book,[1] and has been referred to by Sterne and Spencer. For other aspects of these tracts of thought, see Nicholls and his anonymous antagonist. But Cangiamila and his colleagues—Gerike, Kaltschmied, etc.—are only of decorative importance to our present theme, and for fuller information regarding them, reference must be made to the treatise of Witkowski.[2] It is interesting to note that as late as 1913, 182 days was fixed as "perfection-time," whatever that may be, by Moriani.

6. Ovism and Animalculism

We must now return to the beginning of the century in order to pick up the thread of the main trend of thought. By 1720 the theory of preformation was thoroughly established, not only on the erroneous grounds put forward by Malpighi and Swammerdam, but on the experiments of Andry, Dalenpatius[3] and Gautier, who all asserted that they had seen exceedingly minute forms of men, with arms, heads and legs complete, inside the spermatozoa under the microscope.[4] Gautier went so far as to say that he had seen a microscopic horse in the semen of a

[1] *Histoire des Accouchements*, pp. 133 ff.
[2] Cf. the discussion on Cleopatra (p. 65). It is of interest that prenatal baptism, even including the use of syringes, to this day forms part of official Latin theology at any rate in the Church of France (Ortolan). In literature, we catch an echo of these controversies in the essay of Donne (1633), "That virginity is a Vertue."
[3] Dalenpatius' drawings, reproduced from Leeuwenhoek in Fig. 23, were almost certainly a hoax; see F. J. Cole, pp. 68 ff.
[4] Hartsoeker's drawing, illustrated in Fig. 24, represented not what he had seen himself but what he supposed spermatozoa would look like if they could be seen sufficiently clearly.

horse (he gave a plate of it) and a similar animalcule with very large ears in the semen of a donkey; finally, he described minute cocks in the semen of a cock. Haller remarks gently that he has searched for these phenomena in vain. Vallisneri asserted the same kind of thing about the mammalian ovum, though he admitted that, in spite of long searching, he had never seen one. Besides the main distinction between preformationists and epigenesists, then, there arose a division among the former group, so that the ovists regarded all embryos as being produced from smaller embryos in the unfertilised eggs, while the animalculists re-

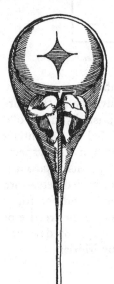

garded all embryos as being produced from the smaller embryos provided by the male in his spermatozoa. The animalculists thus afforded a singular example of a return to the ancient theory mentioned by Aeschylus in the *Oresteia* (see p. 43). Their usual view was that of Hartsoeker[1] and Andry, who pictured each egg as being arranged like the Cavorite sphere in which H. G. Wells' explorers made their way to the moon, i.e. with one trap-door. The spermatozoa, like so many minute men, all tried to occupy an egg, but as the eggs were far fewer than spermatozoa, there were, when all was over, only a few happy animalcules which had been lucky enough to find empty eggs, climb in and lock the door behind them.

Other followers of Leeuwenhoek[2] asserted that there were spermatic animalcules of both sexes, as one could see by a slight difference near their tails, that they copulated, that the females became pregnant and gave birth to little animalcules,

Fig. 24. Hartsoeker's drawing of a human spermatozoon.

that young and feeble ones could be seen, that they shed their skins, and finally that some had been observed with two heads. Haller, who made good use, on the whole, of his strong vein of scepticism, characterised all these remarks as "only conjectures."

The whole controversy was intimately bound up with the question of spontaneous generation, for, whatever the case might be in the higher animals, if it were true that the lower ones could arise *de novo* out of slime, mud or meat infusion, for instance, then *their* parts at least must have been made by epigenesis and not in any other way, for it could hardly be held that a homogeneous infusion had any structure of that kind. And if epigenesis could occur in the lower animals, then the thin

[1] *Essay*, sect. 88.   [2] See p. 175 above.

end of the wedge had been driven in, and it might occur among the higher ones as well. It was in this way that the spontaneous generation controversy came to have a peculiar importance for embryology in the eighteenth century.

Driesch[1] has essayed to make the generalisation that all the supporters of epigenesis were vitalist in their tendencies, while those who adhered to the preformation theory were not. But there are too many exceptions to this rule to make it helpful. In so far as it applies, the association doubtless arose from the fact that the continual production in epigenesis of new organs and new relationships between organs already formed seemed to require an immanent formative force of some kind, such as the *vis essentialis* of Wolff, while on the preformation hypothesis, where embryogeny was little more than a swelling up of parts already there, it could be explained simply as nutrition. But the failure of the "short-cut" mechanistic philosophers such as Gassendi and Descartes led to preformationism just as much as to epigenesis. A remark of Cheyne's throws some light on this question, for in 1715 he wrote, rallying to Gassendi's line of thought for different reasons, "If animals and vege-tables cannot be produced from matter and motion (and I have clearly proved that they cannot), they must of necessity have existed from all eternity."[2] Preformationism thus became the only resource if the uni-versal validity of the mechanical theory of the world was to be retained. Stahl, and later Wolff, saw no point in retaining it, and carefully joined together what Descartes had with equal care put asunder.

Von Haller affords some interesting evidence against the identification of epigenesis with vitalism and preformation with mechanism, for he says, "Various authors have taught that the parts of the human body are formed by a mechanism depending on general laws" (i.e. laws not simply of biological validity), "or by the virtue of some ferment, or by heat and cold making crusts out of the different juices, or in other ways. All these [mechanical] systems have some resemblance to that of M. Wolff." Haller also always speaks of Wolff's *vis essentialis* as "blind."

The original discoveries of de Graaf and Stensen were extended by Tauvry in 1690 to the tortoise, and by Lorenzini[3] in 1678 to the *Tor-pedo*: so that the eighteenth century began with an excellent basis for ovistic preformationism. The greatest names associated with this school were Swammerdam, Malpighi, Bonnet, von Haller, Winslow, Vallis-neri,[4] Ruysch and Spallanzani.[4] But there were many others, some of whom did valuable work, such as Bianchi,[5] Bourguet, Bussière,

---

[1] And Bilikiewicz; see pp. 214 and 219 hereafter.
[2] *Philosophical Principles*, ch. 2, sect. 10 ff., p. 61.
[3] See p. 167.   [4] See Franchini.   [5] *De Nat. Gen.*, pp. 417 ff.

Coschwitz, Fizes, Perrault, Sterre, Teichmeyer, Vercelloni, Vidussi and Weygand. The treatises of Imbert and Plonquet were written from this point of view, as was the bright little dialogue of de Houpeville. J. B. du Hamel asserted that he could see the chick embryo in the egg before fertilisation, and Jacobaeus made a like affirmation in the case of the frog.[1]

On the other side, that of animalculistic preformationism, the contestants were fewer. Their greatest names were Leeuwenhoek, Hartsoeker, Leibniz and the cardinal de Polignac.[2] In England the physicians Keil and Cheyne supported this position, in France Geofroi and the obstetrician la Motte, in Germany Withof and Ludwig, and in Belgium Lieutaud. De Superville wrote in favour of it in the *Philosophical Transactions of the Royal Society*, and an anonymous Swedish work of some fame supported it. To the argument of Vallisneri that the existence of so many animalcules must be an illusion, since Nature could hardly be so prodigal, the animalculists retorted by instancing such observations as that of Baster, who had taken the trouble to count the eggs of a crab and had found that they amounted to 12,444. James Cooke later elaborated a theory[3] of a world of the unborn to which the spermatozoa could retire between each attempt to find a uterus in which they could develop—this avoided Vallisneri's argument.

All those other attending Animalcula, except that single one that is then conceived, evaporate away, and return back into the Atmosphere again, whence it is very likely they immediately proceeded; into the open Air, I say, the common Receptacle of all such disengaged minute sublunary bodies; and do there circulate about with other Semina, where, perhaps, they do not absolutely die, but live a latent life, in an insensible or dormant state, like Swallows in Winter, lying quite still like a stopped Watch when let down, till they are received afresh into some other Male body of the proper kind, to

---

[1] Ch. 3, p. 38.   [2] *Anti-Lucretius*, sect. 8.
[3] Supported by Wollaston. Actually a similar argument had been evolved some seventy years previously by F. M. van Helmont, who was worrying, not, like Cooke, about the lost spermatozoa, but about the ovulated eggs which failed to get fertilised. In his strange discourse on metempsychosis, he says (p. 153): "Question no. 33. Moreover, when we find that Children in the womb be formed out of Eggs, of which there are so great a number in every woman, that we do not find one that bears so many Children as she hath Eggs, which she brought into the World with her: Must we not therefore conclude, that the rest of these Eggs were created in vain, in case they should not at some time or other attain to their full perfection? Now to remove this difficulty, must we not conclude, that the Life of these Eggs doth propagate itself another way, to the end that what doth not arrive at perfection one time, may attain it at another? And that therefore the remaining Eggs must necessarily be revolved in order to their perfection, at which in the production of them, Nature had directed her intention? In like manner what can we suppose to be the reason of that express command of God, which we read, Deut. 23, 2, That no bastard should enter into the congregation of the Lord to the tenth generation; but this, that by means of ten Revolutions, the evil might be wrought out?"

be again set on Motion, and ejected again in Coition as before, to run a fresh chance for a lucky Conception; for it is very hard to conceive that Nature is so idly luxurious of Seeds thus only to destroy them, and to make Myriads of them subservient to but a single one.

But Cooke's attractive hypothesis, published in 1762, came too late, as Punnett says, to save the animalculists.

The idea that human seed, or spermatozoa, floated everywhere in the air (obviously derived by Cooke from the Stoic-Talmudic-Kabbalistic line of thought described on pp. 66, 79) led to the amusing satire of Sir John Hill in 1750 mockingly addressed to the Royal Society, *Lucina sine Concubitu*. He affected to have invented a machine for trapping the seminal animalcules borne on the West wind.

Accordingly after much Exercise of my Invention, I contrived a wonderful cylindrical, caloptrical, rotundo-concavo-convex Machine (whereof a very exact Print will speedily be published for the Satisfaction of the Curious, designed by Mr H-y-n, and engraved by Mr V-rtu), which, being hermetically sealed at one End, and electrified according to the nicest Laws of Electricity, I erected in a convenient Attitude to the West, as a kind of Trap to intercept the floating Animalculae in that prolific quarter of the Heavens. The Event answered my Expectation; and when I had caught a sufficient number of these small original unexpanded Minims of Existence, I spread them out carefully like Silk-worm's Eggs upon White-paper, and then applying my best Microscope, plainly discerned them to be little Men and Women, exact in all their Lineaments and Limbs, and ready to offer themselves little Candidates for Life, whenever they should happen to be imbibed with Air or Nutriment, and conveyed down into the Vessels of Generation.[1]

On the experimental side, Garden came forward with descriptions of little men inside the animalcules, thus "confirming" the work of Gautier and Hartsoeker. It is fair to add, however, that Garden held quite enlightened views of the mutual necessity of egg and spermatozoon. So did Massuet, whose dissertation appeared in 1729 at Leiden. An animalculist, he yet believed both egg and sperm to be needed in generation, the former rather as a nidus. He reversed the Malpighian view. *Si ovum gallinae*, he said, *non foecundatum microscopio inspexeris, nulla in eo animalis forma apparebit*. He gave the correct explanation of Nuck's experiment (see p. 163), saying that *seminis aura seu animalcula* had first passed up the Fallopian tube. In his plate he figured spermatozoa, chick embryos and tadpoles all together, confusing the former with the primitive streak.

Another adherent of enlightened common sense was Hugh Chamberlen, one of the famous obstetrical family. In his English translation

---

[1] See p. 45.

(1683) of Mauriceau's midwifery (1668) he took exception to the double-seed (Epicurean) opinions of the French writer, and added the following as a footnote:

> Our author lying under a Mistake, in his notions concerning the Testicles in this chapter, I shall here give my sentiments. We find that the Testicles of a Woman are no more than, as it were, two Clusters of Eggs, which lie there to be impregnated by the Spirituous Particles, or Animating Effluviums, conveyed out of the Womb through the two Tubes, called by our Author, Deferent Vessels. . . . Some days after the impregnation of the Egg, or Eggs, as in Twins, they decid through those two Tubes into the Womb, where being placed, the Embrio takes up its quarters.

But la Motte maintained that the egg (which he identified with the Graafian follicle) was too big to go down the Fallopian tube, and Sbaragli, another writer on the animalculist side, agreed with him.

As for the supporters of epigenesis, they were few, but they included Descartes, de Maupertuis, Antoine Maître-Jan and John Turberville Needham. Minor writers on the same side were Tauvry, Welsch, Dartiguelongue, Böttger, Drelincurtius and Mazin. After 1750 C. F. Wolff brought an abiding victory to their opinion.

Among the arguments brought forward against the preformationists were:

(1) That it is impossible to explain the production of monsters on a preformation theory. Brunner first brought this point forward in 1683, but its classical statement was that of Étienne Geoffroy de St Hilaire, in his work of 1826 on experimental teratology. On its history, see Strohl and Dareste.

(2) That preformation is incompatible with the facts of regeneration. An intelligence, argued Hartsoeker in 1722, that can reproduce the lost claw of a crayfish, can reproduce the entire animal. This point much impressed Erasmus Darwin.[1] The whole subject was much to the fore in the eighteenth century owing to the brilliant observations of de Réaumur and Trembley.[2]

(3) That the extraordinary resemblance between small embryos of mammals, birds, reptiles, etc., discredits preformation. This was the view of Prévost & Dumas, 1834–1838.

Some maintained a quite independent position, such as Buffon, who welded together an epigenetic theory of fertilisation with a preformationist theory of embryogeny. Pascal (not the great Jansenist) put for-

---

[1] *Zoonomia*, I, 482–537.   [2] See Baker.

ward the chemical view that fertilisation consisted in a combination between the acid semen of the male and the "lixivious" semen of the female, perhaps because in chemistry acids had been regarded as male and alkalis female.[1] Claude Perrault[2] and Connor also suggested that the formation of the embryo was a fermentation set up in the egg by the spermatic animalcule. In this they were following the example of van Helmont, who had originally suggested such a theory.[3] In 1763 Jacobi discovered how to fertilise fish eggs with milt; a practical matter which had a good deal of influence on biological theory. De Launay alone still held to the Aristotelian conception of form and matter.

7. Spontaneous Generation

There is no need here to do more than glance at the spontaneous generation controversy itself, for it has long been well known in the history of biology, especially in connection with the subsequent work of Pasteur. J. T. Needham's books, *New Microscopical Discoveries* of 1745 and *Observations upon the generation, composition, and decomposition of Animal and Vegetable Substances* of 1749, exercised a considerable influence. They were written concisely after the French fashion (Needham had been educated at Douai), and with some brilliance of style, and it is hardly true to say, as Rádl does, that their experimental foundation was meagre. That it was inadequate was proved definitively as events turned out by Spallanzani. De Kruif's picture of the controversy is false and misleading, especially in its estimate of Needham, who is much more truly described in the words of Louis Pasteur.[4]

Needham's case rested upon the statement that if meat broth was placed in a sealed vessel and heated to a high temperature so that all life in it was destroyed, it would yet be found to be swarming some days later with microscopical animals. All depended, therefore, upon the sureness with which the vessel had been sealed and the efficacy of the heat employed to kill all the animalcules initially present; and in the ensuing controversy Needham lost to Spallanzani entirely on the question of technique. It may be remarked here without irrelevance that the problem is still in a sense unsolved, for what the experiments of Spallanzani proved was that animals the size of rotifers and Protozoa do not

---

[1] Cf. Gregory's interesting essay on the animate and mechanical models of reality.

[2] *Oeuvres diverses de Physique et Mécanique* (1721), vol. 2, p. 480.

[3] *Ortus*, I, 21. How interested these men would have been in modern researches on the changes at fertilisation of respiration, glycolytic activity, and enzyme action in the protoplasm of the egg cell.

[4] For an accurate and detailed account of the controversy, see Prescott.

originate spontaneously from broth, and what was proved by those of Pasteur was that organisms the size of bacteria do not originate *de novo* in that way. The knowledge which has been acquired in recent years of "filter-passing organisms," such as the mosaic virus of the tobacco-plant, and phenomena such as the bacteriophage of Twort and d'Herelle, has re-opened the whole matter, so that of the region between, for example, the semi-living particles of the bacteriophage (10^{-15} gram) and the larger-sized colloidal aggregates (10^{-18} gram) we know remarkably little. The possibility of the new formation of viruses without specific ancestry, in the cells of living hosts, is to-day an open question, and we still have no proof that their origin from non-living organic material can never occur. Recently it has proved possible to "synthesise" infective viruses from separate protein and nucleic acid constituents of other viruses, constituents some of which alone are incapable of reproduction.[1] The dictum *omne vivum ex vivo*, accepted with such assurance by the biologists of the early twentieth century, may thus turn out not to mean quite what they thought.

But to dwell further on this would be a digression. The important point was that Spallanzani's victory was a victory not only for those who disbelieved in spontaneous generation, but also for those who believed in the preformation theory of embryogeny.[2] By 1786, indeed, that viewpoint was so orthodox that Senebier, in his introduction to an edition of Spallanzani's book on the generation of animals and plants, could treat the epigenesists as no better than atheists.

Spallanzani's views on embryology were largely drawn from his study of the development of the frog's egg (see Fig. 19). Here he went far beyond Bose, but in spite of many careful observations he thought he saw the embryo already present in the unfertilised ovum. This led him to claim that Amphibia ought to be numbered among viviparous animals. His principal step forward was his recognition of the semen as the actual agent in fertilisation on precise experimental grounds—the narrative of his artificial insemination of a bitch is too famous to quote; he said it gave him more intellectual satisfaction than any other experiment he had ever done. This demonstration finally disposed of the *aura seminalis* which Harvey had found himself obliged to adopt on the grounds of his dissections of does. But Spallanzani failed to convince himself that the spermatozoa themselves were the active agents.

[1] Fraenkel-Conrat has given a good description of this work. There now seems no reason why it should not be possible in the foreseeable future to synthesise a nucleic acid from other organic chemical substances which when introduced into a host cell would show infectivity, i.e. a self-replication or reproduction within the metabolic stream.

[2] This was realised at the time especially by Patrin, who came to Needham's defence in 1778 (see Bilikiewicz, p. 147). See on, p. 218.

8. Preformation and Epigenesis[1]

Of all the preformationists Charles Bonnet was the most theoretical.[2] He was an adherent of that way of thinking mainly on the theoretical ground that the organs of the body were linked together in so intimate a manner that it was not possible to suppose that there could ever be a moment when one or two of them were absent from the ranks.

One needs [he said] no Morgagni, no Haller, no Albinus to see that all the constituent parts of the body are so directly, so variously, so manifoldly, intertwined as regards their functions, that their relationship is so tight and so indivisible, that they must have originated all together at one and the same time. The artery implies the vein, their operation implies the nerves, which in their turn imply the brain and that by consequence the heart, and every single condition a whole row of other conditions.

Bonnet compared epigenesis to crystal-growth, in which particles are added to the original mass independently of the plan or scheme of the whole, i.e. in contrast with the growth of an organism, in which particles are added on only at certain places and certain times under the guidance of "forces de rapport." Przibram has recently discussed the question of how far such a comparison is admissible, but in Bonnet's time at any rate it became very famous. Bonnet referred to von Haller's discovery of the intimate relationship between embryo and yolk as evidence for his theory. The embryo begins, according to him, as an exceedingly fine net on the surface of the yolk; fertilisation makes part of it beat and this becomes the heart, which, sending blood into all the vessels, expands the net. The net or web catches the food particles in its pores, and Bonnet supposed that if it were possible to abstract all the food particles at one operation from the adult animal, it would shrivel and shrink up into the original invisible web from which it originated.

Bonnet was no more afraid of the *emboîtement* principle than was Haller; indeed, he called it "one of the greatest triumphs of rational over

---

[1] White's *The Phlogiston Theory* will interest those who wish to study the rather striking parallel between chemistry and biology in the eighteenth century. Broadly speaking, rationalism in science had too much got the upper hand of empiricism. The traces of preformationism remaining in modern biology are well reviewed by Huxley & de Beer. Whitman distinguished between "predetermination," a physiological or potential preformation not capable of microscopic resolution, and "predelineation," which is the old morphological or visible preformation. Modern embryology might therefore be called "predetermined epigenesis." Waddington has recently (1952) introduced the term "epigenetics" to include everything concerned with the causal analysis of development, that is to say, with the genes and their effects in embryonic life as well as the morphogenetic mechanisms themselves.

[2] Bonnet's practical contributions to science were not numerous but rather important. He confirmed in 1745 (1779, p. 36) Leeuwenhoek's discovery of the parthenogenesis of aphids (1702), and he announced the formation of new individuals after the cutting of worms into segments (see the paper of Erhard). The value of the former observation as a support for ovism is evident. For further details concerning him, see Lemoine and Whitman.

sensual conviction." Many of his arguments were reproductions of Haller's, and he says in his preface that he had written his book some time before Haller's papers on the chick appeared, but then, finding his own views confirmed by the experimentally better founded ones of Haller, he determined to publish what he had set down. Thus in one place he says,

I shall be told, no doubt, that the observations on the development of the chick in the egg, and the doe in the maternal uterus, make it appear that the parts of an organised body are formed one after another. In the chick for instance it has been observed that during the early part of incubation the heart seems to be outside the animal and has a very different form to what it will have. But the feebleness of this objection is easy to apprehend. Some people wish to judge of the time when the parts of an organised body begin to exist by the time when they become visible to us. They do not reflect that minuteness and transparency alone can make these parts invisible to us although they really exist all the time.

Bonnet was therefore what might be called an "organic preformationist," for his objection to epigenesis lay in the fact that it did not seem to allow for the integration of the organism as a whole. His mistake was that he assumed the capacities of the adult organism to be present all through foetal life, whereas the truth is that they grow and differentiate in exactly the same way as the physical structure itself does. Bonnet's philosophical position, which has been analysed by Whitman, again contradicts the generalisation of Driesch[1] that all the epigenesists were vitalists and all the preformationists mechanists. For Bonnet an epigenetic and a mechanical theory were one and the same; he hardly distinguished, as Rádl says, between Descartes and Harvey; and it was just the neo-vitalist idea of the organism as a whole that he could not fit in with epigenesis. Needham and Wolff were undoubtedly epigenesist-vitalists, and Bonnet was undoubtedly a preformationist-vitalist, but Maupertuis was equally clearly an epigenesist-mechanist.

G. L. Leclerc, Comte de Buffon, the most independent figure in the controversy, stood alone as much because of his erroneous experiments as because of his originality of mind. As has so often been observed, Buffon was not really an experimentalist at all; he was a writer, and preferred other people to do his experiments for him. The volume on generation in his *Histoire Naturelle* begins with a very long historical account of the work which had been done in the previous centuries on embryology. At the beginning of the section on reproduction in general he said,

[1] And of Bilikiewicz.

The first and most simple manner of reproduction is to assemble in one body an infinite number of similar organic bodies, and to compose the substance in such a manner that every part shall contain a germ or embryo of the same species, and which might become a whole of the same kind with that of which it constitutes a part.

Such an idea resembles the ancient atomistic speculations, and was explained by W. Smellie, the obstetrician, who translated Buffon into English, as follows:

The intelligent reader will perceive that this sentence, though not very obvious, contains the principle upon which the whole theory of generation adopted by the author is founded. It means no more than that the bodies of animals and of vegetables are composed of an infinite number of organic particles, perfectly similar, both in figure and substance, to the whole animal or plant of which they are the constituent parts.

This conception explains Buffon's curious attitude to the preformation question. An embryo was preformed in its germ because all the parts of the germ were each a model of the animal as a whole, but it was also formed by epigenesis because, the sexual organs being first formed, all the rest arose entirely by a succession of new origins. Buffon's "organic living particles" bear some resemblance to the "biogen molecules" which later generations were to discuss,[1] and he says that an exactly similar but simpler structure is present in dead matter.

In his discussion of former theories he resolutely rejects the *emboîtement* aspect of preformationism, giving various calculations to show its impossibility and maintaining that

every hypothesis which admits an infinite progression ought to be rejected not only as false but as destitute of every vestige of probability. As both the vermicular and ovular systems suppose such a progression, they should be excluded for ever from philosophy.

He completely destroys the theory which the ovists and animalculists had set up in order to explain resemblance to parents, namely that although the foetus might originate either from egg or spermatic animalcule originally, it was moulded into the form of its parents by the influence of the maternal organism during pregnancy. This field,[2] which was more than once disturbed by the contestants during the course of the century, received systematic attention from time to time by medical writers. There was a memorable dispute on the point between Turner and Blondel, whose polemics, written in an exceedingly witty manner, are still very pleasant and amusing to read. Blondel was the sceptic and

[1] And even more to the atoms of Anaxagoras and the Stoic-Kabbalistic "seeds."
[2] See p. 29.

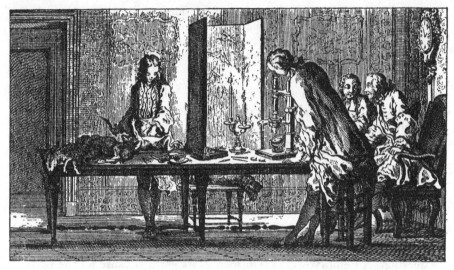

Fig. 25. G. L. L. de Buffon and his friends studying mammalian generation.

This picture appears as a vignette in Buffon's "Histoire Naturelle" at the head of Chapter I of Vol. II (edition of 1750). Buffon himself (1707–1788) is seated at the end of the table, conversing with the Abbé John Turberville Needham, F.R.S. (1713–1781), while Louis Daubenton (1716–1799) looks down the microscope. The surgeon in attendance may be either Guéneau de Montbéliard (1720–1785) or T. F. Dalibard (1703–1779), two other collaborators of Buffon. All these workers were epigenesists and animalculists, and owing to some mistake which has never been explained, they were convinced that they had found spermatozoa in the Graafian follicles of the female ovary. The scene shows them examining the mammalian generative organs (see pp. 168 and 202 of the "Histoire Naturelle," Vol. II, 1750). The ingenious identification of the persons is due to Professor R. C. Punnett. On Guéneau de Montbéliard, see Brunet and Manquat.

Turner the defender of the numerous extraordinary stories which passed for evidence on this subject. It is interesting to note that Turner believed in the continuity of foetal and maternal blood-vessels. Krause and Ens later supported the opinions of Turner, while Okes, in a Cambridge disputation, argued against them.[1]

Buffon's sixth chapter, in which he relates the progress of his own experiments, is unfortunate, in that his main result was to discover spermatozoa in the *liquor folliculi* of ovaries of female animals (see Fig. 25). The explanation of how he came to make such an egregious mistake has never been satisfactorily given, and it was not long before the truth of the observation was questioned by Ledermuller.[2] It led him naturally to the assertion that the ovaries of mammalia were not egg-producing organs but animalcule-producing organs, and to the view

[1] It is not generally known that the philosopher Hegel committed himself to some remarkable assertions on the "psychic unity" of maternal and foetal organism (*Philosophy of Mind*, pp. 28ff.).

[2] *Versuch*, p. 13.

that the beginning of embryonic development lay in the fusion of the male with the female spermatic animalcules—a curious revival of Epicureanism.[1] But it is to be observed that he does not mean one male animalcule with one female animalcule, but rather all with all, in a kind of pangenesis.

All the organic particles which were detached from the head of the animal will arrange themselves in a similar order in the head of the foetus. Those which proceeded from the backbone will dispose themselves in an order corresponding to the structure and position of the vertebrae.

And so on for all the organs. The fact that for the organs common to both sexes a double set of animalcules will thus be provided does not give Buffon any difficulty and is fully admitted by him. Accordingly he could only agree to the aphorism *omne vivum ex ovo* in the sense of Harvey namely as referring to the egg-shaped chorion of Vivipara, and definitely not in the sense of von Baer, namely in the modern sense.

Eggs, instead of being common to all females, are only instruments employed by Nature for supplying the place of uteri in those animals which are deprived of this organ. Instead of being active and essential to the first impregnation, eggs are only passive and accidental parts destined for the nourishment of the foetus already formed in a particular part of this matrix by the mixture of the male and female semen.

Biology at this period was still labouring in the dark without the illumination of the cell-theory, and therefore unable to distinguish between an egg and an egg-cell.[2]

In spite of his leanings towards epigenesis, Buffon repeated precisely the error of Malpighi.

I formerly detected [he says] the errors of those who maintained that the heart or the blood were first formed. The whole is formed at the same time. We learn from actual observation that the chicken exists in the egg before incubation. The head, the backbone, and even the appendages which form the placenta are all distinguishable. I have opened a great number of eggs both before and after incubation and I am convinced from the evidence of my own eyes that the whole chicken exists in the middle of the cicatrix the moment the egg issues from the body of the hen. The heat communicated

---

[1] It is interesting that the rejection of the Epicurean theory of female seed by the Latin theologians led, in eighteenth-century moral theology, to a very unequal emphasis on masturbation as a sin in males and females. The male (cf. the influence of the animalculists) was to be regarded as little short of a murderer if *effusio seminis* occurred; the female could not thus sin *quia verum semen in mulieribus non datur*; see Capellmann, pp. 88 ff.

[2] In 1778 W. Cruikshank found blastocysts in the Fallopian tubes of the rabbit on the third day after coitus, but his accurate observations were not published till 1797.

to it by incubation expands the parts only. But we have never been able to determine with certainty what parts of the foetus are first fixed, at the moment of its formation.

The experiment of taking a look at the cicatrices of eggs on their way down the parental oviduct seems so obvious that Buffon may well have thought of it, and it would be really interesting to know what factor in the intellectual climate made him regard such an observation as not worth attempting. His observations on the embryo itself were good and in some ways new; thus he noticed that the blood first appears on the "placenta" or blastoderm, and for the first few days seems hardly to enter the body of the embryo. He gave an extremely good account of the whole developmental process in the chick and in man, and his opinions on the use of the amniotic liquid and the functions of the umbilical cord were advanced.

J. T. Needham, however, spoke very clearly in favour of epigenesis, though he himself did no embryological experiments.[1] His *Idée sommaire* of 1776, written against Voltaire, who had called him a Jesuit and who had drawn materialistic inferences from his writings, contain the following passage:

The numerous absurdities which exist in the opinion of pre-existent germs, together with the impossibility of explaining on that ground the birth of monsters and hybrids, made me embrace the ancient system of epigenesis, which is that of Aristotle, Hippocrates, and all the ancient philosophers, as well as of Bacon and a great number of savants among the neoteriques. My observations also led me directly to the same result.

Needham's embryology is mostly contained in his *Observations nouvelles sur la Génération* of 1750. He was explicitly a Leibnizian and postulated a vegetative force in every monad.

Needham was not the only thoroughgoing epigenesist of this period. Maupertuis, whose *Vénus Physique* was published anonymously in 1746, came out very clearly in favour of this doctrine.[2] He wrote:

I know too well the faults of all the systems which I have been describing to adopt any one of them, and I find too much obscurity in the whole matter to wish to form one of my own. I have but a few vague thoughts which I propose rather as thoughts to be examined than as opinions to be received, and I shall neither be surprised nor think myself aggrieved if they are

---

[1] His valuable biological discoveries have been somewhat overshadowed by the spontaneous generation controversy. In fact he made admirable contributions on the complicated physiology, sexual and general, of cephalopods and cirripedes, he studied pollen grains as analogues of spermatozoa and was the first to see Brownian motion in them, and he described the horned eggs of elasmobranch fishes.

[2] See Brunet.

rejected. It seems to me that the system of eggs and that of spermatic animalcules are both incompatible with the manner in which Harvey actually saw the embryo to be formed. And one or the other of these systems seems to me still more surely destroyed by the resemblance of the child, now to the father and now to the mother, and by hybrid animals which are born from two different species. . . . In this obscurity in which we find ourselves on the manner in which the foetus is formed from the mixture of two liquors, we find certain facts which are perhaps a better analogy than what happens in the brain. When one mixes silver and spirits of nitre with mercury and water, the particles of these substances come together themselves to form a vegetation so like a tree that it has been impossible to refuse it the name.

This was the *Arbor Dianae*, which played a great part in the embryological controversies of the eighteenth century. It has much interest for us, for it was perhaps the first occasion on which a non-living phenomenon had been appealed to as an illustration of what went on in the living body. It is true that Descartes long before had said that the movements of the living body were carried out by mechanisms like clocks or watches, and that they resembled the statues in certain gardens which could be made to perform unexpected functions by the pressure of a manipulator's foot on a pedal, but these instances were all artificially constructed mechanical devices, whereas the *Arbor Dianae* was a natural phenomenon quite unexplained by the chemists of the time, and the lineal forerunner of Lillie's artificial nerve, and Rhumbler's drop of chloroform. We know now that its formation is a simpler process than anything which occurs in the developing embryo, but the growth of knowledge has made it undeniably clear[1] that the same forces which operate in the formation of the *Arbor Dianae* are at work also in the developing embryo. To this extent Maupertuis is abundantly justified, and Driesch's comments on him are not in agreement with the facts. Maupertuis continues:

Doubtless many other productions of a like kind will be found if they are looked for, or perhaps if they are looked for less. And although they seem to be less organised than the body of most animals, may they not depend on the same mechanics and on similar laws? Will the ordinary laws of motion suffice, or must we have recourse to new forces? These forces, incomprehensible as they are, appear to have penetrated even into the Academy of Sciences at Paris, that institution where so many opinions are weighed and so few admitted.

Maupertuis goes on to speak of the contemporary deliberations on the subject of attraction.

[1] See for example Rinne or Przibram.

Chymistry has felt the necessity of adopting this conception and attractive force is nowadays admitted by the most famous chymists who have carried the use of it far beyond the point which the astronomers had reached. If this force exists in nature, why should it not take part in the formation of animals ?

Maupertuis was thus an epigenesist and a mechanist at the same time. His opinions have an extremely modern ring, and his only retrograde step was in suggesting that the spermatic animals had nothing else to do except to mix the two seeds by swimming about in them. But that legacy of ovism was common all through the eighteenth century, and thirty years later Alexander Hamilton could still say, "From the discovery of Animalcula in *semine masculino* by Leeuwenhock's Glasses, a new Theory was adopted which is not yet entirely exploded."[1]

But the real middle point and fulcrum of the whole period lay in the controversy between von Haller and Caspar Friedrich Wolff, the former at Göttingen and the latter at St Petersburg in the academy of Queen Catherine. Kirchhoff has described this polemic. Wolff's *Theoria Generationis*, which was a defence of epigenesis on theoretical and philosophical grounds, written in a very formal, logical and unreadable manner, appeared when he was only twenty-six years old, in 1759. Leibniz, as Rádl points out, had borrowed from the earlier preformationists the conception of a unit increasing in bulk in order to become another kind of unit, but Wolff, following Needham, borrowed from Leibniz the idea of a monad developing into an organism by means of its own inherent force, and to this he joined the Stahlian notion of a supra-physical generative force in nature. On the practical side, Wolff's work was indeed of the highest importance. If the embryo pre-exists, he argued, if all the organs are actually present at the very earliest stages and only invisible to us even with the highest powers of our microscopes, then we ought to see them fully formed as soon as we see them at all. In other words, at the moment at which any given organ comes into view, it ought to have the form and shape, though not the size, of the same organ when fully completed in the embryo at birth. On the other hand, if this is not the way in which development goes on, then one ought to be able to see with the microscope one shape changing into another shape, and in fact a series of appearances, each one different from that which immediately precedes it, or in other words a series of advancing adaptations of the various parts of the primitive embryonic mass. Wolff chose as his first test case the blood-vessels of the blastoderm in the chick, for he saw that at one moment this apparatus was in existence, while the moment before it had not been. His microscopical researches led him to the conclusion that the homogene-

[1] *Elements*, p. 43.

ous surface of the blastoderm partially liquefies and transforms itself at these points into a mass of islands of solid matter, separated by empty spaces filled with a colourless liquid but afterwards with a red liquid, the blood. Finally, these spaces are covered with membranes and become vessels. Consequently it was demonstrable that the vessels had not been previously formed, but had arisen by epigenesis.

Haller replied to this new experimental foundation of morphogenesis without delay, for he was working on the development of the chick at the same time, and held closely to the opposite theory. We have already seen what his one and only argument against Wolff was. He used it time after time in all its possible variations, maintaining stoutly that the chick embryo was so fluid in the early stages that Wolff had no right to deny the presence of a given structure simply because he could not see it. Haller's explanation of Wolff's results was that the blood-vessels had been there all the time but that they had not become visible until the moment at which Wolff saw the islands forming.

After I had written the above [said Haller], M. Wolff made new objections against the demonstration. Instructed by new researches, he denies absolutely that the yolk-membranes, which he makes two in number, exist before incubation. He pretends that they are new and that they are born at the beginning of incubation, and consequently that the continuity of their vessels with the embryo does not in the least prove that in the body of the mother the yolk received vessels from the foetus. I have compared the observations of this great man with my own and I have found that the yolk never has more than one pulpy and soft membrane, part of which is called the umbilical area, and that the fine exterior membrane does not belong to the yolk but to the inner part of the umbilical membrane. . . . I do not believe that any new vessels arise at all, but that the blood which enters them makes them more obvious because of the colour which it gives them, and so by the augmentation of their volume they become longer.

Wolff replied by another extensive piece of work, which he called *De Formatione Intestinorum,* and which appeared in one of the publications of the Russian academy for 1768. It ruined preformationism. In it he demonstrated that the intestine is formed in the chick by the folding back of a sheet of tissue which is detached from the ventral surface of the embryo, and that the folds produce a gutter which in course of time transforms itself into a closed tube. The intestine, therefore, could not possibly be said to be preformed. From this as a starting-point Wolff went on to propose an epigenetic theory which applied the same process to all organs. It is interesting to note that the facts brought forward by Wolff have never been contradicted, but have been used as a foundation to which numberless morphological embryologists have added facts discovered by themselves. It is noteworthy too that although Wolff's second general principle, that of increasing solidification during embryonic development, led to no immediate results, it has been abundantly confirmed since then. His observations on the derivation of the parts of the early embryo from "leaf-like" layers were even more important, and acted as a very potent influence in the work of Pander and von Baer.

It happened, however, that Haller had much the greater influence in the biological world at the time, so that Wolff's conceptions did not immediately yield fruit in any general advance. Looking back over the second half of the seventeenth and the first two-thirds of the eighteenth centuries, it is remarkable how little theoretical progress was made in view of the abundance of new facts which were discovered. Punnett, in an interesting paper, has vividly brought this out.

The controversy between the Ovists and Animalculists had lasted just a century, and it is not uninteresting to reflect that the general attitude of science towards the problem of generation was in 1775 much what it had been in 1675. When the period opened, almost all students of biology and medicine were Preformationists and Ovists; at its close they were for the most part Ovists and Preformationists.

Ovism sprang in the first instance from de Graaf's discovery of the mammalian "egg," which gave a new and precise meaning to Harvey's aphorism. Preformationism, already old as a theory, acquired an apparent factual basis in the work of Malpighi and Swammerdam, and allied itself naturally with ovism. With Leeuwenhoek and his spermatozoa, animalculism came upon the field. The main outlines of the battle which went on between the two viewpoints have already been drawn, but it is worth remembering that there were independent minds who were impressed by the obvious facts of heredity and found it difficult to call one sex essential rather than the other. Among these Needham and Maupertuis[1] may be counted. Among the lesser writers, James Handley with his *Mechanical Essays on the Animal Oeconomy* of 1730 ought to receive a mention. Though fond of theological arguments, he upheld the common-sense attitude against ovists and animalculists alike—"We dissent in some things," he said, "both from Leeuwenhoeck and Harvey. . . . Both the semen and ova (notwithstanding all that can be said) we believe to be a *causa sine qua non* in every Generation." But what finally killed animalculism was the discovery in so many places of small motile living beings, flagellates, Protozoa, large vibrios. It was difficult to maintain in the face of this new evidence that the sperma-

[1] See the excellent review of Glass which describes, *inter alia*, Maupertuis' pioneer investigation of polydactyly in man.

tozoa were essential elements in generation, though the seminal fluid itself might very well be, as of course was Spallanzani's opinion. The preformation theory was what was holding up further progress, and when Wolff's arguments prevailed in the very last years of the eighteenth century, the way was open for the recognition of the true value of the spermatozoa.

The physician d'Aumont, otherwise unknown, who wrote the article on "Generation" in Diderot's famous *Encyclopaedia*, brought this out in an interesting way; for himself an ovist he summarised the arguments which in 1747 were destroying the animalculist position, and reducing rapidly the number of its adherents.

1. Nature would never be so prolific as to produce such millions of spermatic animalcules, each one with its soul, unnecessarily.
2. The spermatic animalcules of all animals are the same size, no matter how large the animal is; how therefore can they be involved in its generation?
3. They are never found in the uterus after coitus, but only in the sperm.[1]
4. How do they reproduce their kind?
5. What evidence is there that they are any different from the animalcules (of similar shape, etc.) which are to be found in hay infusion, scrapings from the teeth, and many other places? No one supposes that these have relation to reproduction (Bourguet).[2]

9. The Closing Years

The last forty years of the century were not marked by any great movement in a fruitful direction for morphological embryology, an iconographic wave of some merit due to Albinus, W. Hunter, Tarin, Senff, Rosenmuller, Danz and Sömmering[3] excepted; and it was not until 1812 that J. F. Meckel the younger translated Wolff's papers into German. This was one of the principal influences upon Pander and von Baer. In his introduction, Meckel describes how Wolff's work had been disregarded, and points out that Oken, writing in 1806, had apparently never even heard of it. In the very early years of the nineteenth century morphological embryology received a great impetus however. One of the most interesting figures of the new period was de Lézérec, a Breton, whose father had been in the Russian naval service. The son, as a Russian

[1] Loss of motility, and agglutination, doubtless disguised their presence from the investigators of this period.
[2] Von Baer himself (1827) believed in the extraneous nature of the animalcules, and attempted to express it by the name "spermatozoa" which he gave them. Not until Kölliker's work in 1841 was their histogenesis as normal tissue-elements demonstrated.
[3] See Bast.

naval cadet, no doubt stimulated by the writings of Wolff, who had lived at St Petersburg, used to incubate eggs on board ship. He eventually left the sea, studied medicine at Jena, and in 1808 wrote an excellent dissertation on the embryology of the chick, which Stieda has recently brought to light. He then went to Paris, and taking a medical appointment at Guadeloupe, was lost to science. Very much more important was the work of Pander in 1817 and von Baer in 1828,[1] but it belongs to the modern period,[2] and must be left for the next volume. Here it will suffice to say that these great investigators established firmly the conception of the germ-layers (our now familiar ectoderm, mesoderm and endoderm) and clearly distinguished between their formation ("primary differentiation") and the subsequent processes of histological and morphological differentiation. At the same time the mammalian egg was at last discovered, and before long recognised as a single cell.[3] The nucleus of the egg-cell had been seen in molluscs as long ago as 1791 by Poli in Italy, but not clearly described until the work of the Czech Purkyně on the "germinal vesicle" of the hen's egg in 1825. In this way the road lay open for the triumphs of the mid-nineteenth century, when a Kowalevsky could reveal (1867) that such fundamental processes as germ-layer formation and gastrulation were common to all animal phyla.[4]

It is interesting to note, however, that the recapitulation theory, which was first clearly formulated by von Baer, was already taking shape in various minds during the closing years of the eighteenth century.[5] Lewes has thus described the thesis of Goethe's *Morphologie*, written in 1795:

The more imperfect a being is the more do its individual parts resemble each other and the more do these parts resemble the whole. The more perfect a being is the more dissimilar are its parts. In the former case the parts are more or less a repetition of the whole, in the latter case they are totally unlike the whole. The more the parts resemble each other the less subordination is there of one to the other: and subordination is the mark of high grade of organisation.[6]

William[7] and John Hunter belong also to the end of the century.

[1] For information on von Baer, see Kirste; Addison; A. W. Meyer; and Stieda. His autobiography is of great interest.
[2] To this time also belongs Steinheim's work on the development of Amphibia (J. Pagel).
[3] This was the work of Schwann in 1839. Cf. E. S. Russell.
[4] Cf. Dogelb; Oppenheimer; E. S. Russell; and the classical treatise of Frank Balfour.
[5] The history of the concept of recapitulation has recently been gone into with some thoroughness by A. W. Meyer (1935), who is strangely reluctant to find any traces of it earlier than Hunter. On the other hand, I am glad to see that Balss (1936) agrees with me regarding Aristotle on this matter (see p. 49 of the present book).
[6] *Life*, p. 358.   [7] See Duncan.

CHART III

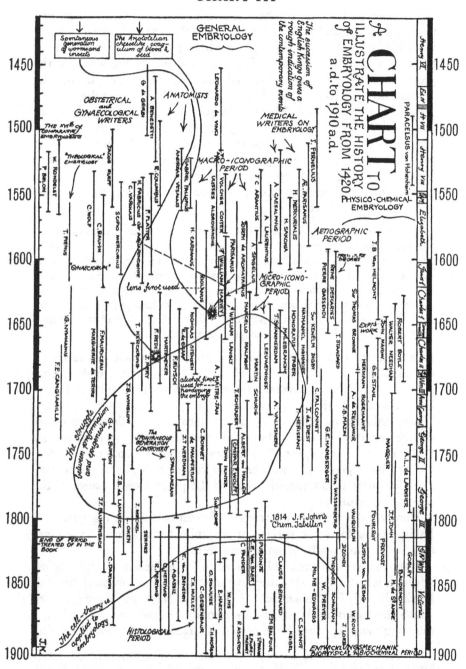

The former, in his book on the anatomy of the gravid uterus, proved finally and completely the truth of the view that the maternal and foetal circulations are distinct. His injections left no shadow of doubt about the matter, and the way was clearly opened up for the study of the properties of the capillary endothelial membranes separating the bloods, a study which is still vigorously proceeding both in its histological and physico-chemical aspects. There was a quarrel between the brothers over the priority of this demonstration. John Hunter's *Essays and Observations* also contain material important for embryology.[1] His drawings of the chick in the egg were very beautiful, and are still in the archives of the Royal College of Surgeons. He adopted Mayow's theory of the office of the air-space, and anticipated von Baer's theory of recapitulation much as did Goethe.

If we were capable of following the progress of increase of the number of parts of the most perfect animal as they were first formed in succession, from the very first to its state of full perfection, we should probably be able to compare it with some one of the incomplete animals themselves, of every order of animals in the creation, being at no stage different from some of the inferior orders. Or in other words, if we were to take a series of animals, from the more imperfect to the perfect, we should probably find an imperfect animal corresponding with some stage of the most perfect.

It is interesting to reflect on the curious course which was taken by the essence of the idea of recapitulation in the history of embryology. As first formulated by Aristotle it was as much bodily as mental, but all his successors until the eighteenth century treated it as a psychological rather than a physiological or morphological theory, and lost themselves in speculations about the vegetative, sensitive and rational souls. Yet the other aspect of the theory was only asleep, and was destined to be of great value as soon as investigators began to direct their attention more to the material than to the psychological aspect of the developing organism.

Hunter did not absolutely reject preformationism, but regarded it as holding good for some species in the animal kingdom; he therefore attached no philosophical importance to it.

Although Wolff's work did not lead to the immediate morphological advances which might have been expected, it was in many ways fruitful. It stimulated J. F. Blumenbach's *Über den Bildungstrieb* of 1789, a work which elaborated the Wolffian *vis essentialis* into the *nisus formativus*, a directing morphogenetic force peculiar to living bodies. It is interesting

---

[1] Detailed and interesting surveys of John Hunter's contributions to embryology have been published by A. W. Meyer (1935, 1936), and Lewis has added to this by his address at the Harvard Bicentenary Celebrations of Hunter.

to note that Blumenbach passed through an exactly opposite succession of opinions to that of Haller, for he was first attracted by preformationism, but being convinced by Wolff's work,[1] abandoned it in favour of epigenesis. Blumenbach compares his *nisus formativus* with the force of gravity, regarding them as exactly similar conceptions and using them simply as definitions of a force whose constant effects are recognised in everyday experience. Blumenbach says that his *nisus formativus* differs from Wolff's *vis essentialis* because it actively does the shaping and does not merely add suitable material from time to time to a heap of material which is already engaged in shaping itself. Wolff was still alive at this time, but made no comment on Blumenbach's ideas. He may well have thought the differences unimportant. Both Blumenbach and Wolff were mentioned by Kant in the *Critique of Judgment*, where he adopted the epigenetic theory in his discussion of embryonic development.

A word must be said at this point about the opinions of the eighteenth century on foetal nutrition. At the beginning of it there was, as has been shown, a welter of conflicting theories, and though later on writers on this subject were fewer, the progress made was no more rapid. In 1802 Lobstein was supporting the view (which had been defended by Boerhaave[2]) that the amniotic liquid nourished the embryo *per os*, though Themel had shown forty years before from a study of acephalic monsters that this could be at most the very slightest source of material. These workers had obviously learnt nothing from Herissant and Brady, who had been over precisely the same ground fifty years earlier. On the other hand, Good and Osiander reported the birth of embryos without umbilical cords, so that the solution of this question became, in the first years of the nineteenth century, balanced, as it were, between the relative credibility of two kinds of prodigy. Nourishment *per os* was defended by Kessel, Hannes and Grambs, and was attacked by Vogel, Bernhard, Glaser, Hannhard and Reichard. The idea lingered on right into the modern period, and as late as 1886 von Ott, who was much puzzled about placental permeability, decided that a great part in foetal nutrition must be played by the amniotic liquid. Weidlich, a student of his, fed a calf on amniotic liquid for some days, and as it seemed to thrive on this diet reported the amniotic liquid to have nutritive properties. The appeal to monsters was still resorted to at the end of the nineteenth century, for Opitz, in order to negative von Ott's conclusions, drew attention to a specimen in the Chemnitz Polyklinik in which the oesophagus of a well-nourished normal infant was closed

[1] And by experiments of his own on the regeneration of hydroids.
[2] *Institutiones*, sect. 382.

at the upper third without the development of the body having been in any way restricted. The fuller possibilities of biochemistry itself have sometimes been exploited in favour of the ancient theory of nourishment *per os*; thus Köttnitz in 1889 collected some data about the presence of peptones and protein in the human amniotic liquid with this object in view. That the foetus swallows the liquid which surrounds it towards the end of gestation in all amniota can hardly be disputed, and as there are known to be active proteolytic enzymes in the intestinal tract, no doubt some of the protein which it contains is digested—but to maintain that any significant part is played in foetal nutrition by this process, has become steadily more and more impossible since 1600.

But to return to the eighteenth century; all was not repetition, occasionally someone brought forward a few facts. Thus the deglutition of the amniotic liquid was discussed by Flemying in 1755 in a paper under the title "Some observations proving that the foetus is in part nourished by the amniotic liquor." "I believe," he said, "that very few, if any at all, will maintain now-a-days with Claudius de la Courvée and Stalpart van-der-Wiel, that the whole of its nourishment is conveyed by the mouth." But he himself had found white hairs in the meconium of a calf embryo with a white hide. Both Aldes and Swammerdam had found the same thing, but Aldes did not think it of any significance, and Swammerdam merely remarked that the calf must lick itself *in utero*.

More interesting was W. Watson's "Some accounts of the foetus *in utero* being differently affected by the Small Pox." This was the earliest investigation of the permeability of the placenta to pathological agents. "That the foetus," said Watson, "does not always partake of the Infection from its Mother, or the Mother from the Foetus, is the subject of this paper." Two of his cases, he said,

evince that the Child before its Birth, though closely defended from the external Air, and enveloped by Fluids and Membranes of its own, is not secure from the variolous Infection, though its Mother has had the Distemper before. They demonstrate also the very great Subtility of the variolous Effluvia.

But other cases

are the very reverse of the former, where though from Inoculation the most minute portion of Lint moisten'd with the variolous Matter and applied to the slightly wounded Skin, is generally sufficient to propagate this Distemper; yet here we see the whole Mass of the Mother's Blood, circulating during the Distemper through the Child, was not sufficient to produce it. . . . From these Histories it appears that the Child before its Birth ought to be consider'd as a separate, distinct Organization; and that though wholly nourish'd by the Mother's Fluids, with regard to the Small Pox, it is liable to be affected in a very different Manner and at a very different Time from its Mother.

Doubtless the modern explanation of Watson's discordant results would be that in one case there were placental lesions, destroying the perfect barrier between the circulations, and in others there were not.

In the last year of the century (but the seventh of the Republic) Citizens Léveillé & Parmentier contributed an interesting paper to the *Journal de Physique* in which they observed the increase in size of the avian yolk on incubation and spoke of a current of water yolkwards.

CONCLUSION

WHEN the contents of this book was given in the form of lectures at University College, it bore the title "Speculation, Observation and Experiment as illustrated by the History of Embryology." Of the first two of these factors we have seen enough, but the third would have necessitated the continuation of the story down to the end of the nineteenth century, and this must still await our projected second volume. The true science of experimental embryology did not come into being until the time of Wilhelm Roux.[1] The early chemical observations on the embryonic liquors (p. 159) were indeed observations rather than experiments, and there was no systematic study of the changes which the liquors undergo during the development of the foetus; this was not done till the time of John Dzondi (1806). Harvey's segregation of does at Hampton Court (p. 146) merits perhaps the name of an experiment, involving as it did the use of "controls;" and an outstanding instance is the ligature of Nuck in 1691 (p. 163). As in Nuck's case, experiment in the hands of both Spallanzani and J. T. Needham led to error. Spallanzani confuted his adversary on the question of spontaneous generation and the vegetative force by what amounted to rigid criticism of experimental conditions, but later on denied their proper function to the spermatozoa on exactly the same methodologically faulty grounds.

But on the whole, experimentation, active interference with the course of Nature and subsequent observation of the resulting system in comparison with systems in which no such interference has taken place, was a characteristically nineteenth-century product as far as biology and embryology are concerned. Only at the present day, indeed, are we beginning to appreciate the statistical and other difficulties attending upon the full application of the experimental method to living organisms, and the manifold obstacles which prevent obedience to the rule that only one variable be modified at one time. But this is no matter of reproach against the older embryologists. Knowledge of form must necessarily precede knowledge of change of form and the factors producing it, and so we see during the last seventy years the production of

[1] 1850–1924. He founded the *Archiv f. Entwicklungsmechanik* in 1894, thus naming the modern discipline of experimental morphology and causal embryology.

"Normaltafeln" or tables of morphological pictures showing normal development; these are the essential basis for experimental studies.

Probably the best way to summarise the influences which have operated in the history of embryology is to concentrate attention on what may be called, borrowing a phrase from general physiology, the "Limiting Factors" of advance. We may thus regard the progress of knowledge about generation as governed by a reaction-chain, one link in which may at any given time be slower than all the others, and hence may set the speed for the whole.

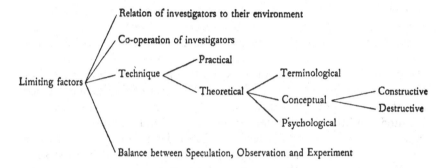

Of these limiting factors the first which may be mentioned (though I do not wish to pronounce here upon their relative importance) is the relation of investigators to their environment. The Carlylean tendency to regard the history of science as a succession of inexplicable geniuses arbitrarily bestowing knowledge upon mankind has now been generally given up as quite mythological. A scientific worker is necessarily the child of his time and the inheritor of the thought of many generations. But the study of his environment and its conditioning power may be carried on from more than one point of view. We have already seen (p. 115) what a sharp distinction the culture-historians (Sigerist, Bilikiewicz, etc.) make between the mental atmosphere of the Renaissance, the Baroque, the Rococo, the "Aufklärung" period, and so on. There is doubtless much to be learnt from historical investigations carried on in this light, but it may sometimes lead to a hypostatisation of abstractions, and as in the case of ovism and feminism (p. 116) its results may border on the fantastic. The social and political ruling ideas of a distinguishable epoch play, on this view, an overwhelmingly important part in the scientific thought of the time, and may act as limiting factors to further advance. Thus the political absolutism of the Baroque period is thought to have mirrored itself in the extreme rationalism of seventeenth-century biology. There is much more to be done in working out the internal relations of successive intellectual climates and their connections with contemporary social situations.

The other principal point of view which may be taken regarding the environment of the scientific worker as a limiting factor is that which emphasises his existence as an economic unit, and seeks to show how his position in a society with such and such a class structure influences the development of his thought. Some reference to this point of view has already been made in the introduction (p. 14). It seems to offer more chance than the preceding method for new discoveries in the history of science, for it directs its attention upon those aspects of human society (trades and techniques, labour conditions, the everyday life of the mine, the factory, the barber-surgeon's shop) which, precisely because of their assumed inferiority, have not been discussed in the majority of books, written inevitably by members of the governing classes, or by those who aspired to imitate gentility. Thus the rather sharp cleavage between the philosophic biologist of the Hellenistic age and the contemporary medical man, who might often be a slave, contributed doubtless to the sterility of ancient Mediterranean medicine, including obstetrics and gynaecology. In the later Christian West there was not much incentive to embryological study so long as the process of childbirth was left to the charms and incantations of barbarous midwives. But for a better insight into the economic position of embryologists in past ages nearly all the work remains to be done.

Next comes co-operation of scholars. In the civilisation of the Hellenistic age, it may be said, a considerable measure of such co-operation had been attained; the works of Aristotle and Hippocrates were fairly readily available in written form, and evidence has been brought forward (pp. 64, 78), particularly with regard to Jewish thought, that this was well used. But we must beware here of suffering a distortion of perspective in the contemplation of antiquity, for it is easy to exaggerate the co-operation of ancient thought. A single idea could consider itself lucky if it passed once in twenty-five years between Greece and India after Alexander (cf. p. 27). Among the conflicting influences that gave rise to the civilisation of the later West, this co-operation, hampered by enormous linguistic difficulties on the one hand, and by the diversion of interest from scientific to ethical and theological channels on the other, sank to a very low level. Hence we have the remarkable spectacle of a Leonardo, many years ahead of his contemporaries, and able to earn a living only as a designer of fortifications, finding it impossible to communicate his discoveries to any living person, and reduced to burying them in notebooks only by a mere chance available to scholars of after ages.

Among the most important of limiting factors we must reckon technique, extending the term to cover mental as well as material methodology. The part which the latter has played in the history of embryology can hardly be overrated. Thus until the introduction of hardening agents, especially alcohol, by Boyle (p. 158), the examination of the early stages of embryos was bound to remain crude, and we have seen (p. 185) how embryology attained an entirely different level immediately afterwards in the hands of Maître-Jan. The parallel case of the microscope is too familiar to dwell on, but the work of Malpighi obviously marked a turning-point in the science (p. 163). It may here be noted, however, that even when methods are available, the workers of the time do not necessarily use them, and although Harvey could have employed an early form of microscope, he restricted himself to the weak lenses, *perspicilia*, or "perspectives," which had already been used by Riolanus.[1] A still more striking instance is that of artificial incubation. Carried on in Egypt since the remotest antiquity (p. 22), this process must have been at the disposal of Egyptian physicians, Alexandrian biologists and Arabic scholars for a period of three thousand years, yet so far as we know, no embryological use of it was ever made. In eighteenth-century France and England the technique of the process had to be painfully rediscovered at a time when biologists were only too eager to make use of such assistance. Let us mention, as other instances of the effect of material technique on embryology, the burst of knowledge which followed the invention of the automatic microtome by Threlfall and others about 1883, and the great advance which in our own century has followed the successful mastery of grafting technique in operations on amphibian embryos by Gustav Born and Hans Spemann.

Just as important, however, as material technique is mental technique. And first with respect to words; on several occasions we have had to notice a standstill on account of the lack of a satisfactory terminology.

[1] As this statement about Harvey may seem surprising to some, it is worth while to recapitulate briefly the facts about the invention of the microscope. For the detailed evidence the classical papers of Singer may be consulted. The introduction of convex lenses as spectacles for presbyopia may now be dated very soon after A.D. 1286 in Italy, according to the exhaustive researches of Rosen. Concave lenses for myopia came into use much later, about 1500, and the first bilenticular system was probably due to Leonard Digges (d. 1571), who invented (but never fully described) a rudimentary telescope. The first lens combination for a microscope was mentioned, again obscurely, by Giambattista della Porta (1540–1615) in his *Magiae Naturalis* (1589), but no practical application was made of it. The microscope really begins with Zacharias Jansen (1580–*ca.* 1630) of Middelburg in Holland, who put together two convex lenses some time between 1591 and 1608, as we know from the detailed account of Pierre Borel. Cornelius Drebbel of Alcmaar, mathematician to King James in 1619, brought one of these instruments into England, i.e. thirty years before the conclusion of William Harvey's researches on generation. Perhaps Harvey made efforts to acquire and use one, perhaps he was too conservative and sceptical—we do not know.

Thus in the thirteenth century Albertus of Cologne had arrived at a point beyond which progress was impossible in the absence of new words. When, for example, there was no other means of describing the sero-amniotic junction in the hen's egg than by speaking of "the hole on the left side of the vessel which runs above the membrane on the right hand of something else" accuracy was difficult and speed impossible. A precisely similar position was occupied by Boerhaave in the eighteenth century, only now in the case of biochemical words. Faced with some substance such as a "greasy, streaky yellow oil, smelling of alkaline salt," Boerhaave was unable to describe it except in these common-sense terms; and lacking the means either to submit it to further analysis or to characterise it by accurate physico-chemical units, he was forced to admit a large number of ultimates into his schemes which were not ultimate at all.

Mental technique as a limiting factor in embryological history goes deeper than words, however, for it involves the concepts of the investigator. What the Germans call "Begriffsbildung" or the construction of concepts congruent with certain sorts of natural phenomena, though never conscious in the history of biology, has none the less been operative. In this field we may remember the doctrine of Galen concerning the natural faculties ($\delta\upsilon\nu\acute{\alpha}\mu\epsilon\iota\varsigma$, p. 70), and the immense length of time which was required for biologists to see that it was nothing more than a concise statement of the phenomena themselves. Not until it was "seen through" as an explanation was post-Renaissance biology possible. Similarly, the peculiar contribution of Leonardo to embryology was his realisation that embryos could be measured, not merely as to dimensions at one moment but as to dimensions at a succession of moments. The application of the concept of change in weight and size with time, a concept which, as modern biology shows, admits of much accuracy when properly worked out, was thus first made by Leonardo. In the same way Boyle was the first to see clearly that a problem of *mixture* is presented by the developing embryo (though Hippocrates had stated it dimly some two thousand years before). If the embryo is made up of mixed things, some definite proportion and way of mixture must exist. And no hope of finding out what this was could be obtained from the Aristotelian elements (heat, cold, moisture and dryness) or from the alchemical principles (salt, sulphur and mercury). Hence Boyle's emphasis on the corpuscularian or mechanical hypothesis, and all its historical implications (p. 176).

Besides this creation of concepts, and the choice of which of them to apply, the mentality of the scientific workers of the past often differed greatly with regard to a fundamental quality which can only be

234

called audacity. Probably Aristotle's greatest claim to our respect is that alone of his contemporaries and predecessors he had the audacity to suggest that animal form is not limitlessly manifold or infinite in its manifestations, but that given industry and intelligence, a classification was possible. This alone marks him out above all subsequent biologists. On a smaller scale, we find the same mental audacity in Kenelm Digby, whose discussions of the development of the chick are remarkable for their naturalistic tone (p. 122), for their conviction that the processes of development are not beyond the reach of the reason and imagination of man. It is most ironic that Digby, who did little or nothing himself to advance our knowledge, should have spoken thus, while his great contemporary, William Harvey, to whom we are indebted for so many advances in embryology, was led to despair of understanding development. Another interesting point that emerges from the same period is that such mental audacity can go, perhaps, too far, as when Descartes and Gassendi built up an embryology *more geometrico demonstrata*, in which the facts were relegated to an inferior position and the theory was all.

But not only must the right concepts be chosen, the wrong ones must be abandoned. One of the principal necessities which has faced investigators since the earliest times has been the recognition of silly questions in order to leave time for the examination of serious ones. It was presumably inevitable that the pseudo-problems concerning the entry of the soul into the embryo should be taken seriously until a very late date. But a more typical instance of a meaningless question may be found in the dispute about what parts of the egg *form* the chick and which *feed* it. The tacit assumption here was that since to commonsense food and flesh are different things, there must be in the hen's egg, besides sufficient provision of food, some sort of pre-flesh out of which the embryo can be made. Not until 1651 did this pseudo-problem go out of currency in the light of Harvey's demonstration of the unsoundness of the assumption.

The expulsion of ethics from biology and embryology forms another excellent example. That good and bad, noble and ignoble, beautiful and ugly, honourable and dishonourable, are not terms with biological meaning, is a proposition which it has taken many centuries for biologists to realise.

Ideas of good and bad entered biology partly under the concept of "perfection." In 1260 Albertus was maintaining that male chicks always hatched from the more spherical eggs and female chicks from the more oval ones, because the sphere is the most perfect of all figures in solid geometry, and the male the more perfect of the two sexes (p. 87).

We realise to-day that to ask which is the more perfect of the two sexes is a meaningless question, for we have expelled ethics from science and cannot regard any one thing as being more perfect than anything else. Again, describing the course of the arteries in the developing chick, Albertus says: "One of the two passages which spring from the heart branches into two, one of them going to the spiritual part which contains the heart, and carrying to it the pulse and subtle blood from which the lungs and other spiritual parts are formed; and the other passing through the diaphragm to enclose the yolk of the egg, around which it forms the liver and stomach." This distinction between the organs above the diaphragm, the lungs, heart, thymus, etc., called "spiritualia," and the organs below, the stomach, liver, intestines, spleen, etc., runs through the whole of the early anatomy. It was as if the organs of the thorax were regarded as a respectable family living at the top of an otherwise disreputable block of flats. To us it seems absurd to call one organ more "spiritual" than another, but that is because we realise the irrelevance of ethical issues in biology. Thomas Aquinas, about the same time, dealt in passing in his *Summa Theologica* with human generation (p. 93).

The generative power of the female is imperfect compared to that of the male; for just as in the crafts, the inferior workman prepares the material and the more skilled operator shapes it, so likewise the female generative virtue provides the substance but the active male virtue makes it into the finished product.

This is really the pure Aristotelian doctrine, but St Thomas gives it the characteristically mediaeval twist. Aristotle might make a distinction between form and matter in generation, but the mediaeval mind, with its perpetual hankering after value, would at once enquire which of the two, male or female, was the higher, the nobler, the more honourable.

In the eighteenth century the same frame of mind persisted. It was maintained that in every detail of the visible world some evidence could be found for the central dogma of natural religion, the belief in a just and beneficent God. Biology was thus not free from the mental bias associated with theology.[1] Between 1700 and 1850 a multitude of books were written which purported to reveal the wisdom and goodness of God in the natural creation. The theologians took what suited their purpose and left the rest. It is instructive to see how Goethe, who was deeply committed to the theological interpretation of phenomena, re-acted to the ornithological anecdotes of his secretary Eckermann on 18th Oct., 1827. He said little while Eckermann told him about the

---

[1] For a striking example of this, see Edmund Gosse's *Father and Son*.

habits of the cuckoo and other birds, but when Eckermann related how he had liberated a young wren near a robin's nest and how he had found it subsequently being fed by the robins, Goethe exclaimed:

That is one of the best ornithological stories I have ever heard. I drink success to you and your investigations. Whoever hears that, and does not believe in God, will not be aided by Moses and the prophets. That is what I call the omnipresence of the Deity, who has everywhere spread and implanted a portion of His endless love.

And so it always was with the theological naturalists; they hailed with enthusiasm the discovery of monogamy in tortoises, or mother-love in goats,[1] but they had nothing to say concerning the habits of the hook-worm parasite[2] or the appearance of embryonic monsters in man. Not until the beginning of the nineteenth century did it become clear that Nature cannot be divided into the Edifying, which may with pleasure be published, and the Unedifying, which must be kept in obscurity. Experimental embryology then contributed to this clearer vision of the living world by its manifold demonstrations that in spite of the apparently deeply teleological character of normal embryonic development, once the individual morphogenetic processes have been experimentally "derailed," they laboriously continue their operations so as to imitate (and therefore ultimately to explain) all the possible varieties of naturally occurring monstrosities.[3] Of course the riddle of normal integration remains.

In the end we may say that the progress of a branch of natural science such as embryology depends on a delicate balance of three things, speculative thought, accurate observation and controlled experiment. Any modification of the optimum balance will act as a powerful limiting factor on progress. Speculative thought, in particular, has shown a tendency to crystallise too readily into doctrines which, by way of attachment to some philosophical or theological issue, live a longer life than they deserve. Thus the Aristotelian theory of the formation of the embryo by the coagulation of the menstrual blood, built in the first

[1] One finds striking parallels for this interest in animal behaviour among the neo-Confucian school of philosophers in mediaeval China (see *Science and Civilisation in China*, vol. 2). In so far as it contributed to a conviction of the reality of an evolutionary process, which for the Chinese thinkers it certainly did, it was useful and commendable. But then they were never committed to the idea of a special creation by an all-beneficent personal deity. For them therefore "gleams of righteousness" in ants and otters were presages of that human community which the impersonal Order of Nature (the Tao) would in due time produce, pieces of evidence about a social evolution, not about a personal Creator.
[2] The guinea-worm (*Dracunculus medinensis*) had been given a dramatic description by Velsch in 1674—and indeed by Avicenna long before him. Ankylostomiasis had been known and described in ancient Egypt.
[3] On lethal genes and their action, see the brilliant book of Hadorn.

instance upon a faulty deduction, became incorporated in the Aristotelian tradition of *forma* and *materia*, and although quite repugnant to observation, remained the official theory throughout the European Middle Ages, and apparently in perpetuity in India. So powerful was the rationalism of a medical education round about 1630 that the physicians to whom Harvey demonstrated the empty uteri of the king's does preferred to believe their books rather than the evidence of their senses. And precisely parallel to this attitude, as we have seen (p. 213), was that of the preformationists in the following century, who, having decided, like Bonnet, that epigenesis was inconceivable, only accepted such observations as confirmed their *a priori* view.

Preformationism as a manifestation of rationality merits further examination. The dogmatic manner in which preformationism was held during the eighteenth century would not perhaps have been so fatal if the biologists of that time had been able to take mathematical reasoning more seriously. There was Harvey's very convincing argument about the circulation of the blood, and Freind's equally convincing, but unfortunately erroneous, deductions about the quantity of menstrual blood and the weight of the newborn foetus (p. 150). If these could have been accepted, it was a pity that Hartsoeker's argument about preformation could not. In 1722 Hartsoeker calculated that $10^{100,000}$ rabbits must have existed in the first rabbit, assuming that the creation took place 6000 years ago and that rabbits begin to reproduce their kind at the age of six months. But to this Bonnet merely answered that it was always possible, by adding zeros to units, to crush the imagination under the weight of numbers, and he described the preformation theory as one of the most striking victories of the understanding over the senses. It would have been better described as one of the most striking victories of the imagination over the understanding.

The fact is that the biologists of the eighteenth century, carried away by preformationist theory, took embryology on to a plane where observation became superfluous. They would have found acceptable the sentiment satirised by Boyle that " 'tis much more high and philosophical to argue *a priori* than *a posteriori*," and were eventually debarred from looking at developing embryos by their conviction that structure and organisation would certainly be there, whether they could see it or not. The preformationist controversy was, in fact, a repetition in biology of the controversy between the rationalists and the empiricists in philosophy. The contemporary rationalists were people who held that

human beings were in possession of certain principles of interpretation which were not simply generalisations from experience, but could nevertheless be used as major premises in arguments concerning Nature. If observations were not in accordance with expectations founded on such reasoning, they were dismissed as illusions. The empiricists, on the other hand, held that there was no knowledge independent of observation, and that the rationalists' principles, in so far as they were admissible at all, *were* generalisations from experience.[1]

It is obvious that nearly all the preformationists were rationalists. They thought that Reason was in a position to decide the issue whatever might be the results of observation. "It is remarkable," as Cole says, in his book on this period, "that the preformationists did not realise that if the point to be established is assumed at the outset all further discussion is superfluous." In this example, then, we have a disturbance of the balance towards the side of rationalistic speculation.

It would be a mistake, however, to regard this tendency as confined to the eighteenth century. Ample examples of its presence can be collected from nearly every period in biological history. "We plume ourselves," says Cole, "on that aspect of our work which is vain and argumentative, and condescend to the more modest but enduring labour of observation." There can be no doubt that this state of affairs, so unfortunate for science, is one aspect of that contempt for manual labour which has run through the stratified structures of all societies in the history of civilisation. The manipulator of paper and ink, educated in the classical traditions of his time, has always seemed, by reason of his superficial similarity to the political administrator, a superior being to the empirical mechanic engaged in the manual work of the arts and industries. The tradition is as old as civilisation, yet for the advance of science it must be broken. Not until the manual worker and the audacious theorist are combined in one person will the fullest development of scientific thought be possible.

On the other hand, there can be no doubt that a plethora of observation and experiment is also bad for scientific progress. Modern biology is the crowning instance of this fact. What has been well called a "medley of *ad hoc* hypotheses" is all that we have to show as the theoretical background of a vast and constantly increasing mass of observations and experiments. Embryology in particular has been theoretically threadbare since the decay of the evolution theory as a mode of explanation. Embryologists of the school of F. M. Balfour thought that their task was accomplished when they had traced a maximum number of evolutionary analogies in the development of an animal. Wilhelm His, perhaps the first causal embryologist, struggled successfully to end this state of affairs.

[1] Woodger.

My own attempts [he wrote in 1888 in a famous passage] to introduce some elementary physiological or mechanical explanations into embryology have not been generally agreed to by morphologists. To one it seemed ridiculous to speak of the elasticity of the germinal layers; another thought that by such considerations we put the cart before the horse; and one recent author states that we have something better to do in embryology than to discuss tensions of germinal layers, etc., since all embryological explanation must necessarily be of a phylogenetic nature.

But this strictly evolutionary dominance in embryology did not last on into the twentieth century. The unfortunate thing is that nothing has so far been devised to put in its place. Experimental embryology, Morphological embryology, Physiological embryology, and Chemical embryology form to-day a vast range of factual knowledge, without one single unifying hypothesis, for we cannot yet dignify the axial gradient doctrines, the field theories and the speculations on the genetic control of enzymes, with such a position. We cannot doubt that the most urgent need of modern embryology is a series of advances of a purely theoretical, even mathematico-logical, nature. Only by something of this kind can we redress the balance which has fallen over to observation and experiment; only by some such effort can we obtain a theoretical embryology suited in magnitude and spaciousness to the wealth of facts which contemporary investigators are accumulating day by day.

BIBLIOGRAPHY

ibn al-'Abbās. See al-Majūsī.

Abderhalden, E. & Hunter, A. *Zeitschr. f. physiol. Chem.* 1906, **48**, 505.

Achillini, A. *Annotationes Anatomiae.* (Bologna, 1520.)

Adams, F. D. *Bull. Geol. Soc. Amer.*, 1934, **45**, 411.

Addison, W. H. F. "The Centenary of the Discovery of the Mammalian Ovum," *Medical Life*, 1927, **34**, 305.

Adelmann, H. B. See Coiter.

Adelmann, H. B. *The Embryological Treatises of Hieronymus Fabricius ab Aquapendente; The Formation of the Egg and of the Chick [De Formatione Ovi et Pulli] (and) the Formed Foetus [De Formato Foetu]; a Facsimile Edition, with an Introduction, a Translation, and Commentary* . . . (Cornell Univ. Press, Ithaca, 1942.)

Adet, P. A. *Grundzüge d. Chemie.* (Basel, 1805.)

Aelianus, Oppianus, & Nicander. *De Natura Animalium*, etc., etc. (Paris, 1858.)

Aeschylus. *Eumenides*, tr. and ed. A. W. Verrall. (Macmillan, London, 1908.)

Akenside, Mark. *Dissertatio Medica Inauguralis . . . De Ortu et Incremento Foetus Humani.* (Potvliet, Leiden, 1744.) See Samuel Johnson's remarks on him in his *Lives of the Poets* (World's Classics ed., II, p. 468).

Akhnaton, Nefer-Kheperu-Ra, Ua-En-Ra, Amen-Hetep IV. "Hymn to Aton," *ca.* 1400 B.C., tr. J. H. Breasted, *Cambridge Ancient History*, vol. 2, p. 118. (Cambridge, 1926.)

Albertus [Magnus], O.P., of Cologne. *De Animalibus*, Libri XXVI, ed. Stadler, H., 2 vols. (Munster i./W., 1916–1921.)

Albertus [Magnus], O.P., of Cologne. *De Secretis Mulierum.* (Cologne, 1475 (?); Venice, 1478.) In Osler, pp. 71, 100.

Albertus [Magnus], O.P., of Cologne. *Secreta mulierum et virorum, cum expositione Henrici de Saxonia.* (Adam von Rottweil, Venice, 1478.) Henry of Saxony died *ca.* 1378.

Albertus [Magnus], O.P., of Cologne. *Secreta mulierum et virorum.* (Printer unknown, Lyon, *ca.* 1498.)

Albertus [Magnus], O.P., of Cologne. *De Secretis Mulierum Libellus, Scholiis auctus & à Mendis repurgatus.* (Leiden, 1560.)

Albertus [Magnus], O.P., of Cologne. *De secretis mulierum.* (Zetzner, Strasbourg, 1601.)

Albertus [Magnus], O.P., of Cologne. *De secretis mulierum.* (H. & T. Boom, Amsterdam, 1669.)

Albertus [Magnus], O.P., of Cologne. *Von Weibern und Geburten der Kinder sampt ihren Artzneyen.* (D. Apollinarem, Erfurt, 1671.)

Albertus [Magnus], O.P., of Cologne. *Les Admirables Secrets d'Albert Le Grand, contenant plusieurs Traitéz sur la Conception des Femmes.* (Cologne, 1712.) (Réimpression, Lyon, 1744–1745.) See also Alletz.

Albertus, M. *Systema jurisprudentiae medicae.* (Halle, 1725.)

Albinus, B. S. *Icones Ossium Foetus humani.* (J. & H. Verbeek, Leiden, 1737.)

Albinus, B. S. *Tabulae septem Uteri Mulieris gravidae cum jam parturine mortuae.* (Leiden, 1748.)

Alcmaeon of Crotona. See Diels.

Aldes, Theodore (Matthew Slade's pseudonym). *Dissertatio epistolica contra D. G. Harveium.* (van den Berge, Amsterdam, 1667.) See also ab Angelis.

Aldes, Theodore (Matthew Slade's pseudonym). "Observationes in ovis factae et skiagraphia nutritionis pulli in ovo et foetu in utero." (MS. bound in Brit. Mus. 1175 *a*, 18.) Title of printed version: *Observationes Naturales in Ovis factae.* (Amsterdam, 1673.) Aldobrandino of Florence. See del Garbo, D.

Aldrovandus, Ulysses. *Ornithologia,* 3 vols. (de Fransiscis, Bologna, 1599.)

Aldrovandus, Ulysses. *Ornithologia, hoc est de Avibus Historia.* (Bologna, 1681.)

Alexander Aphrodisiensis. *Super nonnullis Physicis Quaestionibus solutionum liber.* (Andreas Cratander, Basel, 1520.)

Alexander Aphrodisiensis. *Quaestiones Naturales.* (Scot, Venice, 1541.)

Alexander Philalethes. See Allbutt.

Allbutt, Sir Clifford. *Greek Medicine in Rome.* (Macmillan, London, 1921.)

Alletz, Pons Augustin. *L'Albert Moderne, ou Nouveaux Secrets éprouvés et licites, recueillis d'après les Découvertes les plus récentes,* 1770.

Amatus Lusitanus. *Curationum Medicinalium Centuriae Quatuor.* (Basel, 1556; Venice, 1557, Constantius, Venice, 1559.)

Ammanus, P. *Irenicum Numae Pompilii.* (Leipzig, 1689.)

Anaxagoras of Clazomenae. See Diels.

Andry, Nicolas. *De la génération des vers dans le corps de l'homme.* (Paris, 1700; Lombrail, Amsterdam, 1701; reprinted Paris, 1741.)

ab Angelis, Johannes. *Vindiciae ab epistolica Theodori Aldes dissertatione contra Gul. Harveium auctore Johannes ab Angelis medico Hullensi.* (Schagen, Amsterdam, 1667.)

Anonymous. *A defence of Dr Pocus and Dr Malus against the petition of the unborn babes.* (Cooper, London, 1751.)

Anonymous. "Portraits of Dr William Harvey," pub. by Hist. Sect., Roy. Soc. Med., Oxford, 1913.

Anonymous (Swede). *De Orig. Animalium.*

Antinori, V. *Notizie istoriche relative all' Accademia del Cimento.* (Florence, 1841.)

Antonius Liberalis. (2nd century) *Transformationes,* ed. E. Martini, p. 124. (Teubner, Leipzig, 1896.)

Aquinas. See Thomas of Aquino.

Arabian Nights. See Lane.

Arantius (Aranzi), Julius Caesar. *De Humano Foetu Opusculum.* (Rome, 1564, Carampellum, Bologna, 1595.)

Arendt, H. *Deutsch. med. Presse,* 1910, 14, 167.

Aristophanes. *The Birds,* tr. J. T. Sheppard and A. W. Verrall. (Bowes, Cambridge, 1924.)

Aristotle. *De Generatione Animalium,* tr. and ed. A. Platt. (Oxford, 1912.) Tr. and ed. A. L. Peck. (Loeb Classics, Heinemann, London, 1943.) See also Johannes Philoponus.

Aristotle. *Historia Animalium,* tr. and ed. d'A. W. Thompson. (Oxford, 1910.) See also Camus.

Aristotle. *De Partibus Animalium,* tr. and ed. W. Ogle. (Oxford, 1912.) Tr. and ed. A. L. Peck. (Loeb Classics, Heinemann, London, 1937.)

Aristotle. *Physica.* (Loeb Classics, London, 1929.)

"Aristotle." *Aristotle's book of problems, with other astronomers, astrologers, physicians and philosophers: wherein are contained divers questions and answers, touching the state of man's body.* 29th ed. (London, 1775.)

"Aristotle." *Aristotle's compleat master piece.* 32nd ed. (London, 1788.)

"Aristotle." *Aristotle's complete and experienc'd Midwife.* Made English by W— S—, M.D. 12th ed. (London, n.d.)

"Aristotle." *Aristotle's last legacy. Unfolding the mystery of nature in the generation of man.* (Hitch, London, 1761, 1776.)

"Aristotle." *Book of problems, touching the state of man's body.* 26th ed. (London, 1749, 1750.)

"Aristotle." *Complete and experienc'd midwife.* 9th ed. (London, n.d. *ca.* 1750.)

"Aristotle." *Complete master piece.* ([London], 1751.)

"Aristotle." *Last legacy, unfolding mysteries of the nature of man.* (London, 1749.)

"Aristotle." *Master-Piece or the Secrets of Generation displayed in all the parts thereof.* (How, London, 1684.)

"Aristotle." *The Works of Aristotle, the famous philosopher, containing his complete Masterpiece and family physician, his experienced midwife, his book of problems, and his remarks on physiognomy.* (Camden Pub. Co. London, n.d. [1930?].)

"Aristotle." See d'Arcy Power.

Aromatari, Joseph de. *Disputatio De Rabia Contagiosa cui praeposita est Epistola De Generatione Plantarum ex Seminibus.* (Sarcina, Venice, 1625.) Reprinted in Joachim Jungius' *Opuscula botanico-physica* (Otton, Coburg, 1747), and in *Phil. Trans. Roy. Soc.* 1693.

Asaph ha-Yehudi, MS. work described by Gottheil in *Jewish Encyclopaedia,* 1902, vol. 2, p. 162. See Sarton, vol. 1, p. 614; also Simon.

Ashley Montagu, M. F. "Adolescent Sterility," *Quart. Rev. Biol.* 1939, 14, 13 & 192. Also separately pub., Thomas, Springfield, Illinois and Ryerson, Toronto, 1946.

Ashley Montagu, M. F. *Coming into Being among the Australian Aborigines; an Examination of all the Evidence bearing upon the Procreative Beliefs of the Native Tribes of Australia.* (London, 1937.)

Ashley Montagu, M. F. (ed.). *Studies and Essays in the History of Science and Learning* (Sarton Presentation Volume). (Schuman, New York, 1944.)

Ashley Montagu, M. F. "Embryological Beliefs of Primitive Peoples," *Ciba Symposia*, 1949, **10** (no. 4), 994.

Asclepiades of Parion. See Diels.

Asmundson, V. S. *Scientific Agric.* 1931, **11**, 590; *Ber. ü. d. ges. Biologie*, 1931, **9** and subsequent vols.

Athenaeus. *The Deipnosophists.* (Bohn, London, 1854.)

Aubert, M. A letter appended to J. de Méry (1711).

Aubrey, John. *Brief Lives*, ed. A. Clark. (Oxford, 1898.)

Augerius, H. *De Sanguinis Missione.* (Frankfurt, 1598.)

Augustine of Hippo. *De Immortalitate Animae* and *De Quantitate Animae*, in Migne's *Patrologia*, Paris.

Aulus Gellius. *Noctes Atticae.* (Loeb Classics edition.)

d'Aumont, M. Article "Génération" in Denis Diderot's *Encyclopédie, ou Dictionnaire Raisonée des Sciences, des Arts, et des Métiers*, vol. 7. (Paris, 1757.)

Ausonius. *Opera.* (Loeb Classics, London, 1919.)

Avicenna. See ibn Sīnā.

Baas-Becking, L. G. M.. *Scientific Monthly*, 1924, **18**, 547.

Bachofen, J. J. *Mutterrecht u. Urreligion.* (Kröner, Leipzig, 1927.) See also Turel.

Bachofen, J. J. *Ur-religion u. antike Symbole.* (Reclam, Leipzig, 1926.)

Bacon, Sir Francis (Lord Verulam). *De Augmentis Scientiarum*, ed. Ellis & Spedding. (Routledge, London, 1905.)

von Baer, Karl Ernst. *De Ovi Mammalium et Hominis Genesi.* (Leipzig, 1827.)

von Baer, Karl Ernst. "Commentar zu der Schrift: *De Ovi Mammalium et Hominis Genesi*; Epistola ad Academiam Scient. Petropolitanum." *Zeitschr. f.d. organische Physik (Heusinger's)*, 1828, **2**, 125.

von Baer, Karl Ernst. *Ueber Entwickelungsgeschichte der Thiere, Beobachtung und Reflexion.* (Königsberg, 1828–1837–1888.) The preface to the second volume explains that as the Königsberg publisher failed to get replies to his letters to von Baer, who had moved to St Petersburg, he publishes the MS. of vol. 2 in its unfinished state, eleven years after vol. 1. Von Baer died in 1876. Twelve years later and fifty-one years after the appearance of vol. 2 Stieda published the remaining embryological notes of von Baer. This, therefore, really forms vol. 3 of von Baer's masterpiece. The three volumes are very seldom found together.

von Baer, Karl Ernst. *Untersuchungen über die Gefässebindung zwischen Mutter und Frucht.* (Voss, Leipzig, 1828.) Presented as "Glückwunsch zur Jubelfeier" to S. T. von Soemmering.

von Baer, Karl Ernst. *Nachrichten uber Leben u. Schriften des Herrn Geheim-*

raths Dr K. E. v. B. mitgetheilt von ihm selbst. (Vieweg, Bruanschweig, 1886.)

Baker, J. *Abraham Trembley; Scientist and Philosopher*, 1710–1784. (Arnold, London, 1954.)

Balfour, F. M. *A Treatise on Comparative Embryology*, 2 vols. (Macmillan, London, 1880.)

Ballantyne, J. W. *Teratogenesis; an Enquiry into the Causes of Monstrosities; History of the Theories of the Past.* (Oliver & Boyd, Edinburgh, 1897.)

Ballantyne, J. W. "The *Byrth of Mankinde*; its Author, Editions and Contents," *Journ. Obstet. & Gyn. Brit. Emp.*, 1906 and 1907, also separately pub. Sherratt & Hughes, London (n.d.).

Balss, H. On preformation and epigenesis in Greek philosophy. *Archeion* (*Archivio d. Storia d. Sci.*), 1923, **4**, 319.

Balss, H. *Albertus Magnus als Zoologe.* (München, 1928.)

Balss, H. "Über die Vererbungstheorie des Galenos," *Archiv. f. Gesch. d. Med. u. d. Naturw.*, 1934, **27**, 229.

Balss, H. "Die Zeugungslehre and Embryologie in der Antike"; *Quellen u. Studien z. Geschichte d. Naturwiss. u. d. Med.*, 1936, **5**, 1.

Baranov, P. A. *Istoria Embriologii Rastenii.* (Acad. Sci., Moscow, 1955.)

Barbado. "L'Embryologie Scholastique," *Revue Thomiste*, 1931.

Barbatus, Hieronymus. *De formatione, conceptione, organizatione, et nutritione foetus in utero Dissertatio Anatomica.* (Bodi, Padua, 1676.)

Barbour, A. H. F. "Soranus on Gynaecological Medicine," in *Proceedings of the XVIIth International Congress of Medicine*, 1913, Section of the History of Medicine, p. 269. (London, 1914.)

Barcroft, J. *Features in the Architecture of Physiological Function.* (Cambridge, 1934.)

Barcroft, J. *The Brain and its Environment.* (Yale Univ. Press, New Haven, 1938.)

Bartels, M. See Ploss & Bartels.

Barth, L. G. *Embryology.* (Dryden, New York, 1953.)

Barthold, G. T. *Opera medica tripartita.* (Frankfurt, 1717.)

Bartholinus, Caspar (the Younger). *De ovariis mulierum et generationis Historia epistola anatomica.* (Rome, 1677, Westen, Amsterdam, 1678; also Nürnberg, 1679.)

Bartholinus, Caspar (the Younger). *Exercitationes Miscellaneae.* (Hackiana, Leiden, 1675.)

Bast, T. H. *Ann. Med. Hist.* 1924. **6**, 369.

Baster, J. *Natuurkundige Uitspanningen, behelzende eene Beschrijving, van meer dan vier hondert Planten en Insekten keurig naar het leven afgebeeld.* (van Paddenburg & van Dijk, Utrecht, n.d. *ca.* 1750.)

Baster, J. *Opuscula de animalibus et plantis marinis.* (Haarlem, 1761.)

Bauhin, Caspar (ed.). *Gynaeciorum sive de mulierum affectibus Comment. graecorum, latinorum, barbarorum, iam olim & nunc recens editorum.* (Basel, 1586.) 1. Fel. Plater, *De mulierum partibus generationi.* 2. Moschion, *De passionibus muliebrum*, ed. Conr. Gesner & C. Wolph. 3. Cleopatra, Moschion, Priscianus, *Incerti cujusdam muliebrum libri*, in unam red. p. Casp. Wolphium. 4. Trotula sive potius Erotis, muliebrum; medici liberti Juliae, Muliebrium liber. 5. Nic. Rochel, *De morbis mulierum curandis*. 6. Lud. Banaciolus, *Enneas muliebris*. 7. Jac. Sylvius, *De mensibus muliebribus*. 8. Joa. Ryff, *De conceptu & generatione hominis*.

Baumann, B. *Filosofické Názory Jana Marka Marci* (Č.S.A.V., Prague, 1957).

Baÿ, M. *Bull. de l'Instit. Égypt.* 1912 (sér. 5), 5.

Bayen, M. Cit. in Fourcroy's *System d. chem. Kenntnis*, vol. 4, 476.

Bayon, H. P. "Ancient Pregnancy Tests in the Light of Contemporary Knowledge," *Proc. Roy. Soc. Med.*, 1939, 32, 1527.

Bayon, H. P. "Trotula and the Ladies of Salerno," *Proc. Roy. Soc. Med.*, 1940,

Bayon, H. P. "William Harvey, Physician and Biologist; his Precursors, Opponents and Successors," *Ann. of Sci.*, 1938, 3, 59, 83 & 435; 1939, 4, 65.

Beccher, J. *Physica Subterranea*. (Gleditsch, Leipzig, 1703.)

Beckher, D. *Medicus microcosmus*. (Leiden, 1633.)

Beddoes, T. *Analysis of Mayow's Chemical Opinions*. (Oxford, 1790.)

Beguelin, L. "Memoire sur l'art de couver les œufs ouverts." In *Histoire de l'Acad. des Sciences et Belles-Lettres de Berlin*. (Berlin, 1749.)

Bellinger, F. *Tractatus de foetu nutritio; or, a discourse concerning the Nutrition of the Foetus in the Womb, demonstrated to be by ways hitherto unknown, in which is likewise discover'd the use of the gland Thymus*. (Innys, London, 1717.)

Belon, Pierre. *Histoire naturelle des estranges poissons marins avec la vraie peincture et description du daulphin et de plusieurs autres de son espèce*. (Chaudière, Paris, 1551.)

Belon, Pierre. *La nature et diversité des poissons avec leurs porctraits*. (Estienne, Paris, 1555.)

Belon, Pierre. *Histoire de la nature des oyseaux avec leurs descriptions et naifs porctraits retirez du naturel*. (Cavellat, Paris, 1555.)

Benedictus, A. "De principatu cordis," in *De humani corporis*. (Basel, 1527.)

Berger, J. G. *Physiologia medica*. (Wittenberg, 1702.)

Bernhard, C. *De nutritione foetu per fune umbilicale*. (Hendel, Magdeburg, 1732.)

Berniard, C. *Journ. de physique* (*Rozier's*), 1780, 15, 447.

Berthelot, Marcelin. *La Chimie au Moyen Age*. (Paris, 1893.)

Berthier, A. G. On Descartes' embryology. *Isis* (*Sarton's*), 1914, 2, 86.

Bertuch, J. M. *Dissertatio anatomica de Ovario Mulierum*. (Krebs, Jena, 1681.)

Berzelius, P. P. *Journ. f. Chem. u. Physik* (*Gehlen's*), 1807, 7, 581.

Beseke, J. M. G. *Versuch einer Geschichte der Hypothesen über die Erzeugung der Thiere*. (Mitau, 1797.)

Bianchi, B. *De Natura Generationis*. (Turin, 1741.)

Bidloo, G. *Anatomia Humani Corporis*. (Amsterdam, 1685.)

Bierling, C. T. *Thesaurus theoretico-practicus*. (Jena, 1690.)

Bigelow, M. See Redi, Francesco.

Bilikiewicz, Thaddeus. *Die Embryologie im Zeitalter des Barock und des Rokoko*.

(Thieme, Leipzig, 1932.) (Arbeiten d. Inst. f. Gesch. d. Med., Univ. Leipzig, no. 2.)

Birch, Thomas. *History of the Royal Society*. (London, 1756.)

Blacher, L. A. *Istorii Embriologii v Rossii, XVIII–XIX v.v.* (in Russian). (Acad. Sci., Moscow, 1955.)

Blampignon, E. A. *Étude sur Malebranche* (Douniol, Paris, 1862.)

Blancard, S. *Opera medico-theoretico-practica*. (Leiden, 1702.)

Blasius, Gerardus. *Observata Anatomica*. (Gaasbeck, Leiden & Amsterdam, 1674.) Cit. in von Haller, q.v.

Blersch, K. *Wesen u. Entstehung des Sexus im Denken der Antike*. (Kohlhammer, Stuttgart, 1937.) (Tübinger Beitr. z. Altertumswiss. no. 29.)

Bligh, E. W. *Sir Kenelm Digby and his Venetia*. (Sampson Low, London, 1932.)

Bloch, Bruno. *Die geschichtlichen Grundlagen der Embryologie bis auf Harvey*. (Karras, Halle, 1904.) (Reprinted from *Nova Acta; Abhandl. d. kaiserl. Leopold-Karol. deutsch. Akad. d. Naturforscher*, 1904, **82**, 217.)

Bloch, Bruno. *Zoologische Annalen*, 1905, **1**, 51.

Bloch, I. Art. "Byzantinische Medizin," in Neuburger-Pagel, q.v.

Blondel, J. A. *The Strength of the Imagination in pregnant women consider'd*. (London, 1726.)

Blondel, J. A. *The Power of the Mother's Imagination over the Foetus examin'd in answer to Doctor Daniel Turner's Book intitled 'A defence of the XIIth chapter of the 1st part of a treatise De Morbis Cutaneis.'* (Brotherton, London, 1729.)

Blondel, J. A. *Sur la force de l'imagination des Femmes enceintes sur le Fetus*. (Leiden, 1737.)

Blumenbach, J. W. *Handbuch d. vergleichenden Anatomie* (Dieterich, Göttingen, 1815.) Ch. xxv deals with viviparous; and ch. xxvii with oviparous, development.

Blumenbach, J. W. *Ueber den Bildungstrieb (nisus formativus) und seinen Einfluss auf die Generation und Reproduction*. (Göttingen, 1781.) (Engl. tr. *An Essay on Generation*, London, 1792.)

Boerhaave, Hermann. *Institutiones Medicae*. (Leiden, 1727.)

Boerhaave, Hermann. *Elementa Chemiae, quae anniversario labore docuit in publicis privatisque scholis Hermannus Boerhaave*. (Isaacus Severinus, Leiden, 1732.)

Boerhaave, Hermann. *Praelectiones Academiae*. . . . See von Haller, A.

Bohnius, J. *Circulus anatomico-physiologicus*. (Leipzig, 1686.)

du Bois, A. M. "The Development of Genetics," *Ciba Symposia*, 1939, **1** (no. 8), 234, French tr. *Revue Ciba*, 1939, **1** (no. 3), 66.

Boldrini, B. On Cangiamila. *Riv. di Storia d. Sci. Med. e Nat.* 1927, **18**, 1.

Bonaciolus, L. *De conformatione foetus*. (Moyaert, Leiden, 1650.) With Pinaeus, q.v.

Bonnemain, L. *Observations de faire éclore et élever la volaille sans le secours des poules*. (Paris, 1816.)

Bonnet, Charles. *Traité d'Insectologie*. (Paris, 1745.)

Bonnet, Charles. *Considérations sur les Corps Organisés*. (Rey, Amsterdam, 1762; Fauche, Neuchâtel, 1779.)

Bonnet, Charles. *La Palingénésie philosophique, ou Idées sur l'État passé et sur l'état futur des êtres vivans; Ouvrage destiné à servir de Supplément aux derniers Écrits de l'Auteur et qui contient principalement le précis de ses Recherches sur le Christianisme*. (Claude Philibert et Barthelemi Chirol, Geneva, 1770.)

Bonnet, Charles. *Oeuvres d'Histoire Naturelle et de Philosophie*. (Neuchâtel, 1779.)

Borel, Pierre. *De Vero Telescopii Inventore cum brevi omnium conspiciliorum historia*. (The Hague, 1655.)

Borelli, Giovanni Alfonso. *De Motu Animalium*. (Rome, 1680–1681.)

Borelli, Giovanni Alfonso. *De Motu Animalium; Editio Nova, a plurimis mendis repurgata, ac Dissertationibus physico-mechanicis de Motu Musculorum, et de effervescentia et fermentatione Clarissimi Viri Joh. Bernoullii aucta et ornata*. (Pieter Gosse, Hague, 1743.)

van den Bosch, H. *De Natura et utilitate amnii*. (Utrecht, 1792.)

Bose, Caspar. *Generatio παραδοξος in Rana conspicua*. (Titus, Leipzig, 1724.)

Bose, Caspar. *De obstetricum erroribus*. Inaug. Diss. (Breitkopf, Leipzig, 1729.)

Bostock, J. *Ann. de Chem.* 1808, **67**, 35.

Bostock, J. *Nicholson's Journ.* 1805, **11**, 244; *Journ. Nat. Philos. Chem. and the Arts*, 1806, **14**, 140.

Bostock, J. Cit. in Moleschott's *Physiologie d. Nahrungsmittel*, 1859, vol. 2, p. 84.

Boswell, J. *Life of Samuel Johnson, Esq.* (Cadell, London, 1811.)

Böttger, C. F. *Foetum non ante conceptionem in ovulo praeexistere, sed post eandem formari*. (Brandenburger, Leipzig, 1708.)

Bourguet, Louis. *Lettres philosophiques sur la Formation des Sels et des Crystaux et sur la Génération et le Mechanisme Organique des Plantes et des Animaux à l'Occasion de la Pierre Belemnite, et de la Pierre Lenticulaire*. (Amsterdam, 1729.)

Boyle, Robert. *The Sceptical Chymist; or, chymico-physical doubts and paradoxes, touching the spagyrist's principles commonly called hypostatical, as they are wont to be proposed and defended by the generality of Alchymists* (J. Cadwell for J. Crooke, London, 1661.)

Boyle, Robert. *Phil. Trans. Roy. Soc.* 1666, **1**, 199.

Boyle, Robert. *Continuation of New Experiments Touching the Spring and Weight of the Air and their Effects*. (H. Hall, Oxford, 1669.)

Boyle, Robert. *The Sceptical Chymist; or Chemico-Physical Doubts and Paradoxes, touching the Experiments whereby Vulgar Spagyrists are wont to endeavour to evince their Salt, Sulphur and Mercury to be the True Principles of things, to which in this edition are subjoyn'd divers Experiments and Notes about the Producibleness of Chymical Principles*. (Oxford, 1679.)

Boyle, Robert. *The Sceptical Chymist, or Chymico-physical doubts and para-*

doxes touching the experiments whereby vulgar Spagyrists are wont to endeavour to evince their salt, sulphur, and mercury to be the true principles of things. (Davis, Oxford, 1680.)

Boyle, Robert. *A Continuation of New Experiments Physico-mechanical touching the Spring & Weight of the Aire & their Effects*, p. 99, Exp. VI. (Davis, London, 1682.)

Boyle, Robert. *A Disquisition about the Final Causes of Natural Things. To which are subjoin'd by way of Appendix some uncommon Observations about vitiated Sight.* (J. Taylor, London, 1688.)

Boyle, Robert. *Philosophical Works, abridged, methodized and disposed under the general heads of Physics, Statics, Pneumatics, Natural History, Chymistry and Medicine. With notes by Peter Shaw.* (W. and J. Innys, London, 1725.)

Boyle, Robert. For complete bibliography, *see* Fulton, J. F.

Brachet, J. *Chemical Embryology.* (Interscience, New York & London, 1950.)

Brady, Samuel. *Phil. Trans. Roy. Soc.* 1704, **24**, 2176.

Brand, John. *Observations on Popular Antiquities.* (London, 1810.)

Brendel, A. *De Embryone in ovulo ante conceptum prae-existante.* (Wittenberg, 1703 & 1704.) Reprinted in Haller's *Disputationes Selectae*, 1750.

Briffault, R. *The Mothers.* (Allen & Unwin, London, 1927.)

Brody, S. *Bio-energetics and Growth.* (Reinhold, New York, 1945.)

Browne, E. G. *Arabian Medicine.* (Cambridge, 1921, 1924.)

Browne, Sir Thomas. *Pseudodoxia Epidemica, or enquiries into very many received Tenents and commonly presumed Truths.* (T. H. for Edward Dod, London, 1646.) Ed. Sayle. (Grant, Edinburgh, 1912.)

Browne, Sir Thomas. *Commonplace Books*, ed. Wilkins, in vol. IV of the collected edition. (Pickering, London, 1836.)

Browne, Sir Thomas. *Letters*, ed. Wilkins. (Pickering, London, 1836.)

Browne, Sir Thomas. *Religio Medici*, ed. Sayle. (Grant, Edinburgh, 1912.)

Browne, Sir Thomas. *Hydriotaphia, a treatise on Urn-burial*, ed. Sayle. (Grant, Edinburgh, 1912.)

Browne, Sir Thomas. For complete bibliography, see Keynes, Geoffrey and Leroy, O.

Browne, Sir Thomas. Portraits of, see Tildesley.

Brugsch, H. *Notice raisonné d'un Traité médical datant du XIVème siècle avant notre ère et contenu dans un Papyrus hiératique du Musée royale de Berlin.* (Leipzig, 1863.)

Brunet, P. "Guéneau de Montbéliard" in *Mém. de l'Acad. des Sci. Arts et Belles-lettres de Dijon*, 1925, 125.

Brunet, P. *Maupertuis; son œuvre et sa place dans la Pensée scientifique et philosophique du XVIIIème Siècle.* (Paris, 1929.)

von Brunner, J. C. *Experimenta nova circa Pancreas.* (Amsterdam, 1683.)

von Buddenbrock, W. *Bilder aus d. Geschichte d. biologischen Grundprobleme.* (Bornträger, Berlin, 1930.)

de Buffon, G. L. L., Comte. *Histoire Naturelle.* (Paris, 1749.) (Eng. tr. by William Smellie, Strahan, London, 1785.)

Bühle, C. A. In J. F. Naumann & C. A. Bühle, *Eier der Vögel Deutschlands.* (Halle, 1818.)

Buissière, J. *Phil. Trans. Roy. Soc.* 1694, **18** (no. 207), 11.

Buniva. M. F. See Vauquelin & Buniva.

Burchard, H. *Der Entelechiebegriff bei Aristoteles und Driesch.* Inaug. Diss. (Münster i/W., 1928.)

Burckhardt, R. *Verhandlungen d. naturforsch. Gesellsch. Basel,* 1904, **15**, 377; 1903, **16**, 388; 1910, **20**, 1.

Burnet, J. *Early Greek Philosophy.* 3rd ed. (London, 1920.)

Cabbala. See *Kabbalah.*

Cadman, W. H. "Egyptian Incubators and Methods of Incubation," *Transactions of the 1st World Poultry Congress,* 1921, **2**, 97.

Calepinus, Ambrosius. *Dictionarium,* under "Vitellus." (Bertoch, Reggio in Lombardy, 1502.)

Calkins, L. A. See Scammon & Calkins.

Camerarius, E. *Medicina conciliatrix.* (Frankfurt, 1714.)

Camerarius, R. J. *Specimen Experimentorum physiologico-therapeuticorum circa Generationem hominis et animalium.* In Haller's *Disputationes Selectae,* 1750.

Camus, P. Translation: *L'Histoire des Animaux d'Aristote,* vol. **2**, notes under "Génération" and "Œuf." (Desains, Paris, 1785.)

Candidus, Petrus. *De Genitura hominis.* (Rome, 1474.) See Osler, p. 62.

Cangiamila, F. E. *Embryologia Sacra sive de Officio Sacerdotum Medicorum etc. circa aeternam Parvulorum in Utero existentium Salutem.* (F. Valenza, Palermo, 1745, 1758; German ed., München & Ingolstadt, 1764.)

Cangiamila, F. E. *Embryologia Sacra, sive de Officio Sacerdotum Medicorum, et aliorum, circa aeternam Parvulorum in Utero existentium salutem.* (Walwein, Ypres, 1775.)

Cangiamila, F. E. *Abrégé de l'Embryologie sacrée,* tr. from the Italian by C. Dinouart. (Nyon, Paris, 1762.)

Capellmann, A. *Pastoral-medizin.* (Aachen, 1892.)

Capivaccius, H. "De Formato foetu," in *Opera Omnia,* Sect. 1, lib. 1. (Palthen, Frankfurt, 1603.)

Cardanus, Hieronymus. *De Subtilitate libri XXI.* (Joannes Petreius, Nürnberg, 1550.)

Cardanus, Hieronymus. *Les livres de Hierome Cardanus intitulés de la subtilité et subtiles inventions, ensembles les causes occultes et raisons d'icelles, traduis de Latin en François par Richard le Blanc.* (Jan Foucher, Paris, 1556.)

Cardanus, Hieronymus. *Contradicentium Medicorum,* Tractate 6, section 17. (Macaeus, Paris, 1564.)

Cardelinus, V. *De origine Foetu.* (Amadei, Vicenza, 1628.)

Carmichael, Leonard. "Origin and prenatal growth of behaviour," contrib. to *Handbook of Child Psychology.* (Clark Univ., Worcester, Mass., 1933.)

Case, J. *Compendium Anatomiae.* (Amsterdam, 1696.)

Cassirer, E. *Leibniz' System in seinen wissenschaftlichen Grundlagen.* (Marburg, 1902.)

de Castro, R. *De universa muliebrium morborum Medicina.* (Venice, 1644.)

de Castro, R. *De Natura Mulierum.* (Cologne, 1689.)

Cesana, G. *Archivio di Fisiol.* 1911, **9**, 1.

Cesenas, H. D. Cited in Aldrovandus, q.v.

Chamberlen, Hugh. See Mauriceau.

Chambers, Frank P. *Cycles of Taste.* (Harvard Univ. Press, Cambridge, Mass., 1928.)

Charleton, Walter. *De Catameniis et de Fluore Albo.* (Leiden, 1686.)

Charleton, Walter. *A Ternary of Paradoxes; The Magnetick Cure of Wounds, The Nativity of Tartar in Wine, The Image of God in Man; written originally by Joh. Bapt. van Helmont, Translated, Illustrated, and Ampliated, etc.* (Lee, London, 1650.)

Chattock, A. P. *Phil. Trans. Roy. Soc.* B, 1925, **213**, 397.

Cheyne, G. *Philosophical Principles of Natural Religion, containing the elements of natural philosophy and the proofs of natural religion arising from them.* (Strahan, London, 1715.)

Cheyne, G. *Theory of Acute and Slow Fevers.* (London, 1722.)

Chiarugi, G. On Borelli and the problems of embryology. *Monit. Zool. Ital.* 1929, **40**, 146.

Choulant, Louis. *History of Anatomic Illustration,* tr. M. Frank. (Chicago, 1920.)

Chrysippus of Cnidus. See Allbutt.

Ciccotti, E. *Untergang d. Sklaverei im Altertum.* (Vorwärts, Berlin, 1910.)

Cicero, Marcus Tullius. *De Natura Deorum,* tr. Francis Brooks. (Methuen, London, 1896.)

Clark, Alden. *Atlantic Monthly,* Feb. 1928.

Clement of Alexandria. "Exhortations to the Greeks," in Migne's *Patrologia.*

Cleophantus. See Allbutt.

de Clercq, F. S. A. & Schmelz, J. D. E. *Ethnographische Beschrijving van de West- en Noordkust van Nederlandsch Nieuw-Guinea.* (Leiden, 1893.)

Coghill, G. E. *Journ. Comp. Neurol. & Psychol.* 1909, **19**, 83.

Coghill, G. E. *Anatomy and the Problem of Behaviour.* (Cambridge, 1929.)

Cohen, A. *Everyman's Talmud.* (Dent, London, 1932.)

Coiter, Volcher. "De ovorum gallinaceorum generationis primo exordio progressuque, et pulli gallinacei creationis ordine," in *Externarum et internarum principalium humani corporis partium Tabulae et Exercitationes,* p. 32. (Gerlatz, Nürnberg, 1573.) Translated into English (omitting the last 3 pages) and edited with critical notes by H. B. Adelmann, *Annals Med. Hist.* 1933, **5**, 327, 444. Another portion of the book, of embryological interest—"Ossium tum humani foetus, adhuc in utero existentis, vel imperfecti Abortus, tum infantis dimidium annum nati, brevis Historia atque Explicatio; in qua ossium prima origo, incrementum et discrimen inter tenellulorum ac grandiorum ossa aperte declaratur," p. 57, was reprinted by H. Eysson (without plate) in *Henrici Eyssonii* *med. doct. et prof. Tractatus anatomicus et medicus, de ossibus infantis cognoscendis, conservandis et curandis, accessit V. Coiteri eorundem ossium Historia.* (Cöllen, Groningen, 1659.)

Cole, F. J. Contribution to *Stud. Hist. Meth. Sci.*, vol. 2, 285. (Oxford, 1921.)

Cole, F. J. "Dr William Croone on Generation" in *Studies and Essays in the History of Science and Learning* (Sarton Presentation Volume), ed. M. F. Ashley Montagu, p. 115. (Schuman, New York, 1944.)

Cole, F. J. *Early Theories of Sexual Generation.* (Oxford, 1930.)

Cole, L. J. "The Lay of the Rooster," *Journ. Hered.*, 1927, **18**, 97.

Cole, R. *Annals Med. Hist.* 1926, **8**, 347.

Columbus, Realdus. *De Re Anatomica.* (Venice, 1559.)

Columella, L. Junius. *Husbandry*, anonymous tr. (Millar, London, 1745.)

Connor, B. *Evangelium medicum.* (London, 1697.)

Constantine the African. See Singer, C.

Cook, A. B. *Zeus.*, 3 vols. (Cambridge, 1925 & 1926.)

Cook, S. A. Notes to the 3rd edition of Robertson Smith's *Religion of the Semites.* (Black, London, 1927.)

C[ooke], J. *The New Theory of Generation, according to the best and latest discoveries in Anatomy, farther improv'd and fully display'd.* (Buckland, London, 1762.)

Corner, G. W. "The discovery of the mammalian ovum," in *Lectures on the History of Medicine* (Mayo Foundation, etc.), p. 401. (Saunders, Philadelphia, 1933.)

Cornford, F. M. *Classical Quarterly*, 1930, **24**, 14. (See also Diels on Anaxagoras, Frag. 10.)

Corradi, A. "Dell'antica Autoplastica Italiana," *Atti. Real. Ist. Lombardo*, 1874, 226.

Coschwitz, G. D. *Essays of a society in Edinburgh*, 1730, **5**, 336.

Costaeus, J. *De humani conceptus formatione.* (Bartol, Pavia, 1604.)

Coulton, G. G. *Infant Perdition in the Middle Ages.* (Simpkin Marshall, London, 1922.) Mediaeval Studies, no. 16.

de Craan, Theodore. *Tractatus physico-medicus de Homine, in quo status ejus tam naturalis quam praeternaturalis quoad Theoriam rationalem mechanice demonstratur.* (P. van der Aa, Leiden, 1689.)

de Craan, Theodore. *Oeconomia Animalis.* (Amsterdam, 1703.)

Cramer, M. See Pictet & Cramer.

Crawfurd, R. "Superstitions concerning Menstruation," *Proc. Roy. Soc. Med.* (Hist. Med. Sect.), 1916, **9**, 49.

Crawley, A. E. "Foeticide," contrib. to Hastings' *Encyclopaedia of Religion and Ethics*, vol. **6**. (Clark, Edinburgh, 1913.)

Cremonius, C. *Apologia pro doctrinae Aristoteles de origine et principatu membrorum adversus.* (Venice, 1627.)

Crescentius, Petrus. *De omnibus Agriculturae partibus et de plantarum animaliumque Natura, libri XII.* (Peter, Basel, 1548.)

Crevelt. *Magazin d. Gesellschaft d. Naturforscherfreunde in Berlin*, 1806, **1**, 137.

de la Croix, François Boissier de Sauvages. See Raisin, R. G.

Croone, William. *Phil. Trans. Roy. Soc.* 1672, **7**, 5080. See tr. by F. J. Cole (1944.) See also Birch, *History of the Royal Society,* 1757, vol. **3**, 30.

Cruikshank, W. *Phil. Trans. Roy. Soc.* 1797, **87**, 301.

Culpepper, N. *A Directory for Midwives; or, A Guide for Women, in their Conception, Bearing and Suckling their Children.* . . . (London, 1651.)

Cumston, C. G. "The Finances of Felix Platter, Professor of Medicine at Basel," in *Annals Med. Hist.* 1921, **2**, 265.

Cusanus, Nicholas. See Nicholas of Cusa.

Cuvier, G., Baron. *Edin. New Philos. Journ.* 1836, **20**, 1.

Cyprianus, A. *Epistola de foetu tubario exciso.* (Leiden, 1700.)

Dalenpatius (de Plantade's pseudonym). "Extrait d'une lettre de M. Dalenpatius à l'auteur de ces nouvelles contenant une découverte curieuse, faite par le moyen du microscope," in J. Bernard's *Nouvelles de la République des Lettres,* p. 552. (Amsterdam, 1699.) Abstracted by Leeuwenhoek, *Phil. Trans. Roy. Soc.* 1699, **21**.

Dante Alighieri. *Convivio,* tr. W. W. Jackson. (Oxford, 1909.)

Dante Alighieri. *Divina Commedia,* tr. H. F. Tozer. (Oxford, 1904.)

Danz, D. F. G. *Grundriss der Zergliederungskunde des ungeborenen Kindes.* (Frankfurt, 1792; Giessen, 1793.)

Dareste, Camille. *Recherches sur la production artificielle des Monstruosités, ou essais de Tératogénie expérimentale.* (Reinwald, Paris, 1877.)

Dartiguelongue, J. *Apographe rerum physico-medicarum.* (Amsterdam, 1708.)

Darwin, Charles. *Life and Letters,* ed. F. Darwin. (Murray, London, 1887.)

Darwin, Erasmus. *Zoonomia; or, the Laws of Organic Life.* (London, 1794.)

Dasgupta, S. Chapter "Speculations in the Medical Schools," in *A History of Indian Philosophy,* vol. **2**. (Cambridge, 1932.)

Debrunner, H. "Michel de Montaigne and die Lehre von den Missbildungen," *Gesnerus,* 1946, **3**, 1.

Dehne, J. C. C. *Chem. Ann. (Crelle's),* **3**, 24.

Democritus of Abdera. See Diels.

Descartes, René. MS. "Sur la génération des animaux," in *Œuvres de R. Descartes,* vol. **9**, ed. and tr. V. Cousin. (Levrault, Paris, 1826.)

Descartes, René. *L'Homme, et un traitté de la formation du foetus du mesme autheur.* (C. Angot, Paris, 1664.) The history of this, the first complete treatise on physiology, is peculiar. It is related in the *édition nationale* of Descartes, vol. **10**, by Adam & Tannery (Paris, 1909). Descartes died in 1650. In 1662 appeared at Leiden a quarto volume, *Renatus Des Cartes De Homine,* in which the editor, Florent Schuyl, tells that he had access to a manuscript copy of this unpublished work of Descartes, and had translated it into Latin. His figures were doubtless in part copied from the original but were all redrawn for the editor. In 1664 the Paris printer-publisher, Jacques le Gras, issued *Le Monde de Mr Descartes* in octavo. A little after, namely on the 12th April 1664, the printing of the original French version of Descartes' great treatise on physiology, together with direct copies of the author's own figures, designed to form part of *Le Monde*, was completed by le Gras for Clerselier. This French version, which contains a long preface by Clerselier explaining the history of the authentic MS., is thus the real first edition as designed by Descartes. It is rarer than the earlier Latin edition. At the end of Clerselier's preface is the official *imprimatur*, together with an advertisement to the effect that he has ceded his rights of sale to Jacques and Nicolas le Gras, Charles Angot and Théodore Girard. Most of the copies bear the names of Angot or Girard. The original printer, Jacques le Gras, appears to have acted as publisher only in a minor degree.

Descartes, René. *L'Homme, et la Formation du Foetus, avec les Remarques de Louis de la Forge.* (M. Bobin et N. le Gras, Paris, 1677.)

Detwiler, S. R. *Neuro-embryology.* (Macmillan, New York, 1936.)

Deusingius, A. *Fasciculus dissertationum.* (Groningen, 1660.)

Deusingius, A. *Genesis microcosmi.* (Amsterdam, 1665.)

Deusingius, A. *Historia Foetus extra Uterum in abdomine geniti.* (Cöllen, Groningen, 1661.)

Deventer, J. *Observations importantes sur le manuel des accouchements.* (Paris, 1734.)

Diels, Hermann. *Fragmente der Vorsokratiker.* (Berlin, 1906 & 1922.)

Diels, Hermann. "Wissenschaft und Technik bei d. Hellenen," in *Antike Technik*, pp. 31–33. (Leipzig & Berlin, 1920.)

van Diemerbroeck, I. *Anatomia.* (Utrecht, 1685.)

Diepgen, P. *Frauenheilkunde d. alten Welt.* (Bergmann, München, 1937.)

de Diest, J. *Sui Sanguinis Solus opifex Fetus est.* (Paris, 1735.) Reprinted in Haller's *Disputationes Selectae*, 1750.

Dieterici, F. *Die Philosophie der Araber in IX und X Jahrhunderten n. Chr., aus der Theologie des Aristoteles, den Abhandlungen Alfarabis, und den Schriften der Lauten Brüder* (partial translation of the *Rasā'il Ikhwān al-Ṣafā*, the Treatises of the Brethren of Sincerity). (Hinrichs, Leipzig, 1858–1895.)

Digby, Sir Kenelm. *Two treatises, in the one of which The Nature of Bodies, in the other the nature of Mans Soule, is looked into, in way of discovery of the Immortality of Reasonable Soules.* (Williams, London, 1644.)

Digges, Leonard. *A Geometrical Practise named Pantometria.* (London, 1571.)

Diocles of Carystus. See Allbutt.

Diodorus Siculus. In *Bibliothèque historique*, tr. Miot. (Paris, 1834.) Loeb classics. (Heinemann, London.)

Diogenes of Apollonia. See Diels.

Dionis, P. *Traité des Accouchemens.* (Paris, 1724.)

Dircks, H. *The Life, Times and Scientific Labours of the Second Marquis of Worcester, to which is added a Reprint of his "Century of Inventions" (1663), with a Commentary thereon.* (Quaritch, London, 1865.)

Dittrick, H. *Annals Med. Hist.* 1928, **10**, 90.

Dobell, Clifford. *Antony van Leeuwenhoek and his "Little Animals."* (Bale & Danielsson, London, 1932.)

de Dobrzensky, J. J. Wenc. Biography of Marcus Marci in introductions to Marci's *Liturgia Mentis*. (Regensburg, 1678.)

Dobson, J. F. "Herophilus," *Proc. Roy. Soc. Med.* (Hist. of Med. Sect.), 1925, **18**, 19.

Dobson, J. F. "Erasistratus," *Proc. Roy. Soc. Med.* (Hist. of Med. Sect.), 1927, **20**, 49.

Dogelb, V. A. *A. O. Kovalevsky*. (Biography, in Russian.) (Acad. Sci., Moscow, 1945.)

Dolaeus, J. *Encyclopaedia medica*. (Frankfurt, 1684.)

Donley, J. E. "John Riolan the younger," in *Providence Med. Journ.* 1907, **8**, 246. Review in *Janus*, 1908, **13**, 611.

Donne, John. *Paradoxes and Problems*, first published 1633. (Nonesuch Press, London, 1930, p. 348.)

Drelincurtius, Charles. *Experimenta anatomica, quibus adiecta sunt plurima curiosa super semine virili, foemineis ovis, utero, uterique tubis atque foetu.* (Leiden, 1684.)

Drelincurtius, Charles. *Opuscula de foetus humani conceptione, membranis, umbilico, nutritione atque partu.* (Boutestyn, Leiden, 1685.)

Drelincurtius, Charles. *De Conceptione Conceptus.* (Leiden, 1685.)

Driesch, Hans. *History and Theory of Vitalism.* (Macmillan, London, 1914.)

Duncan, I. M. *Edinburgh Med. Journ.* 1876, **21**, 1061.

Duns Scotus. *De Rerum Principio.* MS., see Harris, C. H. S. and Sharp, D. E.

Duval, J. *Des Hermaphrodits.* (Rouen, 1612.)

Duverney, G. J. "Traité de la Génération," and "Observations sur la Circulation du Sang dans le Foetus," in *Oeuvres Anatomiques*, 2 vols. (Jombert, Paris, 1761.) Vol. **2**, pp. 380, 414 and 458 respectively.

Dzondi, C. H. *Supplementa ad anatomiam et physiologiam potissim. compar.* (Crusius, Leipzig, 1806.)

Dzondi, C. H. *Journ. f. Chem. u. Physik (Gehlen's)*, 1806, **2**, 652.

Ebstein, E. *Mitt. z. Gesch. d. Med. u. Naturwiss.* 1912, **11**, 328.

Ebstein, E., Sticker, G., Feis, and Ferckel, C. *Mitt. z. Gesch. d. Med. u. Naturwiss.*, 1920, **19**, 102, 219, 305.

Eccleshymer, A. C. *St Louis Med. Review*, 1904, **49**, 273.

Eckermann, J. P. *Conversations of Goethe*, tr. J. Oxenford. (London, 1850.)

Eliade, M. *Forgerons et Alchimistes.* (Flammarion, Paris, 1956.)

Ellinger, T. U. H. *Hippocrates on Intercourse and Pregnancy.* (Schuman, New York, 1952.)

Empedocles of Akragas. See Diels.

Engels, F. *L'Origine de la Famille, de la propriété privée, et de l'état.* (Costes, Paris, 1931.)

Ens, A. *Lettres sur l'imagination des femmes grosses.* (Paris, 1745.)

Ent, George. *Opera medico-physica.* (Leiden, 1687.)

Epicurus. See Plutarch and Allbutt.

Epistolae Obscurorum Virorum. Ed. and tr. F. G. Stokes. (Chatto & Windus, London, 1909.)

Erasistratus of Chios. See Dobson.

Erhard, H. "Die Entdeckung der Parthenogenesis durch Charles Bonnet," *Gesnerus*, 1946, **3**, 15.

Esser, A. M. "Moderne europäische und alt-indische Embryologie; eine Vergleichung," *Münch. Med. Wochschr.*, 1925, **72**, 1643.

Ettmüller, M. *Opera medica*. (Rips, Amsterdam, 1696.)

Evans, Joannes. *De Foetus Humani Nutritio Inaug. Diss.* (Balfour & Smellie, Edinburgh, 1788.)

Evelyn, John. *Diary*. (Everyman Edition, Dent, London, 1907.)

Everardus, A. *Novus et genuinus hominis brutique animalis Exortus*. (Kroock, Middelburgh, 1661.)

Everardus, A. *Cosmopolitae historia naturalis, comprehendens humani corporis atomicam et anatomicam delineationem ab ipsis primis foetus rudimentis in utero, usque ad perfectum et adultum statum, lumine praeclaro generationem hominis et efformationem exhibens, dein usum et structuram omnium vasorum in eodem perfecto summa cum arte demonstrans*. (P. van der Aa, Leiden, 1686.)

Faber, Honoratus, S.J. *Tractatus duo quorum prior est de plantis et de generatione animalium, posterior de homine*. (Miguet, Paris, 1666.)

Fabricius ab Aquapendente, Hieronymus. *De Formato Foetu*. (Venice, 1600.)

Fabricius ab Aquapendente, Hieronymus. *De Formatione Ovi et Pulli*. (Padua, 1621.)

Fabricius ab Aquapendente, Hieronymus. *Opera Omnia*. (Goezius, Leipzig, 1687.)

Falconnet, C. *Non est fetui Sanguis Maternus alimento*. (Paris, 1711.) Reprinted in Haller's *Disputationes Selectae*, 1750.

Falckner, L. F. *De Ortu et Propagatione Hominum*. Inaug. Diss. (Sched, Leipzig, 1723.)

Fallopius, Gabrielus. *Observationes Anatomicae*. (Venice, 1561; Cologne, 1562.)

Fasbender, E. *Geschichte der Geburtshülfe*. (Jena, 1906.)

Fasbender, H. *Entwicklungslehre, Geburtshülfe und Gynäkologie in den Hippokratischen Schriften*. (Stuttgart, 1897.)

Favaro, G. *Per la storia dell' Embriologia*. (Padua, 1907.)

Feilchenfeld, W. *Kantstudien*, 1923, **28**, 323.

Feis. "Verwendung d. Menstrualblutes bei Josephus," in *Mitt. z. Gesch. d. Med. u. Naturwiss.*, 1919, **18**, 256; *Isis* (*Sarton's*), 1920, **3**, 319.

Feis. See Ebstein, Sticker, Feis & Ferckel.

Ferckel, C. *Die Gynäkologie des Thomas von Brabant*. (Kühn, München, 1912.)

Ferckel, C. On gynaecology in Ketham. *Archiv. f. d. Gesch. d. Med.*, 1912, **6**, 205.

Ferckel, C. On "De Secretis Mulierum." *Archiv. f. d. Gesch. d. Med.*, 1914, **7**, 47; and *Sudhoff-Festschrift*, 1923, **15**.

Ferckel, C. See Ebstein, Sticker, Feis & Ferckel.

Féré, C. *Journ. d'Anat. et de Physiol. norm. et pathol.* 1897, **33**, 259.

Ferguson, J. *Archiv. f. d. Gesch. d. Math. Naturwiss. u. Technik*, 1913, **6**, 83.

Fernelius, J. *Medicina.* (Andreas Wechel, Paris, 1554.)

Fernelius, J. *Universa Medicina.* (Andreas Wechel, Paris, 1567.) See Sherrington.

Ferrari, H. M. *Une chaire de Médecine au xv* ᵉᵐᵉ *Siècle.* (Paris, 1899).

Ficinus, Marsilius. *Additis argumentis et commentarius Platonis Atheniensis phil. summi.* (Froben, Basel, 1561.)

Fidelis, F. *De relationibus Medicorum.* (Leipzig, 1674.)

Fienus, Thomas. *De Formatrice Foetus, in quo ostenditur animam rationalem infundi tertia die.* (Tong, Antwerp, 1620.)

Fienus, Thomas. *Pro sua de animatione foetus tertia die opinione Apologia adversus Ant. Ponce Santacruz olim Prim. Prof. Vallidol. nunc vero Reg. Hisp. Med. Cubicul. et Protomed. gen.* (Hastenus, Louvain, 1629.)

Fischer, H. & Schopfer, W. "Die Geschichte der Zeugungs- und Entwicklungstheorien im 17, 18 & 19. Jahrhundert," *Gesnerus*, 1945, **2**, 49, 81.

Fischer, I. "Geschichte d. Gynäkologie" in *Biol. u. Pathol. d. Weibes.* (Urban & Schwarzenberg, Berlin, 1926.)

Fischer, I. *Janus*, 1922, **26**, 30.

Fizes, A. *Opera Medica. De Tumoribus, Suppuratione, Cataracta, humani corporis partibus solidis, hominis Liene sano ac secretione Bilis. His accessit De Hominis Generatione Exercitatio a Nicolao Fizes.* (A. et P. Rigaud, Montpellier, 1742.)

Fizes, N. *De Hominis Generatione Exercitatio.* (Delespine, Paris, 1751.)

Flemyng, M. *Phil. Trans. Roy. Soc.* 1755, **49**, 254.

Florian, J. *Nature*, 1932, **130**, 634.

Fludd, Robert. *Opera Omnia.* (Oppenheim, 1617–1619.)

Fog, J. *Acta Obs. et Gyn. Skand.* 1930, **9**, 132.

Forster, J. G. A. See Patrin.

Fourcroy, A. F. *Chem. Ann.* (*Crelle's*), 1795, **2**, 450.

Fourcroy, A. F. *Ann. de Chim.* 1790, **7**, 162.

Fourcroy, A. F. Cit. in Deyeux & Parmentier, *Archiv f. Phys.* (*Reil's*), 1796, **1**, 95.

Fourcroy, A. F. *System d. chem. Kenntnis.* (Königsberg, 1803.)

Fourcroy, A. F. & Vauquelin, L. N. *Ann. de Chim.* 1793, **16**, 113.

Fourier, C. *The Passions of the Human Soul*, tr. J. R. Morell. (London, 1851.)

Fraenkel-Conrat, H. "Rebuilding a Virus," *Sci. American*, 1956, **194** (no. 6), 42.

Franc, G. *Satyrae medicae.* (Leipzig, 1722.)

Franchini, J. Biography of Spallanzani. *Ann. Med. Hist.* 1930 (N.S.), **2**, 56.

Franchini, J. Biography of Vallisneri. *Ann. Med. Hist.* 1931 (N.S.), **3**, 58.

Franklin, K. J. "A Study of the Growth of Knowledge about certain parts of the Foetal Cardio-Vascular Apparatus and about the Foetal Circulation, in Man and some other Mammals," *Ann. of Sci.*, 1941, **5**, 57.

Fraser-Harris, D. F. *Proc. Roy. Soc. Med.* (Hist. of Med. Sect.), 1934, **27**, 1095.

Frazer, Sir J. G. *Folk-Lore in the Old Testament*. (Macmillan, London, 1923.)

Freind, John. *Emmenologia*. (Bennet, Oxford, 1703; Innys, London, 1717; 1720.)

Freind, John. *Emmenologia: Translated into English by Thomas Dale*. (T. Cox, London, 1729.)

Freind, John. *Emmenologie ou traité de l'évacuation ordinaire aux femmes*. (Paris, 1738.)

Fulgentius, Bp. of Ruspe. *De Fide*, in Migne's *Patrologia*.

Fulton, J. F. *Isis (Sarton's)*, 1932, **18**, 77.

Fulton, J. F. *A Bibliography of the Hon. Robert Boyle, F.R.S.* (Oxford, 1932.) Addenda to above. (Oxford, 1933.)

Fulton, J. F. *Proc. & Papers Oxf. Bibliogr. Soc.* 1932, **1**, 1, 339.

Galen of Pergamos. *Opera Omnia*, ed. G. Kühn. (Leipzig, 1828.)

Galen of Pergamos. *On the Natural Faculties*, ed. and tr. A. W. Brock. (Loeb Classics, Heinemann, London, 1924.)

Galilei, Galileo *Opere*, vol. 6. (Florence, 1890.) *Frammenti e Lettere* (1917).

del Garbo, Dino (the elder, d. 1327). *Expositio supra capitulum [Hippocratis] de generatione embrionis*. Printed with Jacobus Foroliviensis, q.v., 1502.

del Garbo, Tommaso. *Supra capitulum de generatione embrionis*. Printed with Jacobus Foroliviensis, q.v., 1502.

Garden, R. *Phil. Trans. Roy. Soc.* 1693, **17** (no. 192), 474.

Garmannus, C. F. *Oologia curiosa, ortum corporum naturalium ex ovo demonstrans*. (Bittorf, Zwickau, 1691.)

Garrison, F. H. *History of Medicine*, 4th edition. (Saunders, Philadelphia, 1929.)

Gassendi, Pierre. *Opera omnia*. (Lyon, 1658.) See also Pinaeus.

del Gaudio, A. Dante on generation. *Archeion (Archivio d. Storia d. Sci.)*, 1924, **5**, 101; 1925, **6**, 121; 1927, **8**, 176.

Gautier d'Agoty. *Zoogénésie, ou génération de l'homme et des animaux*. (Paris, 1750.)

Gaza, Theodore. Commentary on Aristotle's *De Generatione Animalium*. (Aldine, Venice, 1513.)

Geofroi, S. F. *Ergo hominis primordia vermis*. (Paris, 1704.)

Gerber, A. "L'Embryon; Aperçu historique de l'évolution de l'Embryologie," *Revue Ciba*, 1944, **4** (no. 39), 1326.

de Gerbi, G. *Liber Anatomiae corporis humani et singulorum membrorum illius*. (Venice, 1502.)

Gerike, P. *De generatione hominis liber*. (Drimborn, Helmstadt, 1744.)

Gesell, A. & Amatruda, C. S. *The Embryology of Behaviour; the Beginnings of the Human Mind*. (Harper, New York, 1945.)

Gesner, Conrad. *Historia animalium*. (Frankfurt, 1585.)

Gibson, J. "On foetal nutrition," in *Medical Essays*. (Edinburgh, 1726.)

Gibson, Thomas. *The Anatomy of Humane Bodies epitomized*. (London, 1694.)

Gilis, P. "L'Embryologie, son histoire, son rôle dans les sciences anatom-iques," in *Gaz. hebdom. des sci. méd.* (Montpellier, 1887.)

Glanville, Joseph. *Scepsis Scientifica; or, Confest Ignorance the way to Science, in an essay on the Vanity of Dogmatizing and Confident Opinion.* (London, 1665.)

Glanville, Joseph. *Plus Ultra.* (London, 1667.)

Glaser, J. P. *De Nutritione Foetus per solum Umbilicum.* (Gottlob, Wittenberg, 1751.)

Glass, B. "Maupertuis and the Beginning of Genetics," *Quart. Rev. Biol.*, 1947, **22**, 196.

Glenn, W. F. *Southern Practitioner*, 1911, **33**, 117.

Glisson, Francis. *De Ventriculo et Intestinis.* (London, 1677.)

Gmelin, L. & Ebermaier, J. E. C. *Chem. Ann. (Crelle's)*, 1796, **2**, 64.

Gnudi, M. T. & Webster, J. P. *The Life and Times of Gaspare Tagliacozzi, Surgeon of Bologna*, 1545–1599. (Reichner, New York, 1950.)

Gobley, M. *Comptes Rend. Acad. Sci.* 1845, **21**, 766.

Goeckel, H. *Die Wandlungen in der Bewertung des ungeborenen Kindes.* Inaug. Diss. (Heidelberg, 1911.)

Goelicke, A. O. *Medicina forensis.* (Frankfurt, 1723.)

von Goethe, J. W. *Zur Naturwissenschaft überhaupt, besonders Morphologie.* (Stuttgart & Tübingen, 1817–1824.) Also in Collected Works. (Berlin, 1902.)

y Gonzalez, A. W. A. *Anat. Rec.* 1929, **42**, 17; *Proc. Soc. Exp. Biol. & Med.* 1930, **27**, 579.

Good, J. M. *The Nature of Things; a didactic poem. Translated from the Latin of Titus Lucretius Carus.* (London, 1805.)

Good, J. M. *Repertorium d. prakt. Chir. und Med. Abhandlungen für Ärtzte und Wundärtzte*, **3**.

Gosse, Sir Edmund. *Father & Son.* (London, 1909.)

Gotch, Francis. "On some aspects of the scientific method," in *Lectures on the Method of Science*, ed. by T. B. Strong. (Oxford, 1906.)

de Gouey, L. L. *La Veritable Chirurgie établie sur l'experience et la raison, avec des nouvelles decouvertes . . . : et un nouveau Système sur la Génération du Fétus.* (Cabut, Rouen, 1726.) See Hoffman, D.

de Graaf, René. *De mulierum Organis Generationi inservientibus tractatus novus, demonstrans tam homines et animalia, caetera omnia quae vivipara dicuntur, haud minus quam ovipara, ab ovo originem ducere.* (Leiden, 1672.)

de Graaf, René. *Opera omnia.* (Hackiana, Leiden, 1677.)

Grambs, J. *De nutritione et augmento foetus in utero.* (Vulpius, Giessen, 1714.)

Gravel, P. *De Superfoetatione.* (Paris, 1738.) Reprinted in Haller's *Disputationes Selectae*, 1750.

Greenwood, M. *The Medical Dictator, and other biographical Studies.* (Williams & Norgate, London, 1936.)

Gregorovius, F. *The Emperor Hadrian.* (Macmillan, London, 1898.)

Gregory of Nyssa. *De Opificio Hominis*, in Migne's *Patrologia*.

Gregory, J. C. "The Animate and Mechanical Models of Reality," *Journ. Philos. Stud.*, 1927, **2**, 301.

Gregory, J. C. *A Short History of Atomism from Democritus to Bohr.* (Black, London, 1931.)

Grosjean, P., S.J. *Henrici VI Angliae Regis Miracula Postuma.* (Soc. des Bollandistes, Brussels, 1935.)

Grosser, O. *Frühentwicklung, Eihautbildung und Placentation.* (Bergmann, München, 1927.)

Gruner, O. C. *A Treatise on the "Canon of Medicine" of Avicenna, incorporating a translation of the First Book.* (Luzac, London, 1930.)

Guillemaud, C. See Guillemaud, Jacques.

Guillemaud, Jacques. *Child-birth or, The Happy Deliverie of Women.* (Hatfield, London, 1612.)

Guillemaud, Jacques. *De la Grossesse et Accouchement des Femmes. Du gouvernement d'icelles et moyen de survenir aux accidens qui leur arrivent, ensemble de la nourriture des enfans ... avec un traité de l'Impuissance et un autre de la Generation, par Charles Guillemaud.* (Jost, Paris, 1643.) Earlier editions, e.g. Pacard, Paris, 1620, do not contain the treatise on generation.

Günther, F. C. *Sammlung von Nestern und Eyern verschiedener Vögel.* (Nürnberg, 1772.)

Gunther, R. J. *Early Science in Oxford*, 3 vols. (Priv. pub. Oxford, 1925.)

Guttmacher, A. F. *Life in the Making.* (Cassell, London, 1934.)

Haberling, W. On Johannes Müller's nineteenth-century confirmation of Aristotle's discovery of the selachian placenta. *Archiv. f. d. Gesch. d. Math. Naturwiss. u. Technik*, 1927, **10**, 166.

Hadorn, E. *Letalfaktoren in ihrer Bedeutung für Erbpathologie und Genphysiologie der Entwicklung.* (Thieme, Stuttgart, 1955.)

Hadrian, emperor. See Gregorovius.

Haeckel, Ernst. *The Evolution of Man.* (Watts, London, 1906.)

Haeckel, Ernst. *The Riddle of the Universe.* (Watts, London, 1902.)

Haighton, J. *Phil. Trans. Roy. Soc.* 1797, **87**, 159.

Halban, J. *Zeitschr. f. Geb. u. Gyn.* 1904, **53**, 191.

Hall, H. R. Private communication to the author.

von Haller, Albrecht. (ed. et comm.). *Hermanni Boerhaave Praelectiones Academicae in proprias Institutiones Rei Medicae.* (Göttingen, 1744; Leiden, 1758.)

von Haller, Albrecht. *Disputationes selectae*, vol. on "Generatio" (prob. Lausanne, 1750.)

von Haller, Albrecht. *Elementa Physiologiae Corporis Humani*, vols. 7 & 8, "Generatio," Lausanne, 1766. (1st vol. Soc. Typograph. Bern, 1757.)

von Haller, Albrecht. *Sur la formation du cœur dans le poulet.* Mém. II. (Lausanne, 1758); revised and reprinted in *Opera Anatomica Minora*, tom. II, "Ad generationem." (Grasset, Lausanne, 1767.)

von Haller, Albrecht. *La Génération, ou Exposition des Phénomènes relatifs à cette Fonction Naturelle, de leurs mechanisme, de leurs causes respectives, et des effets immédiats qui en resultent, traduites de la physiologie de M. de Haller, augmentée de quelques Notes et d'une Dissertation sur l'Origine des Eaux de l'Amnios.* (Paris, 1774.)

Haly-Abbas. See al-Majūsī.

Hamberger, G. E. *Physiologia medica.* (Jena, 1751.)

Hamburger, V. & Born, W. "Monsters in Nature and Art," *Ciba Symposia*, 1947, **9** (no. 5/6), 666.

du Hamel, J. B. *Historia Regiae Scientiarum Academiae.* (Leipzig, 1700.)

du Hamel, J. B. *Mém. prés. à l'Acad. des Sciences*, 1750, **1**, 345.

Hamilton, A. *Elements of the practice of Midwifery.* (Murray, London, 1775.)

Hamlett, G. W. D. *Quart. Rev. Biol.*, 1935, **10**, 432.

Hammett, F. S. "Heredity Concepts of the Ancient Hindus," *Scientific Monthly*, 1928, **27**, 452.

Handley, James. *Mechanical Essays on the Animal Oeconomy wherein not only the Conduct of Nature in Animal Secretion, but Sensation & Human Generation, are distinctly consider'd & anatomically explain'd, as also the particular manner of the operation of a medicine is accounted for, etc.* (Rivington, London, n.d. prob. 1730.)

Hannes, C. R. *Qua foetum in utero materno per os nutriri demonstratur.* (Straube, Duisburg, 1756.)

Hannhard, J. U. *De nutritione foet. in utero materno.* (Genath, Basel, 1709.)

Hansen, L. *De Termino animationis Foetus Huamni.* Inaug. Diss. (Hendel, Halle, 1724.)

Harnack, A. "Medizinisches aus der ältesten Kirchengeschichte," in Neuburger-Pagel, q.v.

Harris, C. H. S. *Duns Scotus*, 2 vols. (Oxford, 1927.) Cf. rev. by D. E. Sharp, *Journ. Philos. Stud.*, 1928, **3**, 102.

Harris, L. J. *Nature*, 1923, **III**, 326.

Hartland, E. S. *Primitive Paternity.* (London, 1909.)

Hartman, C. G. "On the Relative Sterility of the Adolescent Organism," *Science*, 1931, **74**, 226.

Hartsoeker, Nicholas. *Essay de Dioptrique.* (Paris, 1694.)

Hartsoeker, Nicholas. *Recueil de plusieurs pièces de Physique.* (Utrecht, 1722.)

Harvey, William. *De Motu Cordis et Sanguinis in Animalibus.* (Frankfurt, 1628.)

Harvey, William. *Exercitationes de Generatione Animalium. Quibus accedunt quaedam de partu: de membranis ac humoribus uteri: et de Conceptione.* (Typus Du-Gardianis, impensis Octaviani Pulleyn, London, 1651.)

Harvey, William. *Exercitationes de Generatione Animalium.i Qubus accedunt quaedam de partu: de membranis ac humoribus uteri: et de Conceptione.* (Jan Jansson, Amsterdam, 1651.)

Harvey, William. *Exercitationes de Generatione Animalium.* (P. Frambotti, Padua, 1666.)

Harvey, William. *Anatomical Exercitations concerning the Generation of living creatures*, tr. Martin Llewellyn. (Pulleyn, London, 1653.) Also tr. R. Willis (Sydenham Society, London, 1847.)

Harvey, William. For complete bibliography, see Keynes, G.
Harvey, William. Portraits of, see Anonymous.
Haskins, C. H. *English Hist. Review*, 1921, **36**, 342.
Haskins, C. H. *Isis* (*Sarton's*), 1922, **4**, 264.
Hatchett, Charles. *Phil. Trans. Roy. Soc.* 1799, **89**, 315.
Hatchett, Charles. *Phil. Trans. Roy. Soc.* 1800, **90**, 327.
Hatchett, Charles. *Scherer's Journ.* 1803, **6**, 265.
Hebrew Liturgy. The Authorised daily Prayer Book of the United Hebrew Con-gregations of the British Empire. (Eyre & Spottiswoode, London (5689), 1929.)
Heffter, J. C. *De causis incremento foetu celerrime.* (Hering, Erfurt, 1745.)
Heffter, J. C. *Musei disputatorii physico-medici.* (Leipzig, no date, but pre-sented to the Library of the Royal Society of London, Nov. 10th, 1763.)
Hegel, G. W. F. *Philosophy of Mind*, tr. W. Wallace. (Oxford, 1894.)
Hehl, J. *Observationes quaedam physici de natura et usu aëris ovis avium inclusi.* (Tübingen, 1796.)
Heister, L. *Compendium anatomicum.* (Altdorf, 1718.)
van Helmont, F. M. (son of J. B.) *The Paradoxal Discourses of F. M. van Helmont concerning the Macrocosm and Microcosm, or the Greater and Lesser World, and their Union.* (Kettlewel, London, 1685; German tr., Hamburg, 1691.) This book contains two embryological plates, one taken from Swammerdam, the other from Kerckring (q.v.), but con-tributes nothing to the history of the subject.
van Helmont, J. B. *Ortus Medicinae.* (Elzevir, Amsterdam, 1648, 1652.)
Henke, A. *Über die Entwicklungen und Entwicklungskrankheiten des mensch-lichen Organismus.* (Schrag, Nürnberg, 1814.)
Henneguy, F. *Revue Scientifique*, 1913, **51**, 321.
Henry VI, king of England. See Grosjean.
Henry of Saxony. See Albertus Magnus.
d'Herelle, F. *The Bacteriophage*, tr. G. H. Smith. (Williams & Wilkins, Baltimore, 1926.)
Herissant, F. D. *Secundinæ fetui Pulmonis praestant officia, et sanguine materno Fetus non alitur.* (Paris, 1741.) Reprinted in Haller's *Disputationes Selectae*, 1750.
Heron-Allen, Edward. *Barnacles in Nature and Myth.* (Oxford, 1928.)
Herophilus of Chalcedon. See Dobson.
Herringham, Sir W. *Ann. Med. Hist.* 1932 (N.S.), **4**, 109, 249, 347, 491, 575.
Hertodt, J. F. *Crocologia, seu Curiosa Croci Regis Vegetabilium Enucleatio, continens . . .* (Nisi, Jena, 1671.)
Hertwig, Oskar. *Ältere u. neure Entwicklungstheorien.* (Berlin, 1892.)
Hertwig, Oskar. Contribution to *Handbuch der vergleichenden und experi-mentellen Entwicklungslehre der Wirbeltiere.* (Fischer, Jena, 1906.)
Hertwig, Oskar. *Dokumente zur Geschichte d. Zeugungslehre.* (Bonn, 1918.)
Heussler, Hans. *Der Rationalismus des siebzehnten Jahrhunderts in seinen Beziehungen zur Entwicklungslehre* (Descartes, Spinoza, Leibniz). (Koebner, Breslau, 1885.)

Hieronymus Florentinus. *De hominibus dubii*, 1658.

Highmore, Nathaniel. *The History of Generation, examining the several Opinions of divers Authors, especially that of Sir Kenelm Digby, in his discourse of bodies.* . . . (Martin, London, 1651.)

Highmore, Nathaniel. *Corporis humani disquisitio anatomica in qua sanguinis circulationem prosecutus est.* (The Hague, 1651.)

Hildanus, W. *Opera Omnia.* (Frankfurt, 1646.)

Hildegard, St, of Bingen. *Liber Scivias; Liber Divinorum Operum simplicis hominis.* See Singer, C.; Schulz, H.; and Liebeschütz, H.

Hill, Sir John (pseud. Abraham Johnson). *Lucina sine concubitu. A letter humbly address'd to the Royal Society; in which is proved by most incontestable evidence, drawn from Reason & Practice, that a Woman may conceive and be brought to bed without any commerce with Man.* (Cooper, London, 1750. Repr. Golden Cockerel Press, Reading, 1930.)

Hintzsche, E. "Le Microscope," *Revue Ciba*, 1950, **7** (no. 77), 2674.

Hippocrates of Cos. *Opera Omnia*, ed. E. Littré, 10 vols. (Baillière, Paris, 1839–1861.)

Hippon of Samos. See Diels.

His, Wilhelm. "Die Theorien der geschlechtlichen Zeugung," *Archiv. f. Anthropologie*, 1870, **4**, 197, 317; 1871, **5**, 69.

His, Wilhelm. *Unsere Körperform und das physiologische Problem ihrer Entstehung.* (Vogel, Leipzig, 1874.)

His, Wilhelm. *Proc. Roy. Soc. Edinb.* 1888, **15**, 294.

Hoboken, Nicholas. *Anatomia Secundinae Humanae.* (Ribbium, Utrecht, 1669, 1675.)

Hoffmann, D. *Annotationes in hypotheses Goueyanas.* (Frankfurt, 1719.)

Hoffmann, F. *Medicina rationalis systematica.* (Halle, 1718.)

Hoffmann, J. M. *Idea machinae humanae anatomico-physiologica.* (Altdorf, 1703.)

van Hohenheim, Theophrastus (called Paracelsus). *Opera. Erster bis zehnter Theil der Buecher und Schriften . . . jetzt auffs new auss den Originalen, und Theophrasti eigner Handschrift, soviel derselben zubekommengewesen . . . an tag gegeben: durch Johannem Huserum.* (Conrad Waldkirch, Basel, 1589–1590.) The first collected edition.

von Hohenheim, Theophrastus (called Paracelsus). *Hermetic and Alchemical Writings*, tr. Engl. and ed. A E. White. (Elliot, London, 1894.)

von Hohenheim, Theophrastus (called Paracelsus). *Sämtliche Werke in zeitgemässer Kurzer Answahl*, 5 vols. (Zollikofer, St. Gallen, 1944–.)

Holler, J. *De Morborum Internorum curatione.* (Paris, 1567.)

Hommel, H. *Archiv f. Gesch. d. Med.*, 1927, **19**, 105.

Hopf, L. "Die Anfänge der Anatomie bei den alten Kulturvölkern," in *Abhandl. zur Gesch. d. Med.* 1904, **9**, 1.

Hoppe, E. "Marcus Marci de Kronland, ein vergessener Physiker der 17 Jahrhundert," in *Archiv f. Gesch. d. Math. Naturwiss. u. Technik*, 1927, **10**, 288.

Hopstock, H. "Leonardo as Anatomist," in *Stud. Hist. Meth. Sci.* vol. **2**, 188. (Oxford, 1921.)

Horace (Q. Horatius Flaccus). *Satires, Epistles, and Art of Poetry*, tr. S. Dunster. (Brown, London, 1719).

van Horne, J. *Prodromus* . . . (Leiden, 1668.)

van Horne, J. *Microcosmographia et Microtomia.* (Leipzig, 1707.)

de Houpeville, W. *La génération de l'homme par le moyen des œufs, defendue par Eudoxe et Philotime contre Antigène.* (Lucas, Rouen, 1676.)

Houssay, F. See Licetus, F.

Hübotter, F. "Die Sūtras über Empfängnis u. Embryologie," in *Mitt. d. deutsch. Gesell. f. Natur. u. Volkerkunde Ostasiens*, **36**, c. (Tokyo & Leipzig, 1932.)

Hughes, A. F. W. "Studies in the History of Microscopy, I; The Influence of Achromatism," *Journ. Roy. Microscop. Soc.*, 1955, **75**, 1.

Hughes, H. *New York Med. Journ.* 1905, **82**, 963.

Hunter, John. "Progress and Peculiarities of the Chick" (the MS. accompanying the Hunterian drawings), "Generation of Fish, Shell-fish and Insects," "Notes and Queries on Generation," "On Monsters," in *Essays and Observations.* Ed. R. Owen, 2 vols. (van Voorst, London, 1861.) Vol. **1**, pp. 199, 216, 227 and 239 respectively.

Hunter, William. *Anatomia uteri gravidae.* (Birmingham, 1774.)

Hurd-Mead, Kate. "Trotula," *Isis* (*Sarton's*), 1930, **14**, 349.

Hurd-Mead, Kate. *Ann. Med. Hist.* 1933, **5**, 1, 171, 281, 390.

Hureau de Villeneuve, A. *L'Accouchement dans la race jaune.* (Paris, 1863.)

Hutchinson, G. E. *The Clear Mirror; a Pattern of Life in Goa and in Indian Tibet.* (Cambridge, 1936).

Hutton, J. H. *Primitive Philosophies of Life*, Frazer Lecture. (Oxford, 1938.) Cf. *Nature*, 1938, **142**, 1085.

Huxley, J. S. *Problems of Relative Growth.* (Methuen, London, 1932.)

Huxley, J. S. & de Beer, G. R. *Elements of Experimental Embryology.* (Cambridge, 1934.)

Ilberg, J. *Abhandl. d. sächs. Gesellsch. d. Wissenschaften* (*Philol.-histor. Klasse*), 1910, **28**, 122.

Imbert, F. *Generationis Historia.* (Montpellier, 1745.)

d'Irsay, Stephen. *Albrecht von Haller, eine Studie zur Geistesgeschichte d. Aufklärung.* (Thieme, Leipzig, 1930.) (*Arb. d. Inst. f. Gesch. d. Med., Leipzig*, no. **1**.)

d'Irsay, Stephen. "Time-Implied Function; an historical Aperçu," in *Kyklos; Jahrb. d. Instit. f. Gesch. d. Med. a.d. Univ. Leipzig*, 1928, **1**, 52.

Jacobaeus, Oligerus. *De Ranis Observationes.* (Billaine, Paris, 1676; Copenhagen, 1686.)

Jacobi, M. *Hannover Magazin*, 1763. (The article was translated and published in Yarrell, *History of British Fishes*, 1841, vol. **2**, 87.)

Jacobus Foroliviensis. *Supra librum Hippocratis de natura foetus.* Printed with the commentaries of the del Garbos, father and son (14th century). (Bonetus Locatellus for the heirs of Octavianus Scotus, Venice, 1502.) Another edition, 1518, purely Aristotelian commentaries. See Klebs.

Jalāl al-Dīn al-Rūmī. See Browne, E. G. *History of Persian Literature*. (Cambridge.) Also in *Poems from the Persian*, Augustan Books of Poetry (Second Series), No. 10. (Benn, London, 1927.)

James of Forlì. See Jacobus Foroliviensis.

Jenkinson, J. W. *Vertebrate Embryology*. (Oxford, 1913.)

Joannes Philoponus (Johannes Grammaticus). *De Ortu Animae*. See also his commentary on Aristot. *De Gen. An.* (Venice, 1526).

Johannsen, W. *Naturwiss.*, 1917, 5, 389.

John, J. F. *Chem. Untersuch. der Animalien, Vegetab. u. Mineral.* 1811, vol. 3, 22.

John, J. F. *Magazin d. Gesellschaft d. Naturforscherfreunde in Berlin*, 1810, 4.

John, J. F. *Chemische Tabellen des Tierreichs*. (Maurer, Berlin, 1814.)

Johnson, Abraham. See Sir John Hill.

Jones, W. H. S. *The Doctor's Oath: an essay in the history of medicine*. (Cambridge, 1924.)

Jordan, L. *Disquisitio chem. evict. regn. animal.* Cit. in John, J. F.

Jouard, G. *Des monstruosités et bizarreries de la Nature*. (Paris, 1806.)

Kabbalah Denudata, tr. C. Knorr von Rosenroth. (Frankfurt, 1684.) *De Revolutione animarum ex operibus R. Jizchak Lorija*, chs. xxvi, xlix.

Kaltschmied, C. F. *De dist. inter foet. anim. et non anim.* (Jena, 1747.)

Kant, Immanuel. *Critique of Judgment*. (Macmillan, London, 1892.)

Kant, Immanuel. *Critique of Pure Reason*. (Macmillan, London, 1902.)

Keibel, F. *Normaltafeln zur Entwicklungsgesch. d. Schweines*. (Jena, 1897.)

Keil, J. *Anatomy of the human body abridg'd*. (London, 1698).

Keller, R. "L'Hermaphrodisme," *Revue Ciba*, 1943, 3 (no. 26), 870.

Kendrick, T. D. *The Druids*. (Methuen, London, 1927.)

Kerckring, Theodore. *Osteogenia Foetuum*. (Frisius, Amsterdam, 1670.)

Kerckring, Theodore. *Anthropogeniae ichnographia*. (Amsterdam, 1671.)

Kerckring, Theodore. "An account of what hath been of late observed by Dr Kerkringius concerning eggs to be found in all sorts of females," in *Phil. Trans. Roy. Soc.*, 1672 (no. 81), pp. 4018 ff.

Kerckring, Theodore. *Opera Omnia Anatomica*. (Vid. et fil. Corn. Boutesteyn, Leiden, 1717 and 1729.)

Kerr, J. Graham. *Text-book of Embryology: Vertebrata*. (Macmillan, London, 1919.)

Kessel, J. F. *Foetus in utero mat. liq. amn. deglutire*. (Fickelshew, Jena, 1751.)

de Ketham, Johannes. *The Fasciculus medicinae of Johannes de Ketham, Alemannus. Facsimile of the first (Venetian) edition of 1491 with introduction by Karl Sudhoff, transl. and adapted by Charles Singer*. (Lier, Milan, 1924.)

Keynes, Geoffrey. *A Bibliography of Sir Thomas Browne*. (Cambridge, 1924.)

Keynes, Geoffrey. *A Bibliography of the Writings of William Harvey, M.D.* (Cambridge, 1928.)

Keynes, G. *The Personality of William Harvey*, Linacre Lecture. (Cambridge, 1949.)

Kijper, A. "De Generatione Hominis, De prima foetus formatione, De Vita foetus in utero, etc." in *Disputationes Physico-Medicae Miscellaneae.* (Meyer, Leiden, 1655.)

King, F. H. *Farmers of Forty Centuries.* (Cape, London, 1927.)

Kirchhoff, A. *Jenaische Zeitschr. f. Naturwiss.* 1868, **4**, 193.

Kirste, H. *Münch. Med. Wochenschr.* 1927, **74**, 1286.

Klein, G. Rösslin bibliography. *Archiv f. d. Gesch. d. Med.* 1910, **3**, 304.

von Kölliker, R. A. *Beiträge zur Kenntniss d. Geschlechtsverhältnisse und d. Samenflüssigkeit wirbelloser Tiere und d. Bedeutung d. sog. Samentiere.* (Berlin, 1841.)

König, E. *Regnum animale.* (Basel, 1687.)

Köttnitz, E. M. *Deutsche Med. Wochenschr.* 1889, 900, 927, 949.

Krammer, L. History of the Floating Lung test. *Archiv f. d. Gesch. d. Med.* 1933, **26**, 253.

Krause, C. C. *Quae sit causa prox. mutans corp. foet.* (St Petersburg, 1754.)

de Kruif, Paul. *Microbe Hunters.* (Harcourt Brace, New York, 1926.)

Kuhlemann, J. C. *Observationes quaedam circa negotium generationis in ovibus factae.* (Langenheim, Leipzig, 1754.)

Kuo Zing-Yang. "Ontogeny of Embryonic Behaviour in Aves," *Journ. Exp. Zool.*, 1932, **61**, 395; **62**, 453; *Journ. Comp. Psychol.*, 1932, **13**, 245; 1933, **16**, 379; 1937, **24**, 49; *Journ. Neurophysiol.*, 1939, **2**, 488; *Psychol. Rev.*, 1932, **39**, 499; *Amer. Journ. Psychol.*, 1938, **51**, 361.

Kyper, A. See Kijper, A.

Lachs, J. "Die Gynäkologie d. Soranus." *Volksmann's Sammlung klinischer Vorträge N.F.*, no. 385. (Leipzig, 1902.)

Lactantius, Caeli Firmianus, of Nicomedia. *De Opificio Dei*, in Migne's *Patrologia.* "On the workmanship of God," in *Works*, tr. Thomas Fletcher. (Edinburgh, 1871.)

Ladelci, F. *Atti d. Acc. pontif. d. nuovi Lincei*, 1885, **38**, 122.

de Lamarck, J. B. *Philosophie Zoologique.* (Paris, 1809.)

Landauer, W. "Hatchability of Chicken Eggs as influenced by Environment and Heredity," *Storrs Agric. Exp. Sta. Bulletin*, 1948, no. 262 (a revision of nos. 216 and 236). Contains an elaborate account of the history of artificial incubation, pp. 10–44, cf. p. 177.

Lane, E. W. *Manners and Customs of the modern Egyptians.* (Ward Lock, London, 1836.)

Lane, E. W. (ed. and tr.). *The Arabian Nights.* 3 vols. (London, 1839–1841, often re-issued.)

Lang, C. J. *Opera medica.* (Leipzig, 1704.)

Langguth, C. A. *Panegyrin medicam indicit et embryonem trium cum dimidio mensium abortu rejectum qua faciem externam describit.* Inaug. Diss. (Eichsfeld, Wittenberg, 1751.)

Langly, W. See Schrader, J.

de Launay, C. D. *Nouveau système concernant la génération.* (Paris, 1698, 1726.)

Laurentius, A. *Opera omnia.* (Petit-Pas, Paris, 1628.)

Lecky, *History of Rationalism in Europe,* 4 vols. (London, 1865–1869.)

Ledermuller, M. F. *Versuch zu einer gründlichen Vertheidigung deren Saamenthierchen.* (Nürnberg, 1758.)

van Leeuwenhoek, Anton. *Anatomia, seu interiora Rerum, cum Animatarum tum Inanimatarum,* etc. (Boutesteyn, Leiden, 1687.)

van Leeuwenhoek, Anton. *Continuatio Epist. ad Reg. Soc. Londin.* (Boutesteyn, Leiden, 1689.)

van Leeuwenhoek, Anton. *Arcana Naturae detecta.* (Krooneveld, Delft, 1695.) *Continuatio Arc. Nat. detect.* (Krooneveld, Delft, 1697.)

van Leeuwenhoek, Anton. *Epistolae ad Soc. Reg. Angl.,* etc. (Langerak, Leiden, 1719.)

van Leeuwenhoek, Anton. *Epistolae physiologicae.* (Beman, Delft, 1719.)

van Leeuwenhoek, Anton. *Select Works, containing his Microscopical Discoveries translated from the Dutch and Latin editions by Samuel Hoole.* (Whittingham & Arliss, London, 1798, 1807, 1816.) "The only extensive, though very incomplete, English translation of Leeuwenhoek's works is this bowdlerised version." The reverend editor omitted "all passages which to many readers might be offensive," hence spermatozoa are not mentioned at all, and protozoa and bacteria very little.—Dobell.

van Leeuwenhoek, Anton. *Opera Omnia, seu Arcana Naturae,* etc. 4 vols. (Langerak, Leiden, 1722.) "Leeuwenhoek's papers, most of which appeared in the *Phil. Trans. Roy. Soc.,* were collected and reprinted from time to time in small volumes, which, though not issued by the same publisher, are generally found in 4 volumes bearing the misleading title of *Opera Omnia.* Each collection has its own name, pagination, and index. The arrangement is bad and the pagination confused"—Miall. See van Rijnberk.

van Leeuwenhoek, Anton. [& Johan Ham]. "Observationes de natis e semine genetali animalculis," in *Phil. Trans. Roy. Soc.,* 1677, **12** (no. 142), 1040.

von Leibniz, G. W. *Œuvres,* ed. A. Jacques. (Paris, 1842.)

Lemery, Nicholas. *A course of Chymistry,* tr. from the French by Harris. (London, 1686.)

Lemoine, A. *Charles Bonnet de Genève, philosophe et naturaliste.* (Paris, 1850.)

Leonardo da Vinci. *Quaderni d'Anatomia,* 6 vols., ed. Vangensten, Fohnahn, & Hopstock. (Dybwad, Christiania, 1911.)

Leonhardi, J. G. Note in Macquer's *Chym. Wört.* q.v.

Leroy, O. *A French Bibliography of Sir Thomas Browne.* (Harrap, London, 1931.)

Lesky, E. "Die Zeugungs- und Vererbungslehren der Antike und ihr Nachwirken," *Abhdl. d. Akad. d. Wissenschaften u.d. Literatur (Geistes- u. Sozialwiss. Klasse)* no. 19. (Mainz, 1950.)

Léveillé, J. B. F. *Journ. de Physique*, 1799 (An 7), **48**, 386.

Levinus Lemnius. *Occulta naturae miracula.* (Antwerp, 1559.) *De miraculis occultis naturae.* (Frankfurt, 1604.) (Eng. tr. *The Secret Miracles of Nature.* London, 1658.)

Lewes, G. H. *A Chapter from the History of Science, including Analyses of Aristotle's Writings.* (London, 1864.)

Lewes, G. H. *Life of Goethe.* (London, 1875.)

Lewis, F. T. *New England Journ. Med.*, 1929, **200**, 810 ff.

Lewis, F. T. *Science*, July, 1935.

de Lézérec, Louis Sebastian de Tredern. *Dissertatio inaug. med. sistens ovi avium historiae et incubationis prodromum.* (Jena, 1808.)

Licetus, Fortunatus. *De perfecta constitutione hominis in utero.* (Bertelli, Padua, 1616.)

Licetus, Fortunatus. *De Monstrorum causis natura et differentiis libri duo.* (Padua, 1616, 1634.)

Licetus, Fortunatus. *De Monstris, ex recensione Gerardi Blasii, M.D. et P.P.* (A. Frisius, Amsterdam, 1665.) French tr. F. Houssay. (Ed. Hippocrate, Paris, 1937.)

Licht, H. *Sittengeschichte Griechenlands.* (Dresden, 1926.)

Liebeschütz, H. *Das allegorische Weltbild d. hl. Hildegard von Bingen.* (Teubner, Leipzig, 1930.)

Lieutaud, J. *Elementa physiologiae.* (Aix, 1749.)

Lillie, F. R. *The Development of the Chick.* (Holt, New York, 1919.) Ed. completely revised by H. L. Hamilton. (Holt, New York, 1952.)

Lillie, R. S. *Journ. Gen. Physiol.* 1925, **7**, 493; 1931, **14**, 349.

Lillie, R. S. *Archivio di Sci. Biol.* 1928, **12**, 102.

Lillie, R. S. *Amer. Journ. Psychiatr.* 1929, **9**, 461.

Lillie, R. S. *Science*, 1928, **67**, 593.

van Linde, J. A. *Meletemata Medicinae.* (Frankfurt, 1672.)

Linsing, P. E. *Institutiones Medicae.* (Erlangen, 1701.)

von Lippmann, E. O. *Archiv f. d. Gesch. d. Math. Naturwiss. u. Technik*, 1909, **2**, 233.

von Lippmann, E. O. *Urzeugung und Lebenskraft.* (Springer, Berlin, 1933.)

Lischwitz, J. C. *De Ortu et Propagatione Hominum.* (Sched, Leipzig, 1723.)

Lister, Martin. *Dissertatio de Humoribus.* (London, 1709; Amsterdam, 1711.)

Littré, E. See Hippocrates.

Liu, J. L. See Maxwell & Liu.

Llewellyn, Martin. See Harvey.

Lobstein, J. F. *Essai sur la nutrition du foetus.* (Levrault, Strasbourg, 1802.)

Loeb, Jacques. "Über d. chem. Charakter d. Befruchtungsvorganges," in Roux's *Vorträge*, vol. **2**. (Engelmann, Leipzig, 1908.)

Lones, T. E. *Aristotle's Researches in Natural Science.* (London, 1912.)

Longfield, Johannes. *Dissertatio medica de febre hectica.* (Edinburgh, 1759.)

Lorenzini, Stefano. *Osservazioni intorno alle Torpedini.* (l'Onofri, Florence,

1678.) Eng. tr. *The curious observations of Mr S. Lorenzini on the dissection of the Crampfish now done into English by J. Davis.* (Wale, London, 1705.)

Lowe, P. R. *Ibis,* 1929, **5**, 40.

Lu, Gwei-Djen & Needham, Joseph. "A Contribution to the History of Chinese Dietetics," *Isis (Sarton's),* 1951, **42**, 13.

Lucian of Samosata. *Opera Omnia,* tr. A. M. Harmon. (Loeb Classics, Heinemann, London, 1919.)

Lucretius, C. Titus. *De Rerum Natura,* tr. W. E. Leonard. (Dent, London, 1916.)

Ludwig, C. G. *Institutiones physiologiae.* (Leipzig, 1752.)

Lukas, F. *Zeitschrift des Vereins f. Volkskunde,* 1894, **4**, 227.

Maar, V. *Life and Works of Nicolaus Steno (Stensen).* (Copenhagen, 1910.)

Macht, David. *Bull. Johns Hopkins Hosp.* 1911, **22**, 143.

McKay, J. S. *History of Ancient Gynaecology.* (Baillère, Tindal & Cox, London, 1901.)

McMurrich, J. P. *Leonardo da Vinci the Anatomist.* (Williams & Wilkins, Baltimore, 1930.) Leonardo's embryology is discussed on p. 228.

Macquer, P. J. *Chymisches Wörterbuch.* (Leipzig, 1781.)

Macrobius, A. A. *Opera Omnia.* (Griphium, Leiden, 1556.)

Maître-Jan, Antoine. *Observations sur la formation du poulet où les divers changemens qui arrivent à l'œuf à mesure qu'il est couvé sont exactement expliqués et représentés en figures.* (d'Houry, Paris, 1722.)

al-Majrītī, Abū'l-Qāsim Maslama ibn Aḥmad. See Sarton, vol. **1**, p. 668.

al-Majūsī, 'Alī ibn al-'Abbās (Haly-Abbas). *Liber Totius medicinae necessaria continens,* tr. by Stephen of Antioch (A.D. 1127), annotated by Michael de Capella. (Myt, Lyon, 1523.)

Malebranche, Nicolas. *De la Recherche de la Vérité.* (Paris, 1672, 1674, 1675, 1678, 1772.)

Malinowsky, Bronislaw. *Sexual Life of Savages.* (Routledge, London, 1929.)

Malpighi, Marcello. *De Formatione Pulli in Ovo.* (London, 1672.)

Malpighi, Marcello. *De Ovo Incubato.* (London, 1675.)

Malpighi, Marcello. *Opera Omnia.* (Littlebury, London, 1686; Leiden 1687.) For bibliography, see Züno.

Malpighi, Marcello. *La Structure du Ver à Soye, et de la formation du Poulet dans l'œuf; Deux dissertations addressées en forme de Lettre à l'Academie Royale d'Angleterre.* (Villery, Paris, 1686.)

Manquat, M. *Rev. Quest. Scientifiques,* 1927, **11**, 70.

de Marchette, D. *Anatomia.* (Padua, 1656.)

Marci, Marcus, of Kronland. *Idearum Operatricium Idea.* (Prague, 1635.) See Baumann; Dobrzensky; Hoppe; Pagel.

von Martuis, H. *Abhandlung ü. d. Geburtshülfe b. d. Chinesen.* (Freiburg i./B., 1820.)

Massuet, P. *De generatione ex animalculo in ovo.* Inaug. Diss. (Verbeek, Leiden, 1729.)

de Maupertuis, P. L. M. *Venus physique.* (Leiden, 1744, 1745; Bruyset, Lyon, 1745, 1746; Dresden, 1752; Lyon, 1788.)

Mauriceau, François. *Traité des Maladies des Femmes Grosses.* (Paris, 1668.)

Mauriceau, François. *Tractaat van de Siektens der Swangere Vrouwen en der gene, die eerst gebaart hebben.* (Jan Morterre, Amsterdam, 1759.)

Mauriceau, François. *The Diseases of Women with Child & in child-bed; as also the best means of helping them in natural and unnatural labours,* tr. Hugh Chamberlen. (Darby, London, 1683.)

Mauriceau, François. *Von Kranckheiten schwangerer Weiber.* (Nürnberg, 1687.)

Mauriceau, François. *Observations sur la Grossesse.* (Paris, 1695.)

Maxwell, J. P., & Liu, J. L. *Ann. Med. Hist.* 1923, **5**, 95.

May, M. T. "Nicholas Steno on the Passage of Yolk into the Intestine of the Chick," *Journ. Hist. Med. & Allied Sci.,* 1950, **5**, 119.

Mayer, R. *Robert Mayer's kleinere Schriften und Briefe,* ed. Weyrauch. (Stuttgart, 1893.)

Mayow, John. *Tractatus duo, quorum prior agit de Respiratione; alter de Rachitide.* (H. Hall, Oxford, 1669.)

Mayow, John. *Tractatus Duo.* (C. Driehuysen & F. Lopez de Haro, Leiden, 1671.)

Mayow, John. "De Respiratione foetus in utero et ovo" in *Tractatus Quinque Medico-Physici* (e Theatro Sheldoniano, Oxford, 1674.) Eng. tr. A. C. B. & L. D., Alembic Club, Edinburgh, 1907.

Mazin, J. B. *Conjecturae physico-medico-hydrostaticae de Respiratione Foetus.* (Rizzardi, Brixen, 1737.)

Mazin, J. B. *Institutiones medicae-mechanicae.* (Brussels, 1735.)

Meckel, J. F. *Beyträge zur vergleichende Anatomie.* Leipzig, vol. **1**, 1808; vol. **2**, 1811.

Meckel, J. F., *System d. vergleichende Anatomie.* 1821.

de Mendoza, Petrus Hurtado, S. J. *Universa Philosophia,* 2 vols. (Lyon, 1624.)

Mengert, W. F. On the man-midwife movement. *Ann. Med. Hist.* 1932 (N.S.), **4**, 453.

Merat-Gaillot, F. V. *Ann. de Chim.,* 1799 (An VIII), **34**, 68.

Mercato, Luiz. *De mulierum affectionibus libri quatuor.* (F. Valgrisius, Venice, 1587; Società Veneta, Venice, 1602.)

Mercklin, G. A. *De Transfusione Sanguinis.* (Nürnberg, 1679.)

Mercurialis, Hieronymus. *De Hominis Generatione.* (Schönwetter, Frankfurt, 1602.)

Mercurialis, Hieronymus. *De Morbis Puerorum,* esp. bk. 1 (Meietus, Venice, 1587.)

Mercurius, Scipio. *La commare o riccoglitrice.* (Ciotti, Venice, 1595; Venice, 1620–1621; de Rossi, Verona, 1645; Venice, 1680.) Germ. tr. by G. C. Welsch, *Kindermutter oder Hebammenbuch.* (Leipzig, 1653, 1671.)

Merton, E. S. "Sir Thomas Browne's Embryological Theory," *Journ. Hist. Med. & Allied Sci.,* 1950, **5**, 416.

de Méry, J. *Problèmes de Physique.* (Boudot, Paris, 1711.)

de Méry, J. Œuvres, ed. L. H. Petit. (Alcan, Paris, 1888.)

de la Mettrie, Julien Offray. Man a Machine. (G. Smith, London, 1750.)

Metzger, H. "Schelling u.d. Biologie," Archiv f. d. Gesch. d. Math. Naturwiss. u. Technik, 1909, 2, 159.

Meyer, A. W. "Mr John Hunter on Generation," California & Western Med., 1935, 43, nos. 2, 3, 4, 5.

Meyer, A. W. "The Hunters in Embryology," California & Western Med., 1936, 45, nos. 5 & 6; 1937, 46, no. 1.

Meyer, A. W. An Analysis of the 'De Generatione Animalium' of William Harvey. (Stanford Univ. Press, Palo Alto, Calif., 1936.)

Meyer, A. W. "Some Historical Aspects of the Recapitulation Idea," Quart. Rev. Biol., 1935, 10, 379.

Meyer, A. W. "The Elusive Human Allantois in Older Literature," art. in Charles Singer Presentation Volume, Science, Medicine & History, ed. E. A. Underwood, 2 vols. (Oxford, 1954), vol. 1, p. 510.

Meyer, A. W. Essays on the History of Embryology. (Univ. Press, Stanford, Calif., 1931.) Reprinted from California & Western Medicine, 1931, 35–37.

Meyer, A. W. "The Discovery and Earliest Representations of Spermatozoa," Bull. Inst. Hist. Med., 1938, 6, 89.

Meyer, A. W. "Was von Baer's Discovery [of the Mammalian Ovum] an Accident?" Bull. Inst. Hist. Med., 1937, 5, 33.

Meyer, A. W. The Rise of Embryology. (Stanford Univ. Press, Palo Alto, Calif., 1939.) [Errata list in F. T. Lewis' review, Anat. Rec., 1940, 76, 365.]

Meyer, A. W. Human Generation; Conclusions of Burdach, Döllinger and von Baer. (Stanford Univ. Press, Palo Alto, Calif., 1956.) Includes English translations of K. F. Burdach's De primis momentis formationis foetus (Hartung, Königsberg, 1814) and De foetu humano adnotationes anatomicae (Voss, Leipzig, 1828). Also of J. J. I. von Döllinger's Versuch einer Geschichte d. menschlichen Zeugung (1816). Also of K. E. von Baer's "Commentar zu der Schrift: De Ovi," etc. (q.v.).

Meyer, Hans. Der Entwicklungsgedanke bei Aristoteles. (Bonn, 1909.)

Meyer, Hans. Geschichte der Lehre von den Keimkräften von der Stoa bis zum Ausgang d. Patristik. (Hanstein, Bonn, 1914.)

Meyer, Hans. "Das Vererbungsproblem bei Aristoteles," Philologus, 1919, 75, 1.

Meyerhof, M. On the end of the School of Alexandria. Archeion (Archivio d. Storia d. Sci.), 1933, 15, 1.

Miall, L. C. The Early Naturalists; their lives and work. (Macmillan, London, 1912.)

Middlebeek, S. De Incremento foetu humano in utero. (Langerak, Leiden, 1719.)

Migne, J. P. (ed.). Patrologiae cursus completus. (Paris, 1844–64.)

Miller, J. L. "Renaissance Midwifery, 1500–1700," in Lectures on the History of Medicine (Mayo Foundation, etc.), p. 297. (Saunders, Philadelphia, 1933.)

Minot, C. S. *The Problem of Age, Growth and Death.* (Murray, London, 1908.)

Mirskaia, L. & Crew, F. A. E. *Proc. Roy. Soc. Edinburgh.* 1930.

Mitterer, M. A. "Mann und Weib nach dem biologischen Weltbild des hl. Thomas und dem der Gegenwart," *Zeitschr. f. kathol. Theol.*, 1933, **57**, 491.

Moellenbrock, V. *De Varis.* (Leipzig, 1672.)

Moissides, D. *Janus*, 1922, **26**, 59, 129.

de Molière, J. B. P. *Le Malade Imaginaire.* (Hachette, London, 1920.)

Mondière. "Nubilité," art. in *Dict. des Sciences Anthropologiques.* (Paris, 1890.)

Mondino de Luzzi. *Anathomia*, ed. J. Adelphus. (Strassburg, 1513.)

Monro, Alex. "Essay on the Nutrition of Foetuses," 1734, repr. in *Works*, ed. by his son, A. Monro. (Elliott, Edinburgh, 1781), p. 371.

Montalenti, G. "Il sistema aristotelico della generazione degli animali." *Rassegna d. studi sessuali e di eugenica* (Rome), 1926, **6**, 113. Rev. in *Archeion*, 1926, **7**, 137.

Morache, G. *Journ. de Méd. de Paris*, 1904, **2**, 14.

Moraux, P. "À propos du νοῦς θύραθεν chez Aristote," *Bibliothèque philos. de Louvain*, 1955, **16**, 254.

Moriani. *Boll. d. R. Accad. Med. Genova*, 1913.

de la Motte, G. M. *Dissertations sur la génération.* (d'Houry, Paris, 1718.)

de la Motte, G. M. *Traité complet des accouchemens naturels, non naturels, et contre nature.* (Paris, 1721.)

Moubray, B. *A Practical Treatise on Breeding, Rearing and Fattening all kinds of Domestic Poultry . . . with an account of the Egyptian method of Hatching Eggs by Artificial Heat.* (Sherwood, London, 1816.)

Müller, Johannes. *Über d. glatten Hai d. Aristoteles u. ü. d. Verschiedenheiten unter den Haifischen und Rochen in der Entwickelung des Eies.* (Berlin, 1842.)

Müller-Hess, G. "Die Lehre von der Menstruation vom Beginn der Neuzeit bis zur Begründung der Zellenlehre," *Abhdlg. z. Geschichte d. Med. u. Naturwiss.*, 1938, no. 27.

Muraltus, J. *Clavis medicinae.* (Zürich, 1672.)

Murray, M. A. "The Bundle of Life," *Ancient Egypt*, 1930, 65.

Murray, M. A. & Seligman, C. G. *Man*, 1911, **11**, 165.

Nardi, Giovanni. *Noctes geniales.* (Giambattista Ferroni, Bologna, 1655.)

Neale, J. M. *Mediaeval Hymns and Sequences*, 2nd edition, p. 194. (Masters, London, 1863.)

Needham, John Turberville, Abbé. *An Account of some New Microscopical Discoveries, founded on An Examination of the Calamary, and its wonderful Milt-Vessels (each of which tho' they exceed not an Horse-Hair in Diameter, contains a minute Apparatus analogous to that of a Pump, with a fine spiral Spring, Sucker, Barrel, etc.) tending to prove by an accurate Description of their Motion, Action, etc., that the hitherto supposed Animalcules in the*

Semen of Animals, are nothing more than Machines similar, tho' inconceivably less, to those discovered in this Sea-Production—Also, Observations on the Farina Faecundans of Plants; with a new Discovery and Description of the Action of those minute Bodies, analogous to that of the Calamary's Milt-Vessels; And an Examination of the Pistil, Uterus, and Stamina of several Flowers, with an attempt to shew how the Seed is impregnated—Likewise, Observations on the supposed Embryo Sole-Fish fixed to the Bodies of Shrimps; with a new Discovery of a remarkable Animalcule found single on the Tail-Part of each Embryo; (and) A Description of the Eels or Worms in blighted Wheat; and other curious Particulars relating to the Natural History of Animals, Plants, etc. (Dedicated to the Royal Society.) (F. Needham, London, 1745.)

Needham, John Turberville, Abbé. *Observations upon the generation, composition, and decomposition, of Animal and Vegetable Substances.* (London, 1749.) Summarised in *Phil. Trans. Roy. Soc.*, 1750, **45**, 615.

Needham, John Turberville, Abbé. *Nouvelles Observations Microscopiques.* (Ganeau, Paris, 1750.) This is a 2nd edition of the *New Mic. Disc.* of 1745, but contains in addition *Observations nouvelles sur la génération, la composition, et la décomposition, des substances animales et végétales.*

Needham, John Turberville, Abbé. French tr. of, and notes appended to L. Spallanzani's *Nouvelles recherches sur les découvertes microscopiques et la génération des corps organisés.* (Lacombe, Paris, 1769.) The 2nd vol. has a different title and deals with geology and mineralogy.

Needham, John Turberville, Abbé. *Idée sommaire ou vüe générale du systeme physique et metaphysique de Monsieur Needham sur la génération des corps oragnisés.* (Paauw, Brussels, 1776.)

Needham, Joseph. *Chemical Embryology,* 3 vols. (Cambridge, 1931.)

Needham, Joseph. *Biol. Rev.,* 1930, **5**, 142.

Needham, Joseph. *Ann. Rev. Biochem.* 1933, **2**, 346.

Needham, Joseph. *Order and Life.* (Cambridge and Yale, 1936.)

Needham, Joseph, *Biochemistry and Morphogenesis.* (Cambridge, 1942, reprinted 1950.)

Needham, Joseph. *Science and Civilisation in China,* 10 vols. (Cambridge, 1954–.)

Needham, Walter. *Disquisitio anatomica de formato foetu.* (R. Needham, London, 1667; P. le Grand, Amsterdam, 1668.)

Nekrassov, A. D. *Die Befruchtung in d. Tierwelt; die Geschichte d. Problems* (in Russian), 1930. Also in *Archiv f. d. Gesch. d. Med. (Sudhoff's),* 1933, **26**, 89.

Nenterus, G. P. *Physiologia.* (Strassburg, 1714.)

Neuburger, M. *History of Medicine.* (Hodder & Stoughton, London, 1910.)

Neuburger, M. & Pagel, J. *Handbuch d. Geschichte d. Medizin.* (Fischer, Jena, 1902.)

Neumann, A. Cit. in John's *Chem. Tab.* p. 107, q.v.

Nice, M. M. "Incubation-Periods throughout the Ages," *Centaurus,* 1954, **3**, 311.

Nicholas of Cusa. *De Docta Ignorantia* (1440), in *Opera*. (Basel, 1565.)

Nicholls, F. *The Petition of the Unborn Babes to the Censor of the Royal College of Physicians of London*. (Cooper, London, 1751.)

Nicholls, F. *Disquisitio de motu cordis et sanguinis in homine nato et non nato*. (Hughs, London, 1773.)

Nitzsch, F. *Journ. f. Ephemerid. Eruditorum*, 1671.

Nolanus, Ambrosius. *Castigationes adversus Averroem*. (Venice, 1532.)

Noortwyck, W. *Uteri humani gravidi anatomia et historia*. (Verbeek, Leiden, 1743.)

Nuck, A. *Adenographia curiosa et uteri foeminei anatome nova*. (Leiden, 1691.)

Nunn, A. *Qua eversa vasorum rubrorum uteri anastomosi ac communicatione cum placenta saniorem ac naturae institutio magis consentaneum nutritionis foetus modum et mechanismum*. (Hering, Erfurt, 1751.)

Nymmanus, G. *Dissertatio de Vita Foetus in Utero*. (de Haro, Leiden, 1644, with the third edition of Plazzoni's book on the organs of generation; reprinted 1664.)

Ogle, W. *Aristotle on the Parts of Animals*. (Kegan Paul, London, 1882.)

Oken, Lorenz. *Die Zeugung*. (Bamberg & Würzburg, 1805.)

Oken, Lorenz. *Beiträge zur vergleichenden Zoologie*. (Bamberg & Würzburg, 1806.)

Okes, T. *Duae dissertationes in schol. pub. Cantab.; II. Foetuum deformitates non oriuntur ab imaginatione praegnantis*. (Archdeacon, Cambridge, 1770.)

Onymos, J. "De natura Foetus in utero materno situ," in *Fasciculus dissertationum medicarum*. (Bonk, Leiden, 1745.)

Opitz, W. *Centralbl. f. Gyn.* 1887, **11**, 734.

Oppenheimer, J. "Guillaume Rondelet," *Bull. Inst. Hist. Med.*, 1936, **4**, 817.

Oppenheimer, J. "Historical Introduction to the study of Teleostean Development," *Osiris*, 1936, **2**, 124.

Oppenheimer, J. "The Non-Specificity of the Germ-Layers," *Quart. Rev. Biol.*, 1940, **15**, 1.

Oppenheimer, J. "Problems, Concepts and their History [in Embryology]," art. in *Analysis of Development*, ed. B. H. Willier, P. A. Weiss & V. Hamburger. (Saunders, Philadelphia & London, 1955.) p. 1.

Oppenheimer, J. "Methods and Techniques [in Embryology]," art. in *Analysis of Development*, ed. B. H. Willier, P. A. Weiss & V. Hamburger. (Saunders, Philadelphia & London, 1955.) p. 25.

Orcham, Janus. *De generatione animantium conjectura observationi cuidam Harveanae ne vetus pervulgataque omnium gentium opinio per hanc concidat, submissa a Jano Orchamo*. (Schultzyl, Brandenburg, 1667.)

Oribasius of Pergamos. In *Medicae artis principes, post Hippocraticem et Galenum Graeci Latinitate donati; Aretaeus, Ruffus Ephesius, Oribasius, Paulus Aegineta, Aetius, Alexander Trallianus, Actuarius, Nic. Myrepsius, Corn. Celsus, Scrib. Largus, Marcell. Empiricus, aliique praeterea quorum unius nomen ignoratur. Henr. Stephani de hac sua editione tetrastichon.*

(Fugger, 1567.) French tr. by Bussemaker & Daremberg, 6 vols. (Paris, 1851–1876.)

Ornstein, Martha. *The Role of the Scientific Societies in the Seventeenth Century.* (Chicago, 1928.)

Ortlob, J. F. *Physiologia.* (Leipzig, 1697.)

Ortolan, T. "Embryologie Sacrée," art. in *Dictionnaire de Théologie Catholique,* ed. A. Vacant, E. Mangenot, & E. Amann, vol. 4, p. 2405. (Paris, 1924.)

Osiander, M. *Neue Denkw. für Ärtzte u. Geburtshülfer,* 1795, **1,** 184.

Osler, Sir William. *Incunabula Medica.* (Oxford, 1923.)

von Ott, D. *Archiv f. Gyn.* 1886, **27,** 129.

Ottow, B. Introd. to K. E. von Baer, *Über d. Bildung d. Eies d. Säugetiere u. d. Menschen.* (Leipzig, 1927.)

Pagel, J. "S. L. Steinheim," *Janus,* 1903, **8,** 233, 286.

Pagel, J. See Neuburger & Pagel.

Pagel, Walter. *Archiv f. d. Gesch. d. Med.* 1931, **24,** 19. Also *J. B. van Helmont; Einführung in d. philosophische Medizin des Barock.* (Springer, Berlin 1930.)

Pagel, Walter. *Centralbl. f. Pathol.* 1932, **56.**

Pagel, Walter. "Religious Motives in the Medical Biology of the seventeenth century." *Bull. Inst. Hist. Med.* 1935, **3,** 97.

Pagel, Walter. "J. B. van Helmont *De Tempore,* and Biological Time," *Osiris,* 1949, **8,** 346.

Pander, Heinrich Christian. *Dissertatio sistens Historiam metamorphoseos quam ovum incubatum prioribus quinque diebus subit.* (Würzburg, 1817.) *Beiträge zur Entwickelungsgeschichte des Hühnchens im Eye.* (Würzburg, 1818.)

Paracelsus, Philippus Aureolus Theophrastus Bombastus von Hohenheim. See von Hohenheim.

Paré, A. *The Workes of that famous Chirurgeon Ambroise Parey translated out of Latin and compared with the French by Th. Johnson* (dedicated to Lord Herbert of Cherbury). (Clark, London, 1678.)

Paris, J. A. *Phil. Trans. Roy. Soc.,* 1810, 304; *Trans. Linnean Soc. London,* 1811, **10,** 304.

Paris, J. A. *Ann. Philos.* (*Thomson's*), 1821 (2nd ser.), **1,** 2.

Parisanus, Aemilius. *De Subtilitate.* (Deuchin, Venice, 1623.)

Parmenides of Elea. See Diels.

Parmentier. See Léveillé.

Parsons, James. *A mechanical and critical Enquiry into the Nature of Hermaphrodites.* (London, 1741.)

Parsons, James. *Philosophical Observations on the Analogy between the Propagation of Animals and that of Vegetables; in which are answered some Objections against the Indivisibility of the Soul, which have been inadvertently drawn from the late curious and useful Experiments upon the Polypus and other Animals, with an Explanation of the Manner in which each Piece of a divided Polypus becomes another Animal of the same Species.* (Davies, London, 1752.)

Partington, J. R. *Origins & Development of Applied Chemistry*. (Longmans, London, 1935.)

Pascal, Jean. *Nouvelle découverte sur les effets des fermens du corps humain*. (Paris, 1681.)

Pasteur, Louis. "Fermentations et Générations dites spontanées", *Œuvres de Pasteur réunies par P. Vallery-Radot* in vol. 2, pp. 210 ff. (Paris.)

[Patrin, E. L. M.] *Zweifel gegen die Entwicklungstheorie, ein Brief an Herr Senebier von L.P* [*atrin*]. (Göttingen, 1788.) This was translated into German from the original French by J. G. A. Forster, under whose name it has often been quoted. The letter was written from St. Petersburg in Nov. 1778.

Patterson, T. S. *Isis (Sarton's)*, 1931, **15**, 47, 504.

Pauli, J. G. Annotations in van Horne, q.v. (1707).

de Pauw, C. *Recherches philosophiques sur les Égyptiens et les Chinois*, 5 vols. (Berlin, 1774; Bastien, Paris, 1795.)

Pechlin, J. N. *Observationes physico-medicae*. (Hamburg, 1691.)

Peck, A. L. Inaug. Diss. (Cambridge, 1929.)

Peck, A. L. (ed. & tr.) *Aristotle's 'Parts of Animals.'* (Loeb Classics, Heinemann, London, 1937.)

Peck, A. L. (ed. & tr.) *Aristotle's 'Generation of Animals.'* (Loeb Classics, Heinemann, London, 1943.)

de Peramato, Pedro. *Opera medica*. (Barrameda, Sydonia (Cadiz), 1576.)

Perrault, Claude. "Mécanique des animaux," in *Essais de Physique*, 4 vols. (Paris, 1680–1688.)

Perrault, Claude. *Œuvres diverses de Physique et Mécanique*. (van der Aa, Leiden, 1721.)

Perrault, Claude. *Mémoires pour servir a l'Histoire Naturelle des Animaux*. (Paris, 1671, 1676.) Printed at the Royal Press under the personal supervision of Sébastien Mabre-Cramoisy (1585–1669), its first director. Eng. tr. by A. Pitfeild. (London, 1688.)

Colbert secured Louis' recognition of the Academy in 1668. The work of the Academy was done conjointly, but in fact most of the dissections of animals were performed by the polymath architect Claude Perrault (1613–1688), assisted later by the physician, anatomist and naturalist, Joseph Guichard Duerney (1648–1730). The first published result of the joint activity of the Academy was printed in 1667 by Frédéric Léonard as a small quarto, entitled *Observations qui ont este faites sur un grand Poisson dissequé dans la Bibliothèque du Roy . . . et sur un Lion. . . .* It consisted of extracts of two letters to Cureau de la Chambre (1594–1675), the personal medical attendant of the King. One of the letters describes the dissection of a shark in the Bibliothèque du Roy on 24th June, 1667. The other describes the anatomy of a lion which had recently died at Vincennes and was dissected in the Bibliothèque on 28th June, 1667. The letters were unsigned but were the work of Perrault. In 1669 the same printer brought out a small quarto volume entitled *Description anatomique d'un Cameleon, d'un Castor, d'un Dromadaire, d'un Ours et d'une Gazelle*. He says that in doing so "he continues to give to the public the observations made in the dissection of all sorts of animals in the Bibliothèque du Roy." He adds that "these five descriptions are of the animals of which I have secured the blocks. I hope to produce the others as the engraver delivers the blocks." Thus arose the great publication of 1671–1676.

Petersen, J. *Janus*, 1909, **14**, 457.

Philistion of Locri. See Allbutt.

Pictet, A. & Cramer, M. *Helv. Chim. Acta*, 1919, **2**, 188.

Pinaeus, Severinus. *Opusculum physiologicum et anatomicum in duos libellos distinctum. In quibus primum de integritatis et corruptionis virginum notis, deinde de graviditate et partu naturali mulierum, in quo ossa pubis et ilium distrahi tractatur.* (Paris, 1597; Robert Nivelle, Paris, 1598.)

Pinaeus, Severinus. *De virginitatis notis, graviditate et partu.* With *L. Bonaciolus, De conformatione foetus. Plater, De origine partium. Gassendi, De septo cordis pervio.* (Moyaert, Leiden, 1641, 1650.)

Pitcairn, A. *The Works of Dr Archibald Pitcairn wherein are discovered the true foundation and principles of the Art of Physick with cases and observations upon most distempers and medicines.* (Curll, London, 1715.)

de Plantade, F. See Dalenpatius.

Plater, F. See Platter.

Plato. *Alciabiades*, ed. B. Jowett in the *Collected Dialogues*, p. 120. (Oxford, 1892.)

Plato. *Timaeus*, ed. B. Jowett in the *Collected Dialogues*. (Oxford, 1892.)

Platt, A. (tr.) *Aristotle's 'Generation of Animals.'* (Oxford, 1910.)

Platter, Felix. "De origine partium earumque in utero conformatione," in *Quaestiones Medicae*. (Basel, 1625.) And with Pinaeus, q.v. See Cumston.

Plazzoni, F. *De partibus Generatione inservientibus libri duo.* (Pasquati, Padua, 1621; Wittenberg, 1628; de Haro, Leiden, 1644, 1664.)

Plempius, V. F. *Fundamenta medicinae.* (Louvain, 1644.)

Plinius, Gaius Secundus. *Natural History*, tr. Philemon Holland. (Islip, London, 1634.)

Plonquet, B. *De generatione corp. organ. disquisitio.* (Stuttgart, 1749.)

Ploss, H. & Bartels, M. *Das Weib in der Natur- und Völkerkunde.* (Grieben, Leipzig, 1895.)

Plot, Robert. *Natural History of Staffordshire.* (Oxford, 1686.)

Plutarch of Chaeronea. *De placitis philosophorum, hoc est brevis recensio sententiarum de rebus naturalibus*, ed. G. Xylander. (Aubriorum, Frankfurt, 1620.)

Plutarch of Chaeronea. *Moralia*, tr. by Philemon Holland. (Hatfield, London, 1603.)

Poggendorff, J. C. *Geschichte d. Physik.* (Leipzig, 1879.)

de Polignac, Melchior. *Anti-Lucretius, sive de Deo et Natura libri IX*. (Leiden, 1748.) Eng. tr. G. Canning, (London, 1766.)

Polybus. See Hippocrates.

Porphyrius. Cit. in *Grundriss d. Gesch. d. Philos.; I, Philos. d. Altertums*, F. Ueberweg & K. Praechter, 12th ed. (Berlin, 1926.)

della Porta, Giambattista. *Magiae Naturalis, sive de miraculis rerum naturalium* . . . (Cancer, Naples, 1558; Plantin, Antwerp, 1561.) Expanded from four books to twenty (Salviani, Naples, 1589). French tr. of the 1st ed. (Paris, 1913).

Portal, A. *Histoire de l'Anatomie et de la Chirurgie*. (Paris, 1770.)

Pouchet, G. *La Biologie Aristotélique*. (Alcan, Paris, 1885.)

Powdermaker, Hortense. *Life in Lesu*. (Williams & Norgate, London, 1933.)

Power, Sir d'Arcy. *The Birth of Mankynde, or the Women's Book—a bibliographical study*. (Bibliogr. Soc. London, 1927.)

Power, Sir d'Arcy. Chapter "Aristotle's Masterpiece" in *Foundations of Medical History*, p. 147. (Williams & Wilkins, Baltimore, 1931.)

Power, Henry. *Experimental Philosophy in three Books; containing New Experiments Microscopical, Mercurial, Magnetical*. (T. Roycroft for John Martin and James Allestry, London, 1664.)

Praechter, K. *Philologus*, 1927, **83**, 18.

Prescott, F. "Spallanzani on Spontaneous Generation and Digestion," *Proc. Roy. Soc. Med.* (Hist. of Med. Sect.), 1930, **23**, 495.

Preuss, Julius. *Biblisch-Talmudische Medizin*. (Karger, Berlin, 1911.)

Prévost, J. L. & Dumas, J. B. A. *Ann. Sci. Nat.* 1824, **1**, 1, 274; 1824, **3**, 113.

Preyer, W. *Spezielle Physiologie des Embryos*. (Grieben, Leipzig, 1885.) French tr. by M. Wiet (Alcan, Paris, 1887). Eng. tr. of chs. 6, 7 and part of 9 only, by G. E. Coghill & W. K. Legner, *Embryonic Motility and Sensitivity* (Nat. Research Council, Washington, D.C., 1937). Monographs of the Soc. for Research in Child Devel., vol. 2, no. 6 (serial no. 13).

Priestley, Joseph. *Experiments & Observations on different kinds of air*. (London, 1775.)

Proust, L. J. Cit. in John's *Chem. Tab.*, p. 108, q.v.

Prudentius Fortunatus. See Neale.

Przibram, H. *Die anorganischen Grenzgebiete d. Biologie*. (Bornträger, Berlin, 1926.)

Punnett, R. C. "Ovists and Animalculists," *Amer. Nat.* 1928, **62**, 481.

Purkyně, J. E. (Purkinje). *Symbolae ad Ovi Avium Historiam ante incubationem*. (Breslau, 1825; Leipzig, 1830.) Repr. in *Opera Selecta* (*Omnia*), vol. 1, ed. Z. Frankenberger, F. K. Studnička et al. (Spolek Českých Lékařů, Prague, 1948.) Eng. tr. by G. W. Bartelmez, in *Essays in Biology in honour of H. M. Evans* (Univ. of Calif. Press, Berkeley, 1943).

Puteanus, Erycius. *Ovi Encomium*. (Maire, Leiden, 1643.)

Quilletus, Claudius. *Callipaedia; or, The Art of Getting Pretty Children, in Four Books*, tr. from the original Latin by several hands. (McCaslan, Edinburgh, 1768.)

Quinisext Council. In *Compend. of the Councils*, tr. W. Lambert. (London, 1868.)

ibn Qurra, Thābit. See v. Töply, p. 75 and Sarton, vol. ɪ, p. 599.

ibn Rabban. See al-Ṭabarī.

Radbruch, G. *Geburtshilfe und Strafrecht.*

Rádl, Emanuel. *Geschichte der biologischen Theorien.* (Engelmann, Leipzig, 1905.) Eng. tr. E. J. Hatfield. (Oxford, 1930.)

Raisin, R. J. *Embryologia, seu Dissertatio de Fetu; in qua Fetus ab adulto differentiae dilucide exponuntur. Propugnata ad gradum Baccalaureatus consequendum a Rudolfo-Jeremia Raisin e monte Bellicardo, Artium Liberalium Magistro et Medicinae Alumno; Praeside R.D.D. Francisco de Sauvages, Regis Consiliario ac Medico, etc.* (Rochard, Montpellier, 1753.)

Rallius, G. F. *De generatione animalium disquisitio medico-physica in qua celeberrimorum virorum D. G. Harveii et A. Deusingii sententia a nuperis J. Orchami instantium vindicatur, ipsumque generationis opus juxta recentiorum observata succinte exponitur.* (Höffner, Stettin, 1669.)

Rasā'il Ikhwān al-Ṣafā. (Treatises of the Brethren of Sincerity.) See Dieterici.

Rathbone, Eleanor F. *Child Marriage; the Indian Minotaur.* (Allen & Unwin, London, 1934.)

Rathke, Heinrich. "Kiemen bey Säugthieren," *Isis (Oken's),* 1825, 747. "Kiemen bey Vögeln," *Isis (Oken's),* 1825, 1100.

Rau, J. J. *De Ortu et Generatione Hominis.* (Lange, Leiden, 1718.)

Raven, C. E. *John Ray, Naturalist—his Life and Works.* (Cambridge, 1942.)

Ray, John. *The Wisdom of God in Creation,* 6th edition. (London, 1714.)

Raynold, T. *The Byrth of Mankynde.* (London, 1545.) See Roesslin and Rösslin.

de Réaumur, R. A. F. "Sur les diverses reproductions qui se font dans les Écrevisses, les Omars, les Crabes, etc.; et entre autres sur celles de leurs Jambes et de leurs Écailles," in *Mémoires de l'Acad. des Sciences,* 1712 (1731), p. 223.

de Réaumur, R. A. F. *L'Art de faire éclore et élever en toute Saison des oiseaux domestiques de toutes especes soit par le moyen de la chaleur du fumier soit par le moyen de celle du feu ordinaire.* (Imp. Royale, Paris, 1749; 2nd ed. 1751.)

de Réaumur, R. A. F. *The Art of Hatching and Bringing up Domestick Fowls of all Kinds at any Time of the Year, either by means of the heat of Hot-Beds or that of Common Fires.* (Davis, Millar & Nourse, London, 1750.)

Redi, Francesco. *Esperienze intorno alla generazione degl' insetti.* (Florence, 1668.) Engl. tr. M. Bigelow. (Open Court, Chicago, 1909.)

Redi, Francesco. *Osservazioni intorno agli animali viventi che si trovano negli animali viventi.* (Matini, Florence, 1684.)

Reichard, Z. B. *De modo nut. foet.* (Nonnius, Erfurt, 1783.)

de Reies, C. *Campus Elysius jucundarum Quaestionum.* (Frankfurt, 1670.)

Reinhard, F. On Ancient Egyptian obstetrics and gynaecology. *Archiv f. d. Gesch. Med.* 1916, **9**, 315; 1917, **10**, 124.

Remotti, E. *Richerche di Morfol.,* 1931, **11**, 1; *Monit. Zool. Ital.,* 1932, **42** (Suppl.), 219.

Rhades, P. *Disputatio de ferr. sang.* (Leipzig, 1753.)
Rhodion, E. See Raynold, Roesslin and Rösslin.
Rhumbler, L. In Abderhalden's *Handbuch d. biologischen Arbeitsmethoden*, 1923, vol. 5, pt. 3, 219.
Rice, C. H. *Psyche*, 1929, 9, 68.
Richards, O. W. "The History of the Microscope; Selected References," *Trans. Amer. Micros. Soc.*, 1949, 68, 55.
Riddle, Oscar. Numerous papers in *Amer. Journ. Physiol.* and other journals. Bibliography up to 1931 in Needham, J., *Chem. Embryol.* q.v.
van Rijnberk, G. (ed.) *Collected Letters of A. van Leeuwenhoek, edited, illustrated and annotated by a committee of Dutch Scientists.* (Amsterdam, 1929–.)
Rinne, F. *Grenzfragen des Lebens.* (Quelle & Meyer, Leipzig, 1931.)
Riolanus, Johannes (the elder). Sect. "De Anatom. Hum. Foet." in *Opera Omnia.* (Palthen, Frankfurt, 1611.)
Riolanus, Johannes (the younger). *Anthropographia.* (Paris, 1618.)
Ritter, W. E. *Quart. Rev. Biol.*, 1935.
Rituale Sacramentorum Romanum, p. 519. (Rome, 1587.) See also *Liturgy & Worship*, p. 527. (S.P.C.K. 1933.)
Robertson-Smith, William. *Lectures on the Religion of the Semites.* 3rd ed., with notes by S. A. Cook. (Black, London, 1927.)
Robin, P. A. *Animal Lore in English Literature.* (Murray, London, 1932.)
Rodemer, W. *Die Lehre von d. Urzeugung bei Griechen u. Römern.* Inaug. Diss. (Giessen, 1928.)
Roederer, J. G. *De foetu perfecto.* (Strassbourg, 1750.)
Roederer, J. G. *De foetu observationes.* (Göttingen, 1758.)
Roesslin. See Rösslin, Raynold, Rhodion; Power; Klein.
Roesslin, Eucharius. *Schwangerer Frauen und Hebammen Rosegarten.* (Chr. Egenolph, Frankfurt, 1533.)
Romanov, A. L. & Romanov, A. J. *The Avian Egg.* (Wiley, New York, Chapman & Hall, London, 1949.)
Rondelet, G. *Libri de piscibus marinis, in quibus verae piscium effigies expressae sunt.* (B. Bonhomme, Lyon, 1554–1555.)
Rondelet, G. *Methodus curandorum omnium morborum corporis humani.* (Paris, 1575.)
Rooseboom, M. *Microscopium* (an explanatory history of the microscope). (Rijksmuseum voor de Geschiedenis der Natuurwetenschappen, Leiden, 1956.)
Roscher, W. H. *Omphalos.* (Teubner, Leipzig, 1913.)
Roscher, W. H. *Neue Omphalos-studien.* (Teubner, Leipzig, 1915.)
Roscoe, John. *The Baganda.* (London, 1911.)
Rosen, E. "Carlo Dati on the Invention of Eyeglasses," *Isis (Sarton's)*, 1953, 44, 4.
Rosen, E. "The Invention of Eyeglasses," *Journ. Hist. Med. and Allied Sci.*, 1956, 11, 13, 183.
Rosenfeld, L. On Marcus Marci. *Isis (Sarton's)*, 1931, 17, 325.

Rosenmuller, J. C. *Quaedam de ovariis embryonum et foetuum humanorum.* (Tauchnitz, Leipzig, 1802.)

von Rosenroth. See *Kabbalah Denudata.*

Rosenstadt, B. *Archiv f. mik. Anat.* 1912, **79**, 612.

Rosenthal, C. O. On the man-midwife movement. *Janus*, 1923, **27**, 117, 192.

Ross, Alexander. *The Philosophicall Touch-Stone; or, Observations upon Sir Kenelm Digbie's Discourses of the Nature of Bodies, and of the reasonable Soule, in which his erroneous Paradoxes are refuted, the Truth, and Aristotelian Philosophy, vindicated, & the Immortality of Man's Soule briefly, but sufficiently, proved.* (Young, London, 1645.)

Ross, Alexander. *Medicus Medicatus; or, the Physician's Religion cured by a lenitive or gentle Potion; with some animadversions upon Sir Kenelm Digbie's Observations on Religio Medici, by A. R.* (Young, London, 1645.)

Ross, Alexander. *Arcana Microcosmi; or, the hid secrets of man's body discovered; in an anatomical duel between Aristotle and Galen concerning the parts thereof; . . . with a refutation of Dr Brown's Vulgar Errors, the Lord Bacon's Natural History, and Dr Harvy's book De Generatione, Comenius, and others; whereto is annexed a letter from Dr. Pr. to the Author and his answer thereto, touching Dr Harvy's book De Generatione; by A. R.* (Newcomb, London, 1652.)

Rösslin, Eucharius. *Der swangern Frawen und hebammen Rosegarten.* Facsimile of the original edition of 1513, with an introduction by Prof. Gustav Klein. (München, 1910.) See Roesslin.

Rostand, J. *L'Aventure Humaine; du Germe au Nouveau-Né.* (Fasquelle, Paris, 1933.) Eng. tr. by Joseph Needham, *Adventures Before Birth.* (Gollancz, London, 1936.)

Roux, Wilhelm. *Gesammelte Abhandlungen über Entwickelungsmechanik der Organismen*, 2 vols. (Engelmann, Leipzig, 1895.)

Rozière, M. & Rouyer, M. *Description de l'Égypte.* (Publ. by the Emperor Napoleon, Paris, 1809.)

Rueff, Jakob. *De Conceptu et Generatione hominis et iis quae circa haec potissimum consyderantur Libri sex.* (Froschorus, Zürich, 1554.) Tr. W. Haller?, from Rueff's *Tröstbüchle.* (Zürich, 1554.)

Rueff, Jakob. *De Conceptu et Generatione hominis; de matrice et ejus partibus, necnon de conditione infantis in utero, et gravidarum cura et officio; de partu et parturientium infantiumque cura omnifaria; de differentiis non naturalis partus et earundem curis; de mola aliisque falsis uteri tumoribus, simulque de abortibus et monstris diversis, necnon de conceptus signis variis; de sterilitatis causis diversis, et de praecipuis matricis aegritudinibus, omniumque horum curis variis, Libri sex; opera clarissimi viri Jacobi Rueffi, chirurgi Tigurini, quondam congesti. Nunc denuo recogniti et in plerisque locis castigati, picturis insuper convenientissimis foetus primum in utero siti, deinde in paru, mox etiam matricis et instrumentorum ad partum promovendum et extrahendum pertinentium, illustrati, ornati, et in usum earum qui parturientibus, et obstetricibus consulere debent, typis evulgati. (Georgius*

Corvinus for Sigismund Feyerabend, Frankfurt-am-Main, 1580; another edition, 1587.) Eng. tr. *The Expert Midwife*. (London, 1637.)

Rüsche, F. "Blut, Leben, Seele," *Studien z. Gesch. u. Kulturgesch. d. Altertums, Ergänzungsband*, 5. (Paderborn, 1930.)

Russell, E. S. *Form and Function; a contribution to the History of Animal Morphology*. (Murray, London, 1916.)

Ruysch, F. *Thesaurus anatomicus*. (Amsterdam, 1701.)

Ryff, W. *Omnium Humani Corporis partium descriptio, seu ut vocant Anatomia*. (Pistor, Strassbourg, 1541.)

ibn Saʻīd al-Kātib, ʻArīb. See Schrutz.

de St Germain, Bertrand. *Descartes considéré comme physiologiste et comme médecin*. (Paris, 1869.)

de St Hilaire, Étienne Geoffroy. *Mém. Mus. d'Hist. Nat.* 1826, **13**.

de St Romain, G. B. *Physica*. (Leiden, 1684.)

Salmon, W. *General practise of Chymistry*, printed as bk. VI of *Pharmacopoeia Londiniensis*. (Dawks, London, 1678.)

Santayana, George. *Dialogues in Limbo*. (London, 1925.)

Sarsi. Cit. in Harris, L. J.

Sarton, George. *Introduction to the History of Science*, 5 vols. (Williams & Wilkins, Baltimore, 1927-1947.)

Sarton, George. "The Discovery of the Mammalian Egg and the foundation of modern embryology, with a complete facsimile of von Baer's 'De ovi mammalium et hominis genesi' (Leipzig, 1827)," in *Isis* (*Sarton's*), 1931, **16**, 315.

Saxonia, Hercules. *Pantheum Medicinae Selectum*. (Palthen, Frankfurt, 1603.)

Sbaragli, O. *Scepsis de ortu viviparorum*. (Bologna, 1701.)

Scaliger, J. C. *Aristoteles X Libri Hist. Anim. Comment*. (de Harsy, Leiden, 1584.)

Scammon, R. E. & Calkins, L. A. *Growth of the Human Body in the Pre-Natal Period*. (Univ. Press, Minneapolis, 1929.)

Schatz, C. F. *Die griechischen Götter u. d. menschlichen Missgeburten*. (Bergmann, Wiesbaden, 1901.)

Scheel, P. *De liquore amnii aspersae arteriae foet. humanorum, cui adduntur quaedam generaliora de liq. amn.* (Copenhagen, 1798.)

Scheele, C. W. *Physico-chemische Schriften*, vol. 2, p. 57. (Leipzig, 1894.)

Scheele, C. W. *Scherer's Journ.* 1801, **4**, 120.

Schmelz, J. D. E. See de Clercq & Schmelz.

Schmidt, C. W. "Der Entwicklungsbegriff in der Aristotelischen Naturphilosophie," *Archiv f. d. Gesch. d. Math. Naturwiss. u. Technik*, 1917, **8**, 49.

Schoock, Martin. *Dissertatio de ovo et pullo*. (Strick, Utrecht, 1643.) A mere compendium of quotations from Coiter and Aldrovandus-Adelmann.

Schopfer, W. "L'Histoire des Théories relatives à la Génération aux XVIIIème et XIXème siècles," *Gesnerus*, 1945, **2**, 81.

Schott, Gaspar, S.J. *Physica Curiosa, sive Mirabilia naturae et artis*, bk. v: *De Mirabilibus Monstrorum*. (Endter, Würzburg, 1662.)

Schrader, J. *Observationes et historiae omnes et singulae e Guiljelmi Harvei libello De Generatione Animalium excerptae et in accuratissimum ordinem redactae: item Wilhelmi Langly De Generatione Animalium observationes quaedam. Accedunt ovi faecundi singulis ab incubatione diebus factae inspectiones; ut et observationum anatomico-medicarum decades quatuor denique cadavera balsamo condiendi modus studio Justi Schraderi, M.D.* (Wolfgang, Amsterdam, 1674.)

Schrag, L. E. *De Praecipuis Differentiis quae inter Nascendum Natumque Hominem obtinent*. (Teubner, Leipzig, 1827.)

Schrecker, P. "Malebranche et le Préformisme Biologique," *Rev. Internat. de Philos.*, 1938, 1, 77.

Schrutz. "Medizin d. Araber," in Neuburger-Pagel, q.v.

Schultze, B. S. *Jenaische Zeitschr. f. Med. u. Naturwiss.* 1868, 4, 141.

Schulz, H. (tr.) *Hildegard von Bingen; Ursachen und Behandlung d. Krankheiten*. (Gmelin, München, 1933.)

Schurig, Martin. *Parthenologia historico-medica; hoc est virginitatis consideratio, qua ad eam pertinentes pubertates et menstruatio, item varia de insolitis mensium viis, necnon de partium genitalium muliebrium pro virginitatis custodia.—Gynaecologia historico-medica; hoc est congressus muliebris consideratio, qua utriusque sexus salacitas et castitas deinde coitus ipse eiusque voluptas exhibentur.* (Hekel, Dresden & Leipzig, 1729–1730.)

Schurig, Martin. *Embryologia historico-medica; hoc est infantis humani consideratio physico-medico-forensis, qua ejusdem in utero nutritio, formatio, sanguinis circulatio, vitalitas seu animatio, respiratio, vagitus et morbi, deinde ipsius ex utero egressus praematurus et serotinus, imprimis partus legitimus et circa eundem occurrentia, verbi gratia partus difficilis, post matris mortem, numerosus et multiplex, tam puellarum, quam vetularum, item per insolitas vias, et plane insolitus, porro varia symptomata e.g. uteri prolapsus ejusque inversio et resectio, denique partus Caesareus et suppositius cum puerperarum tortura raris observationibus exhibentur.* (Hekel, Dresden & Leipzig, 1732.)

Schwab, M. *The Jerusalem Talmud*. (Maisonneuve, Paris, 1878.)

Schwann, T. *Mikroskopische Untersuchungen ü.d. Übereinstimmung in der Struktur und dem Wachstume d. Tiere und Pflanzen* (1839). Repr. in Ostwald's Klassiker d. exakten Wissenschaften, no. 176. (Engelmann, Leipzig, 1910.)

Scot, Michael. *Liber Introductorius*. MS. See Haskins, C. H.

Scultetus, J. *Armamentarium chirurgicum*. (Frankfurt, 1666.)

Seger, G. *Diss. Anatom. de Hippocratis orthodoxia in doctrina de nut. foet. hum. in ut.* (Decker, Basel, 1660.)

Sellius, B. A. *Anatomica exercitatio de Allantoide*. (Reuther, Kiel, 1729.)

Senebier, Jean. *Ébauche de l'histoire des êtres organisés avant leur fécondation* (1785), printed with Spallanzani's *Expériences pour servir à l'histoire de la génération des animaux et des plantes*. (Chirol, Geneva, 1786.)

Seneca, L. Annaeus. *Quaestiones Naturales*, tr. T. Lodge. (Stansby, London, 1610.) Modern tr. J. Clarke & A. Geikie (Macmillan, London, 1910.)

Senff, C. F. *Nonnulla de incremento ossium embryonum*. (Kümmel, Halle, 1802.)

Senn, C. "Die Entwicklung d. biologischen Forschungs-Methode in der Antike u. ihre grundsätzliche Förderung durch Theophrast von Erasos." (Aarau, 1933.) *Veröfftl. d. Schweiz. Ges. f. Gesch. d. Med. u. Naturwiss.*, no. 8.

Sennertus, D. *Hypomnemata physica*. (Wittenberg, 1636.)

Sennertus, D. *Practica medicinae*. (Wittenberg, 1654.)

de Serres, O. *Théâtre d'Agriculture*. (Paris, 1600.)

Sharp, D. E. *Journ. Philos. Stud.* 1928, **3**, 105.

Shedd, W. G. T. *A History of Christian Doctrine*. (Edinburgh, 1865.)

Sherrington, Sir Charles. *The Endeavour of Jean Fernel*. (Cambridge, 1946.)

von Siebold, E. C. I. *Geschichte der Geburtshülfe*, 2 vols. (Pietzcker, Tübingen, 1901.)

Sigerist, H. E. "William Harvey's Stellung in der europäischen Geistesgeschichte," *Archiv f. Kulturgesch.* 1928, **19**, 166.

Simon, Isidore. *Asaph ha-Jehoudi, Médecin et Astrologue du moyen âge*. (Lipschutz, Paris, 1933.)

ibn Sīnā, Abū 'Alī al-Ḥasan ibn 'Abdallāh (Avicenna). Qānūn fī'l-Ṭibb, Latin tr. *Canon Medicinae*. (Venice, 1608.) See Gruner.

Singer, Charles (ed.) *Studies in the History and Method of Science*, 2 vols. (Oxford, 1917 and 1921.)

Singer, Charles. "The Scientific Views and Visions of St Hildegard," in *Stud. Hist. Meth. Sci.* vol. **1**, p. 1.

Singer, Charles, "The 'Anathomia' of Hieronymo Manfredi," in *Stud. Hist. Meth. Sci.* vol. **1**, p. 80.

Singer, Charles. "Steps leading to the Invention of the First Optical Apparatus," art. in *Studies in the History and Method of Science*, vol. **2**, p. 385.

Singer, Charles. "Notes on the Early History of Microscopy," *Proc. Roy. Soc. Med.* (Hist. of Med. Sect.), 1914, **7**, 247.

Singer, Charles, "The Dawn of Microscopical Discovery," *Journ. Roy. Mic. Soc.*, 1915, 317.

Singer, Charles. *The Evolution of Anatomy*. (Kegan Paul, London, 1925.)

Singer, Charles. See Sudhoff & Singer.

Sinibaldus, J. B. *Geneanthropia sive de Hominis Generatione decateuchnon*. (Caballi, Rome, 1642; Zubrodt, Frankfurt, 1669.)

Slade, M. See Aldes, T.

Smellie, W. *Treatise on the Theory and Practice of Midwifery*, 3 vols. (1751–1764.) Ed. A. H. McClintock, 2 vols. (Sydenham Soc., London, 1876.)

Smellie, W. *A Set of Anatomical Tables with Explanations, and an Abridgment of the Practice of Midwifery, with a view to illustrate a Treatise on that subject, and a Collection of Cases*. (C. Elliot, Edinburgh, 1785.)

Smellie, W. See Buffon.

de Smidt, L. *De ortu et generatione hominis*. (Langerak, Leiden, 1718.)

Smith, Sir F. *History of Veterinary Literature.* (Baillère, Tindal & Cox, London, 1919.)

Snape, Andrew, jun. *The Anatomy of an Horse . . . & an Appendix containing two Discourses, the one, of the Generation of Animals, the other, of the Motion of the Chyle, and the Circulation of the Bloud.* (M. Flesher, London, 1683. Reprinted 1687.)

Snelle, H. *Delineatio theoriae mechanicae.* (Leiden, 1705.)

von Sömmering, S. T. *Icones embryonum humanorum.* (Frankfurt-am-Main, 1799.)

Soranus of Ephesus. *Die Gynäkologie d. Soranus von Ephesus.* Germ. tr. H. Lüneberg. (München, 1894.)

Soranus of Ephesus. *On the diseases of women.* (Teubner, Leipzig, 1882.) French tr. by F. J. Herrgott (Nancy, 1895.) See Sudhoff; Lachs; Ilberg.

Souèges, R. *L'Embryologie Végétale; résumé historique.* (Paris, 1934.)

Spach, Israel. *Gynaeciorum, sive de mulierum affectibus et morbis, libri Graecorum, Arabum, Latinorum, veterum et recentium, quotquot extant, imaginibus exornati.* (Strassbourg, 1597.)

Spallanzani, Lazaro, S.J. *Saggio di osservazioni microscopiche concernenti il sistema della generazione dei Signori di Needham e Buffon.* (Modena, 1766.) Reprinted Soc. Tip. Bari, 1914. French tr. Regley. (Paris, 1769.)

Spallanzani, Lazaro. S.J. *Expériences pour servir à l'histoire de la génération des animaux et des plantes.* (Chirol, Geneva, 1785 & 1786.) See Senebier.

Spallanzani, Lazaro, S.J. *Mémoires sur la Respiration.* (Geneva, 1803.)

Spallanzani, L. *Tracts on the Natural History of Animals and Vegetables,* tr. J. G. Dalyell. (Creech, Edinburgh, 1803.)

Spangenberg, J. *Neues Archiv d. Criminalrechts,* 1908, **2,** 22.

Spemann, Hans. *Experimentelle Beiträge zu einer Theorie der Entwicklung.* (Springer, Berlin, 1936.) Eng. tr. (with the omission of ch. 18), *Embryonic Development and Induction.* (Yale Univ. Press, New Haven, 1938.)

Spencer, Herbert (obstetrician). *William Harvey; Obstetric Physician and Gynaecologist* (Harveian Oration). (Harrison, London, 1921.)

Spencer, Herbert (obstetrician). *The Renaissance of Midwifery.* (Harrison, London, 1924.)

Spencer, Herbert (obstetrician). *The History of British Midwifery from 1650 to 1800.* (Bale & Danielsson, London, 1927.)

Spencer, R. F. "Primitive Obstetrics," *Ciba Symposia,* 1950, **11** (no. 3), 1158.

Spencer, Sir W. Baldwin & Gillen, F. J. *The Arunta.* (Macmillan, London, 1927.)

Spengler, O. *The Decline of the West,* 2 vols. (Allen & Unwin, London, 1926.)

Sperlingen, J. *Tractatus physicus de formatione homine in utero.* (Wendt, Wittenberg, 1641.)

Spielmann. *De optimo recens nati alimento.* (Strassbourg, 1753.)

Spigelius, Adrianus. *De Formato Foetu.* (Merianus, Frankfurt, 1631.)

Sponius, J. *Aphorismi novi ex Hippocratis Operibus.* (Leiden, 1684.)

Sprat, Thomas. *History of the Royal Society.* (London, 1670 & 1722.)

Stahl, G. E. *Theoria medica vera* (1708), ed. L. Choulant. (Voss, Leipzig, 1831.)

Stalpartius van der Wiel, P. *De Nutritione Foetus Exercitatio.* (van der Aa, Leiden, 1687.)

Standard, T. Letter-book B of the Oxford Philosophical Society, *ca.* 1685. MS. Ashmole, 1813, p. 156; in Gunther, vol. 4, p. 120.

Stein, J. B. "Jan Palfyn [1650–1730]," *Med. Record*, 1913, January 11th.

Steinheim, Salomon Levy. "Schreiben betreffend eine Beobachtung ü. d. Lebensverhältnisse d. eingesperrten grünen Kletterfrösche in Winter," in *Litt. Annalen (Hecker's)*, 1831, 20, 266. See Pagel, J.

Steinheim, Salomon Levy. *Die Entwickelung der Frösche. Ein Beitrag zur Lehre der Epigenese.* (Perthes & Besser, Hamburg, 1820.)

Steinheim, Salomon Levy. *Die Entwickelung des Froschembryo's; insbesondere des Muskel- und Genital-system's. Ein neuer Beitrag zur Lehre der Epigenese.* (n.p., n.d.)

Steinschneider, Moritz. *Hebräische Bibliographie*, 1858–1882, vol. 19, p. 35.

Steno. See Stensen.

Stensen, Nicholas. *De Musculis et Glandulis Observationum Specimen.* (Copenhagen, 1664.) See Maar.

Stensen, Nicholas. *De vitelli in intestina pulli transitu Epistola.* Printed with *De Musc. et Gland. Obs. Specimen.* (Copenhagen, 1664.) Also in *Opera*, ed. V. Maar, vol. 1, p. 209. (Tryde, Copenhagen, 1910.)

Stensen, Nicholas. *Elementorum Myologiae Specimen, seu musculi descriptio geometrica. Cui accedunt canis Carchariae dissectum caput et dissectus piscis ex canum genere.* (Florence, 1667.)

Stensen, Nicholas. "In ovo et pullo observationes" and "Observationes anatomicae spectantes ova viviparorum," *Acta Med. Hafniensia*, 1673, 2, 81, 210 (1675).

Sterne, L. *The Life and Opinions of Tristram Shandy* (1759). (Dent, London, 1924).

van der Sterre, D. *Tractatus novus de generatione ex ovo.* (Blancard, Amsterdam, 1687.)

Sticker, G. See Ebstein, Sticker, Feis & Ferckel.

Stiebitz, F. *Archiv f. Gesch. d. Med. u. Naturwiss.* 1930, 23, 332.

Stieda, Ludwig. *Karl Ernst v. Baer, eine biographische Skizze.* (Vieweg, Braunschweig, 1886.)

Stieda, Ludwig. *Der Embryologe Sebastian Graf von Tredern und seine Abhandlungen über das Hühnerei.* (Bergmann, Wiesbaden, 1901.) Also *Anat. Hefte*, 1902, 18.

Stockhamer, F. *Microcosmographia.* (Venice, 1682.)

Stopes, M. *Contraception, Birth Control, its theory, history & practice.* (London, 1931.)

Strachey, Lytton. *Books and Characters.* (London, 1922.)

Straton of Lampsacus. See Allbutt.

Strauss, L. *De ovo galli exercitatio physica.* (Karger, Giessen, 1669.)

Strohl, J. *Missbildungen im Tier- u. Pflanzenreich; Versuch einer vergl. Betrach-*

tung. (Fischer, Jena, 1929.) Rev. in *Mitt. z. Gesch. d. Med. u. Naturwiss.* 1930, **29**, 156.

Studnička, F. K. *Anat. Anz.* 1927 and 1932; *Acta Soc. Nat. Brno* (in Czech), 1927. See Florian.

Stur, J. "Zur Geschichte d. Zeugungsproblem" (the aphorisms of Michael Psellos, 1018–1079), in *Archiv f. d. Gesch. d. Med. (Sudhoff's)*, 1931, **24**, 312.

Sturmius, C. *De plantarum animaliumque Generatione.* (Nürnberg, 1687.) Reprinted in Haller's *Disputationes Selectae*, 1750.

Sudhoff, K. On Paracelsus and the balance. *Archiv f. d. Gesch. d. Math. Naturwiss. u. Technik*, 1908, **1**, 84.

Sudhoff, K. *Archiv f. d. Gesch. d. Med.* 1910, **4**, 109.

Sudhoff, K. *Archiv f. d. Gesch. d. Med.* 1925, **17**, 1.

Sudhoff, K. & Singer, C. "Johannes de Ketham, Alemanus, Fasciculus Medicinae, 1491." Facsimile of the first edition with historical introd. and notes by K. Sudhoff, tr. and adapted by Ch. Singer, in *Monumenta Medica* (ed. H. Sigerist), vol. **1**. (Lier, Milan, 1924.) Rev. in *Isis (Sarton's)*, 1924, **6**, 547.

Suidas. *Lexicon*, ed. A. Adler. (Leipzig, 1928.)

de Superville, Daniel. *Phil. Trans. Roy. Soc.* 1740, **41**, 294.

Swammerdam, Jan. *Natuurbibel* or *Biblia Naturae, sive historia insectorum*, ed. A. v. Haller; see the chapter: "Het eine Dier in het andere of der Kapel verborgen binnen in de Reeps." (Leiden, 1737–1738.)

Swammerdam, Jan. *Miraculum naturae sive uteri muliebris fabrica.* (Leiden, 1672.) Swammerdam's results had already been described by J. van Horne in his *Prodromus* of 1668.

Swenson, E. A. *Anat. Rec.* 1929, **42**, 40.

Sylvius, F. *Opera medica.* (Amsterdam, 1680.)

al-Ṭabarī, Abū'l-Ḥasan 'Alī ibn Sahl ibn Rabban. *Firdaus al-Ḥikma* (The Paradise of Wisdom). See E. G. Browne, *Arabian Medicine* (Cambridge, 1924), p. 37; and Sarton, vol. **1**, p. 574.

Tagliacozzi, Gaspare. *De Curtorum Chirurgia per insitionem, Libri Duo. In quibus ea omnia, quae ad huius chirurgiae, narium scilicet, aurium ac labiorum per insitionem restaurandorum cum theoricen tum practicen pertinere videbantur, clarissima methodo cumulatissime declarantur.* (Bindoni, Venice, 1597.)

Tarin, P. *Ostéographie du foetus.* (Briasson, Paris, 1753.)

Tauvry, D. *Anatomia.* (Ulm, 1694.)

Tauvry, D. *Nouvelle Anatomie raisonnée.* (Paris, 1690.) Eng. tr. *A New Rational Anatomy.* (London, 1701.)

Tauvry, D. *Traité de la génération et de la nourriture du fœtus.* (Girin, Paris, 1700.)

Teichmeyer, H. F. *Elementa anthropologiae.* (Bielck, Jena, 1719.)

Teichmeyer, H. F. *Institutiones medico-legales.* (Jena, 1723.)

Telesius, Bernardinus. *De Natura Rerum* (1565), in *Varii de naturalibus rebus libelli.* (Venice, 1590.)

Telesius, Bernardinus. *De Rerum Natura iuxta propria principia Liber primus & secundus denuo editi.* (Cacchi, Naples, 1570.)

Terelius, Dom. *De Generatione et Partu Hominis.* (Marsilius, Leiden, 1578.)

du Tertre, Marguerite. *Instruction de Sagefemmes.* (Paris, 1677.)

Tertullianus, Q. Septimius. *De Anima,* in Migne's *Patrologia,* q.v.

Teuscher, H. *Fortschritte d. Medizin,* 1888, **6**, 863.

Thābit ibn Qurra. See Qurra.

Themel, J. C. *Commentatio medica qua nutritionem foetus in utero per vasa umbilicalia solum fieri occasione monstri ovilli sine ore et faucibus nato ostenditur.* Contained in *Fasciculus dissertationum anatomico-medicarum.* (Schreuder, Amsterdam, 1764.)

Themistius. *In libros Aristot. de anima periphrasis,* ed. R. Heinze. (Reimer, Berlin, 1899.)

Thibaut, P. *The Art of Chymistry,* tr. into English by an F.R.S. (London, 1675.)

Thomas of Aquino, O.P. *Summa Theologica.* Eng. tr. 10 vols. (London, 1911–1917.)

Thomas, P. F. *La Philosophie de Gassendi.* (Alcan, Paris, 1889.)

Thompson, d'Arcy W. *On Aristotle as a Biologist; with a proemion on Herbert Spencer* (philosopher). (Herbert Spencer Lecture, Oxford, 1913.)

Thompson, d'Arcy W. *Growth and Form.* (Cambridge, 1917.) Revised ed. (Cambridge, 1942).

Thompson, C. J. S. *The Mystery and Lore of Monsters.* (Williams & Norgate, London, 1930.)

Thomson, G. P. *Aeschylus and Athens.* (Lawrence & Wishart, London, 1941.)

Thomson, T. *A System of Chemistry.* (Edinburgh, 1804.)

Threlfall, Sir Richard. *Biol. Rev.* 1930, **5**, 357.

Tildesley, Miriam L. *Sir Thomas Browne; his skull, portraits, and ancestry.* (Cambridge, n.d.) Privately published reprint from *Biometrika,* **15**.

von Töply, R. "Studien zur Geschichte der Anatomie im Mittelalter, "in Neuburger-Pagel, q.v.

Torreblanca, F. *De Magia.* (Leiden, 1678.)

Tradescant, John. *Museum Tradescantianum; or, a collection of rarities preserved at South Lambeth near London.* (Brooke, London, 1656.)

Trembley, Abraham, Abbé. *Mémoires pour servir à l'histoire d'un genre de polypes d'eau douce, à bras en forme de cornes.* (Leiden, 1744.) See Baker.

Tschassovnikov, S. G. *Le Physiologiste Russe,* 1898, **1**, 68.

Tur, Jan. "The concept of Homology from Harvey to de Graaf" (in Polish), in *Archiwum Hist. i Fil. Medyc.* 1930, **10**, 96.

Tur, Jan. "Régnier de Graaf, the last embryologist without a microscope" (in Polish), in *Archiwum Hist. i Fil. Medyc.* 1931, **11**, 56.

Turel, A. *Du Règne de la Mère au Patriarcat; pages choisies.* (Alcan, Paris, 1938.) See Bachofen.

Turner, D. *The force of the mother's imagination further consider'd.* (London, 1730.)

Turner, D. *The force of the mother's imagination upon her foetus in utero still farther consider'd, in the way of a reply to Dr Blondel's last book, to which is added the 12th chapter of the 1st part of a treatise 'De morbis cutaneis' as it was printed therein many years past, in a letter to Dr Blondel.* (Walthoe, London, 1730.)

Valentinius, M. *Nosocomium in praxi medicinae.* (Frankfurt, 1711.)

Vallesius, F. *Controversiarum medicarum et philosophicarum.* (Wechel, Frankfurt, 1582.)

Vallisneri, Antonio. *Considerazioni ed esperienze intorno alle generazioni de' Vermi ordinari del corpo umano.* (Padua, 1710.)

Vallisneri, Antonio. *Istoria della Generazione dell' Uomo e degli Animali, se sia da' Vermicelli spermatici ossia dalle Uova.* (Venezia, 1721.) Reprinted in *Opere fisico-mediche.* (Venice, 1733.) German tr. *Historie von der Erzeugung der Menschen und Thiere.* (Lemgo, 1739.)

Vallisneri, Antonio. *Nuove esperienze sulli svilluppi.* (Padua, 1713.)

Varandaeus, J. *Opera Omnia.* (Leiden, 1658.)

Varolius, C. *Resolutio Corporis Humani.* (Wechel, Frankfurt, 1591.)

Vaughan, A. C. "The Genesis of Human Offspring; a Study in early Greek Culture," *Smith College Classical Studies,* no. 13. (Northampton, Mass., 1945.)

Vauquelin, L. N. & Buniva, M. F. *Horkel's Archiv,* 1800, 1, 32.

Vauquelin, L. N. & Buniva, M. F. *Ann. de chim. et de physique,* 1799 (An VIII), **33**, 269, 275.

Vauquelin, L. N. & Buniva, M. F. *Chem. Ann. (Crelle's),* 1801, 1, 217; **2**, 269.

Vauquelin, L. N. & Buniva, M. F. *Allgemeines Journ. f. Chemie (Scherer's),* 1801, **4**, 671; 1803, **6**, 207.

Velsch, G. H. *Exercitatio de Vena Medinensi ad Mentem Ebsinae, sive de Dracunculo Veterum Specimen exhibens novae versionis ex Arabico cum commentario uberiori, cui accedat De Vermiculis capillaribus Infantium.* (Augsburg, 1674.)

Velsch, G. H. *Sylloge Curationum.* (Augsburg, 1675.)

Velthusius, L. *Tractatus duo medico-physici; unus de liene, alter de generatione.* (Zyll, Utrecht, 1657.)

Venetianer, L. *Asaf Judaeus; der älteste medizinische Schriftsteller in hebräischer Sprache.* 2 pts. (Trübner, Strassbourg, 1916 & 1917.)

Venette, N. *Abhandlung von der Erzeugung der Menschen.* (Woltersdorf, Königsberg & Leipzig, 1762.)

Venusti, A. M. *Discorso generale intorno alla generatione.* (Somasco, Venice, 1562.)

Vercelloni, J. *Ephem. Nat. Cur.* Cent. v, obs. 9.

Verheyen, P. *Anatomia corporis humani.* (Leipzig, 1699.)

Vesalius, Andreas. *De Humani Corporis Fabrica.* (Basel, 1543.)

Veslingius, J. *Syntagma anatomicum.* (Padua, 1641, 1647, 1677.)

Viardel, C. *Observations sur la Pratique des Accouchemens Naturels, contre la*

Nature, et Monstrueux. (Paris, 1671, 1748.) Germ. tr., *Von der weiblichen Geburt.* (Frankfurt, 1767.)

Vicarius, J. J. *Basis Universae Medicinae.* (Ulm, 1700.)

Vidussi, G. M. *Motivi di dubitare intorno la generazione de' viventi sensitivi secondo la commune opinione de' moderni.* (Lovisa, Venice, 1717.)

Vieussens, R. *Novum Vasorum Corporis Humani Systema.* (Amsterdam, 1705.)

Vincent of Beauvais, O.S.B. (fl. 1250). *Bibliotheca mundi, seu Speculum quadruplex naturale, doctrinale, morale, historiale (Speculum Majus).* (Douai, 1624.)

Vinci. See Leonardo da Vinci.

Vogel, J. H. *Commentatio physiologica qua foet. in ut. non liq. amn. sed sang. umb. advecto nutriri.* (Bossiegel, Göttingen, 1761.)

de Voltaire, François Marie Arouet. "Akakia," in *Œuvres.* (Geneva, 1768–1777.)

Vorwahl, H. "Beseelung," in *Archiv f. d. Gesch. d. Med.* 1931, **13**, 126.

Vullers, J. "Altindische Geburtshülfe," in Henschel's *Janus.* (Giessen, 1846.)

Wachtler, J. *De Alcmaeone Crotoniata.* (Leipzig, 1896.)

Waddington, C. H. *Sci. Progr.* 1934, **29**, 336.

Waddington, C. H. *How Animals Develop.* (Allen & Unwin, London, 1935.)

Waddington, C. H. *The Epigenetics of Birds.* (Cambridge, 1952.)

Waddington, C. H. *Principles of Embryology.* (Allen & Unwin, London, 1956.)

Waldschmidt, J. *Praxis Medicinae Rationalis,* pp. 722, 743, 744. (Paris, 1691.)

Waller, R. *Phil. Trans. Roy. Soc.* 1693, **17**, 523.

von Wasserberg, L. *Baldinger's Magazin,* 1780, **2**, 300.

Watson, W. *Phil. Trans. Roy. Soc.* 1749, **46**, 235.

Webb, A. *Pathologica Indica.* (Thacker, Calcutta, n.d. [1846, 1848].)

Weber, F. *Jüdische Theologie.* (Dörffling, Leipzig, 1897.)

Wedel, G. W. *De Morbis Infantum.* (Jena, 1717.)

Weidlich. See von Ott.

Weindler, Fritz. *Geschichte der gynäkologisch-anatomischen Abbildung.* (Zahn & Jaensch, Dresden, 1908.)

Weinrich, Martin. *De Ortu Monstrorum Commentarius, in quo essentia, differentiae, causae et affectiones mirabilium animalium explicantur.* (Breslau (?), 1595.)

Wellmann, M. On Alcmaeon of Crotona and on the relations of Democritus and Hippocrates. *Archeion (Archivio d. Storia d. Sci.),* 1929, **11**, 156, 297.

Wellmann, M. *Die Fragmente der sikelischen Aerzte Akron, Philistion, und des Diokles von Karystos.* (Berlin, 1901.)

Wentscher, E. *Englische Philosophie, ihr Wesen und ihre Entwicklung.* (Leipzig, 1924.)

Weygand, O. *Suppl. der Breslauer Sammlung,* **4**, 53. (No date, *ca.* 1730.)

White, J. H. *The Phlogiston Theory.* (Arnold, London, 1932.)

Whitman, C. O. "Bonnet's Theory of Evolution; a system of negations," in *Biol. Lectures, Woods Hole,* 1894. (Boston, 1895.)

Whittaker, T. *Macrobius*. (Cambridge, 1923.)

Willier, B. H., Weiss, P. A. & Hamburger, V. (ed.) *Analysis of Development*. (Saunders, Philadelphia & London, 1955.)

Willis, R. Edition of Harvey's works, with introduction and prefaces, etc. (Sydenham Society, London, 1847.)

Willoughby, Francis. *Ornithologia*. (Martyn, London, 1676.)

Winkler, Daniel. *Animadversiones in Tractatum, qui inscribitur 'Dissertatio de vita foetus in utero,' qua luculenter demonstratur infantem in utero non anima matris sed sua ipsius vita vivere*, etc. (Steinmann, Jena, 1630.)

Winslow, J. B. *Exposition anatomique de la structure du Corps Humain*. (Paris, 1732.)

Withof, P. L. *De Systema Leeuwenhoekii*. (Leiden, 1746.)

Witkowski, G. J. *Histoire des Accouchements*. (Steinheil, Paris, 1887.)

Wolf, Caspar. *Gynaeciorum; hoc est, de mulierum tum aliis, tum gravidarum, parientum et puerperarum, affectibus et morbis, libri veterum ac recentiorum*. (Guarinus, Basel, 1566.)

Wolff, C. F. *Theoria Generationis*. (Halle, 1759.)

Wolff, C. F. *Über die Bildung des Darmkanals im befruchteten Hühnchen*, tr. J. F. Meckel. (Halle, 1812.) From "De formatione intestinorum praecipue, tum et de amnio spurio, aliisque partibus embryonis gallinacei nondum visis" in *Novi Comment. Acad. Sci. Imp. Petropol.* 1768, **12**; 1769, **13**.

Wollaston. W. *The Religion of Nature delineated*. (London, 1724.)

Wolphius. See Wolf, Caspar.

Woodger, J. H. *Sci. Progr.* 1931, **26**, 300.

Worcester, Henry Somerset, 1st Marquis of. *A Century of the Names and Scantlings of such Inventions as at present I can call to mind to have tried*. (London, 1663.) See Dircks.

Xenophon. *Oeconomicus*, ed. H. A. Holden. (London, 1884.)

Yarrell, W. *Zool. Journ.* 1826, **2**, 433.

Yearsley, M. *Doctors in Elizabethan Drama*. (Bale & Danielsson, London, 1933.)

Zacchias, P. *Quaestiones medico-legales*. (Frankfurt, 1688.)

Zäch, C. *Mitteilungen d. Lebensmitteluntersuchungen*, 1929, **20**, 209.

Zeller, E. *History of Greek Philosophy*. (Longmans, London, 1881.)

Zeller, J. *Infanticidas non absolvit nec a tortura liberat Pulmonum Infantis in aqua subsidentia.* (1691.) Reprinted in Haller's *Disputationes Selectae*, 1750.

Zeller, J. *De Vita humana ex Fune pendente*. (1692.) Reprinted in Haller's *Disputationes Selectae*, 1750.

Zeno of Citium. See Allbutt.

Zervos, S. G. On Babylonian and Assyrian obstetrics and gynaecology. *Archiv f. d. Gesch. d. Med.* 1912, **6**, 401.

Ziegler, H. E. *Lehrb. d. vergl. Entwicklungsgeschichte d. nied. Wirbeltiere.* (Fischer, Jena, 1902.)

Zirkle, Conway. *Isis (Sarton's)* 1936, **25**, 95.

Züno, M. Malpighi bibliography. *Archeion (Archivio d. Storia d. Sci.),* 1929, **11**, 55.

Zypaeus, F. *Fundamenta medica.* (Brussels, 1684.)

The following works remain inaccessible to me in England and I have not yet seen them:

Mantellassi, C. *Diversi Sistemi con la Generazione.* (Florence, 1749.) Reprinted in *Receuil de pièces de Médecine* (Paris, 1763) and in *Pièces intéressantes sur la Médecine.* (Lamy, Paris, 1782.)

le Monnier, P. *De Conceptu et Incremento Foetu.* (Bonk, Leiden, 1742.)

Paitoni, G. B. *Della generazione dell' uomo.* (Recurti, Venice, 1722; Zane, Venice, 1726.)

Scheid, J. V. *Speculum paradoxae circa generationis hominis.* (1694.)

I would like to express my gratitude to the following for the help they have given me in tracing these and other books: Dr S. A. Asdell, Miss Ethel G. Brodie, Dr R. E. D. Clark, Dr E. J. Dingwall, Miss Elinor Gregory, Dr Arnold C. Klebs, Mr W. B. McDaniel, Dr Walter Pagel and Mr H. Zeitlinger.

INDEX

INDEX

INDEX

Vicarius, J. J., 182
Vidussi, G. M., 208
Vieussens, R., 182
Vincent of Beauvais, 94
da Vinci, Leonardo, 36, 77, 96–9, Plate V,
    125, 161, 193, 198, 232, 234
viper, 106
vis essentialis, 202, 207, 226
vitalism, 48, 70, 115, 120 n. 2, 141, 183, 207,
    214
vitellin, 31
vitelline membrane, 101, 199, 200, 221
viviparity, 39, 54
viviparous animals, early work on, 37, 39, 41,
    100, fig. 6 (p. 101), 124, 127, 135 160, 161,
    162, 197, 212, 217
Vogel, J. H., 227
de Voltaire, F. M. A., 203, 218
Volvox, 200
Vorwahl, H., 22 n. 1
Vullers, J., 25 n. 8
vulture, 101

W

Wachtler, J., 30
Waddington, C. H., 12 n. 1, 192, 213 n. 1
Waldschmidt, J., 180
Waller, R., 178
Ward, J., 158
water-content of embryo, 33, fig. 4 (p. 34),
    fig. 7 (p. 102), 123 n. 1, 174, 190
Watson, W., 228–9
Webb, A., 26
Weber, F., 78–9
Wedel, G. W., 181
Weidlich, 227
weight, of embryonic bones, fig. 21 (p. 196)
    of embryonic organs, 191–2
    of parts of egg, 177
Weindler, F., 96 n. 1, 99 n. 1
Wellmann, M., 32 n. 3
Wells, H. G., 206
Welsch, 210
Wentscher, E., 149 n. 1
Weygand, O., 208
White, J. H., 213 n. 1
Whitman, C. O., 213 nn. 1 and 2, 214
Whittaker, T., 69 n. 3

Willier, B. H., 12 n. 1
Willis, Robert, 161
Willis, Thomas, 158
Willoughby, Francis, 175
Winckler, D., 142 n. 2
wind-eggs, 28, 52, 67, 142
Winslow, J. B., 207
Wisdom literature, 64, 78, 85
Withof, P. L., 208
Witkowski, G. J., 205
Wolf, Caspar, 109
Wolff, C. F., 116, 144, 193, 201, 202, 207,
    214, 220–3, 224, 226–7
Wollaston, 208 n. 3
Woodger, J. H., 239 n. 1
Worcester, Henry Somerset, Marquis of, 191
Wren, Christopher, 158

X

Xenophon, 14

Y

Yarrell, W., 103
Yearsley, M., 15
yeast, embryonic development compared with
    action of, 50–1, 55, 91
yolk, 30, 31, 36, 52, 53, 67, 86, 88, 89, 90, 101,
    102, 103, 104, 106, 108, 109, 116, 118,
    127, 131, 132, 135, 136, 137–8, 139, 144,
    161 n. 2, 162, 172–3, 185, 195, 199–200,
    213, 229
"white", 53, 135
yolk-membrane, *see* vitelline membrane
yolk-sac, 36, 53, 90 n. 1, 200

Z

Zacchias, P., 145, 175, 180
Zäch, C., 188 n. 1
Zegarra, 120
Zeller, E., 30
Zeller, Johannes, 194–5
Zeno of Citium, 60
Zervos, S. G., 18 n. 1
Ziegler, H. E., 168, Plate XII
Zirkle, C., 28 n. 1
Zonzinas, 120
Zypaeus, F., 170

Printed in the United States
By Bookmasters